Disorders of Movement: Diagnosis and Treatment

Disorders of Movement: Diagnosis and Treatment

Editor: George Freeman

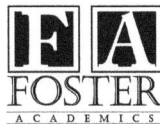

FA
FOSTER
ACADEMICS

www.fosteracademics.com

www.fosteracademics.com

FA FOSTER
ACADEMICS

Cataloging-in-Publication Data

Disorders of movement : diagnosis and treatment / edited by George Freeman.
    p. cm.
Includes bibliographical references and index.
ISBN 978-1-63242-726-7
1. Movement disorders. 2. Movement disorders--Diagnosis.
3. Movement disorders--Treatment. I. Freeman, George.
RC376.5 .D57 2019
616.83--dc23

Foster Academics,
118-35 Queens Blvd., Suite 400,
Forest Hills, NY 11375, USA

ISBN 978-1-63242-726-7 (Hardback)

Contents

Permissions

List of Contributors

Index

Preface

Disorders of movement are the clinical conditions characterized by insufficient voluntary and involuntary movements or excess of movement. These are conventionally divided into hyperkinetic and hypokinetic movement disorders. Hyperkinetic movement disorders refer to dyskinesia, or repetitive, excessive involuntary movements, which intrude with the normal flow of motor activity. Some of such disorders are dystonia, spasmodic torticollis, blepharospasm, myoclonus, etc. Hypokinetic movement disorders may refer to hypokinesia, akinesia, bradykinesia and rigidity. Examples include primary or idiopathic parkinsonism, striatonigral degeneration, Hallevorden-Spatz disease, etc. The first step in the management of such disorders is making a differential diagnosis of the disorder and then confirming the diagnosis through metabolic screening, CSF examinations, and neurophysiological and pharmacological tests. Treatment of each disorder is different and depends on the diagnosis. The objective of this book is to give a general view of the different disorders of movement along with their diagnoses. It elucidates the concepts and innovative models around prospective developments with respect to the management of movement disorders. Those in search of information to further their knowledge will be greatly assisted by this book.

Significant researches are present in this book. Intensive efforts have been employed by authors to make this book an outstanding discourse. This book contains the enlightening chapters which have been written on the basis of significant researches done by the experts.

Finally, I would also like to thank all the members involved in this book for being a team and meeting all the deadlines for the submission of their respective works. I would also like to thank my friends and family for being supportive in my efforts.

Editor

Hydrocephalic Parkinsonism: lessons from normal pressure hydrocephalus mimics

Brian W Starr[1], Matthew C Hagen[2] and Alberto J Espay[1]*

Abstract

Background: Hydrocephalus is an under-recognized presentation of progressive supranuclear palsy (PSP) and dementia with Lewy bodies (DLB).

Methods: We describe four normal pressure hydrocephalus (NPH)-like presentations of pathology-proven PSP (n = 3) and DLB (n = 1) and review the literature on the hydrocephalic presentation of these atypical parkinsonisms.

Results: Despite the presence of ventriculomegaly disproportionate to the extent of parenchymal atrophy, all patients demonstrated early postural impairment and/or oculomotor abnormalities that encouraged a diagnostic revision. Hallucinations were the only early atypical manifestation of the hydrocephalic DLB presentation.

Conclusions: Early postural impairment, falls, oculomotor impairment, and/or hallucinations are inconsistent with the diagnosis of NPH and suggest PSP or DLB as the underlying NPH mimic. We postulate that previously reported cases of "dual" pathology (e.g., NPH *and* PSP) actually represent the hydrocephalic presentation of selected neurodegenerative disorders.

Keywords: Normal pressure hydrocephalus, Ventriculomegaly, Progressive supranuclear palsy, Dementia with Lewy bodies

Background

Hydrocephalus as an imaging finding is commonly interpreted as potentially representing normal pressure hydrocephalus (NPH) largely because of the favorable therapeutic implications [1]. However, NPH is a relatively rare disorder, recently calculated to be 1.19/100,000/year, and reduced further to 0.36/100,000/year when defined as *sustained* improvement at 3 years after ventriculoperitoneal shunt (VPS) placement [1]. Between 1995 and 2003, from 411 patients referred as NPH to the Mayo Clinic, only 41 were tentatively endorsed as such and barely 14 experienced gait improvement after a trial of cerebrospinal fluid removal, the *sine qua non* for the diagnosis. Of the 12 patients who underwent VPS placement, definite gait improvement was present in only 6 by one year and just 4 after 3 years, one third of the original VPS-treated cohort. Remarkably, pathology available in 5 patients in the VPS-treated cohort revealed the presence of neurodegenerative disorders, progressive supranuclear palsy (PSP) and dementia with Lewy bodies (DLB), each accounting for a case.

Because of the large volume of NPH referrals to tertiary care centers, predicting a *sustained* response to VPS placement is paramount to justifying this invasive procedure. We examined four patients referred to us for suspected NPH but whose pathology demonstrated PSP and DLB. The preliminary diagnosis of NPH in these patients was based on the interpretation of imaging features, namely the presence of hydrocephalus judged disproportionate to the extent of surrounding parenchymal atrophy. While a careful neurological examination suggested further NPH work up was unwarranted in three patients, cerebrospinal fluid diversion in one (case 4) supported this diagnosis by yielding subjective benefits in gait and urinary function. In addition to early impairment postural reflexes, other clinical red flags against NPH emerged between 12 and 24 months. We suggest that PSP and DLB, as previously reported for Alzheimer disease (AD), is capable of generating a neuroimaging profile suggestive of communicating hydrocephalus, with ventriculomegaly disproportionate to the extent of parenchymal atrophy, prompting a diagnostic consideration for NPH and potentially misdirecting treatment toward cerebrospinal fluid diversion.

* Correspondence: alberto.espay@uc.edu
[1]Gardner Family Center for Parkinson's Disease and Movement Disorders, Department of Neurology, University of Cincinnati, 260 Stetson St, Suite 2300, Cincinnati, OH 45267-0525, USA
Full list of author information is available at the end of the article

Methods

Case reports

Four consecutive patients referred to our center for suspected NPH for whom brain autopsy was obtained were identified in our center from the years 2007–2012. After evaluation in our center, VPS placement was discouraged for the first three patients but pursued in the fourth to no avail. Written informed consent was obtained from all patients for the publication of patient-related data and videotapes.

Results

Case 1

This 68-year-old woman developed balance impairment followed by falls, mostly forward, urinary incontinence, and intermittently slurred speech over a 2-year period. Head CT demonstrated mild to moderate hydrocephalus

(Figure 1A), prompting referral for VPS placement. On neurological examination, she exhibited a tremorless parkinsonian phenotype with cognitive impairment (MMSE = 19/30) associated with echolalia, growling dysarthria, and hypomimia, prompting a revised clinical diagnosis of PSP. By three years from symptom onset, she developed square-wave jerks, slow saccades, and supranuclear vertical gaze palsy (Additional file 1: Video S1). Donepezil, rivastigmine, and memantine trials provided no benefit. She died after six years from symptom onset. Neuropathological studies confirmed the diagnosis of PSP with concurrent AD neuropathologic changes (Braak stage II; CERAD score A) and mild associated arteriolosclerosis and atherosclerosis (Figure 2A-D).

Case 2

This 79-year-old man developed difficulty with "complex" leg movements, such as those required when walking across

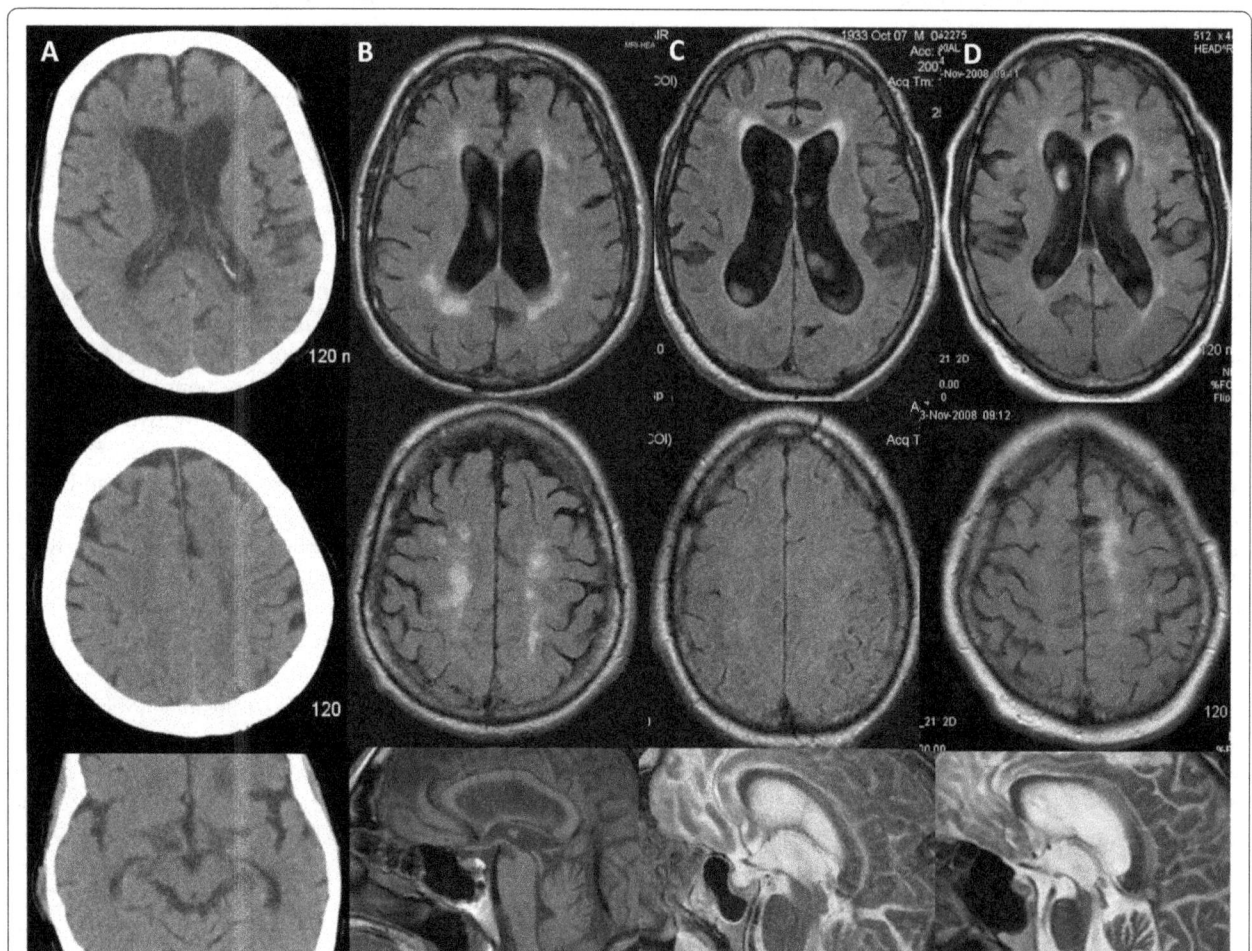

Figure 1 Neuroimaging of the NPH suspected cases. Head CT **(A)** and FLAIR sequences of brain MRI **(B-D)** for cases 1–4 (A-D) showed mild to moderate ventriculomegaly (upper row), with relatively mild or absent (Case 3) associated parenchymal atrophy as judged by the apical axial cuts (middle row). Some degree of midbrain atrophy is appreciable in all cases, including the one ultimately diagnosed as DLB on pathology **(C)** despite a clinical picture that suggested a rapidly progressive form of PSP. Leukoencephalomalacia in the right cerebellar hemisphere and left parasagittal frontal lobe was due to remote stroke in Case 4.

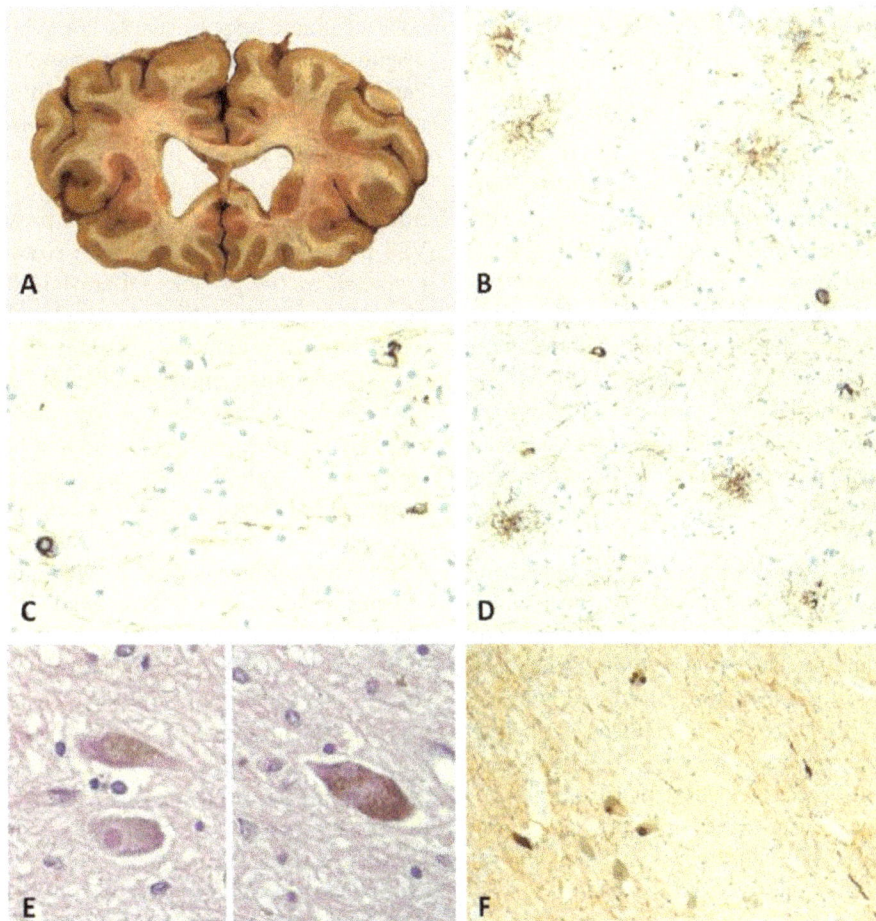

Figure 2 Neuropathology images of selected cases. A. (Case 1) Coronal section demonstrating enlargement of the anterior horns of the lateral ventricles. **B**. (Case 1) Tufted astrocytes and tau positive neurons in the caudate nucleus (tau stain (AT8), magnification 200×). **C**. (Case 1) Coiled bodies in the parietal white matter (tau stain (AT8), magnification 400×). **D**. (Case 1) Tufted astrocytes and tau positive neurons in the parietal cortex (tau stain (AT8), magnification 200×). **E**. (Case 3) Lewy bodies in the substantia nigra (H&E, magnification 400×). **F**. (Case 3) Substantia nigra, Lewy bodies and Lewy neuritis (alpha-synuclein, magnification 200×).

a railroad or stepping on a train wagon. Brain MRI obtained within one year was interpreted as mild hydrocephalus (Figure 1B), prompting a referral for was consideration of VPS placement. His examination showed parkinsonism with marked gait and postural impairment, upgaze restriction, and stimulus-sensitive axial myoclonus (Additional file 2: Video S2), as well as mild dysexecutive impairment (MMSE = 28/30; Frontal Assessment Battery = 14/18; Montreal Cognitive Assessment = 25/30). His revised clinical diagnosis was PSP and VPS placement was discouraged. Death occurred 10 years after symptom onset. Post-mortem studies confirmed the diagnosis of PSP with associated low-grade AD neuropathology (Braak stage II; CERAD score A) and brainstem Lewy bodies.

Case 3

This 73-year-old man initially exhibited falls, visual hallucinations, irritability and combative behavior. Within two months he was unable to ambulate independently and had noticeable memory loss. Brain MRI taken at 3 months from symptom onset demonstrated moderate ventriculomegaly without overt atrophy in the apical cuts, suggesting the diagnosis of NPH (Figure 1C). However, in short sequence he developed dysarthria evolving to anarthria, severe dysphagia, and needed assistance for all activities of daily living. At 5 months, his examination showed retrocollis with axial-predominant rigidity and ophthalmoplegia, taking place at one of his "bad spells" (Additional file 3: Video S3). Cognitive assessment was impossible given marked dysarthria. Rivastigmine provided no benefits but donepezil eliminated his visual hallucinations. A rapidly progressive form of PSP was suspected and shunting was discouraged. Despite the early rapid progression, death from aspiration pneumonia occurred six years after symptom onset. Post-mortem neuropathology unexpectedly revealed DLB (neocortical lewy body type, Braak stage V; high likelihood) (Figure 2E-F) with mild to moderate arteriolosclerosis and mild AD neuropathology (Braak stage II; CERAD score A).

Case 4

This 72-year-old man with progressive gait and balance impairment underwent a brain MRI, which upon presence of hydrocephalus, hyperdynamic fluid signal in the third ventricle, and entrapped sulci in several cortical areas (Figure 1D) prompted a referral to our center. Initial examination 18 months after symptom onset demonstrated mild non-fluent aphasia, visuospatial dysfunction, and delayed recall (MMSE = 24; Montreal Cognitive Assessment = 13/30] in the setting of wide based, unsteady gait. Mild impairment of upgaze with absent vertical optokinetic responses was present at the initial examination (Additional file 4: Video S4). External lumbar drainage provided benefits in gait and urinary function. VPS placement, however, was followed by improvements in gait and urinary function for about 6 months, followed by deterioration of his overall parkinsonism and cognitive function. He developed frontal release signs and disinhibition, with worsening of dysexecutive dementia, mild facial dystonia, greater oculomotor dysfunction (impairment of upgaze, slowed downgaze, square-wave jerks), and marked postural impairment with backward falls. He died from aspiration pneumonia six years from onset of symptoms. Suspected PSP was confirmed on postmortem studies, which also revealed unusually marked and widespread occipital cortical involvement.

Discussion

There are two major shortcomings in the appraisal of NPH as an entity, namely the absence of clinical and pathological biomarkers and the reliance on short-term response to drainage for its definition [2], which often does not "hold water" in the long term [1]. Indeed, the longer the follow up, the lower the frequency of response, and the higher the diagnostic revision rate [1]. Important lessons derived from the suspected NPH patients presented here were that cognitive impairment predated or occurred concurrently with gait dysfunction, and impairment of postural reflexes was universal. This is in keeping with the observation that postural instability at the initial evaluation of a suspected NPH patient predicts the absence of sustained improvement at 3 years from VPS placement [1].

Besides early impairment of postural reflexes, our patients had early cognitive impairment, either predating or occurring concurrently with gait impairment. Cognitive impairment is a regrettable component of the "classic" NPH triad. Of the 8 cognitively impaired VPS-treated patients in the Mayo Clinic series, only 1 continued to benefit at 3 years [1]. This implies that by the time a patient

with hydrocephalus develops cognitive impairment, the odds of shunt responsiveness are substantially low, and diagnostic considerations other than NPH are warranted. Patients may have AD if cognitive impairment predominates [3] and PSP or DLB if parkinsonism is an important clinical manifestation. In the former situation, AD biomarkers may be particularly helpful in discriminating AD from true NPH. In a sample of 37 prospectively followed VPS-treated "NPH" patients, poor sustained response was predicted by the presence of amyloid β plaques, neuritic plaques, and/or neurofibrillary tangles observed in cortical biopsies taken at the time of shunt insertion [3]. Cortical biopsies identified amyloid-β aggregates in over half of presumed NPH patients who had initial response to VPS but eventual progression of dementia [4]. Similarly, 8 out of 9 patients with clinically diagnosed NPH that came to autopsy at the Sun Health Research Institute within a 12-year period, demonstrated AD pathology (one also with DLB) and the other met pathologic criteria for PSP [5].

A major pitfall of the interpretation of these data is to assume that these patients had "co-occurrence" of AD and NPH [5,6], rather than the hydrocephalic presentation of a single, neurodegenerative disorder. This potential misinterpretation is giving rise to reports of NPH patients "evolving" to AD [7], without considering the possibility that NPH may have been an early clinical misdiagnosis. Although the postulation of an "AD-NPH syndrome" [8,9] has already led to a negative clinical trial [10], clinicians continue to offer VPS to patients with hydrocephalus in the setting of dementia, because it is part of the "classic triad" (conversely, some neurosurgeons may be reluctant to shunt if dementia is not present in patients whose hydrocephalus may "only" be associated with gait impairment).

PSP appears to be the most common etiology of suspected NPH with a parkinsonian phenotype (Table 1). It was present in 3 of 4 such cases from the Queen Square Brain Bank, none of whom had, at presentation, any oculomotor dysfunction [11]. However, postural instability and mild dysexecutive impairment were present in all. VPS placement in three resulted in short-term benefits but subsequent deterioration ensued within one year. The early Toronto experience showed that 3 of 5 NPH patients with hydrocephalus and early response to VPS evolved into a parkinsonian phenotype confirmed to represent PSP in two (one with pathology confirmation) and DLB in another [12].

Our cases and the review of the literature highlight several key clinically relevant messages: 1) early cognitive impairment is the most important "cognitive red flag" of the NPH triad and predicts an alternative diagnosis; 2) early impairment of postural reflexes, with or without falls, is the most common "motor red flag" of the NPH triad, and should suggest PSP or DLB; 3) visual hallucinations are a strong clinical biomarker of synucleinopathies [13] and

Table 1 NPH-like presentations for pathology-confirmed PSP and DLB cases: summary of the published literature

Case	Age, gender	Disease duration at presentation	Initial clinical features	Late clinical features	Response to VPS	Pathology
1 [1]	82, F*	1.1 years	GD, CI, UI, postural instability	N/A	Transient improvement in GD/UI; worse at 3 years	PSP
2 [5]	77, M♣	N/A	GD, CI, UI	N/A	VPS placed, outcome data not available	PSP
3 [11]	78, F	2 years	GD, CI, UI, falls, generalized bradykinesia, dysarthria	Restriction of vertical eye movements, hypophonia, frontal release signs	Not placed	PSP
4 [11]	68, M	4 months	GD, CI, UI, gait ignition failure, falls, hypomimia, micrographia	Restriction of vertical gaze, slow saccades, dysarthria, gait freezing	Transient improvement but progressive dementia	PSP
5 [11]	66, F	2 years	GD, CI, falls, micrographia	Restriction of vertical gaze, slow saccades, dysarthria, dysphagia, gait freezing, dementia	Transient improvement in GD/CI but progressive dementia	PSP
6 [12]	69, M	N/A	GD, CI, UI	VSGP, akinesia, rigidity	6-month "marked" improvement in GD, CI, and UI	PSP
7 [1]	66, F♦	3.1 years	GD, CI, UI, postural instability	"Clinical diagnosis of DLB"	Some improvement in GD at 3–6 months; no improvement at 3 years	DLB
8 [5]	80, M♠	N/A	GD, CI	N/A	VPS placed, outcome data not available	DLB
9 [7]	87, F	2 years	GD, CI, UI	Postural instability, falls, rare visual hallucinations	Initial marked improvement in GD/CI – No follow-up data.	DLB

GD: gait disturbance; CI: cognitive impairment; UI: urinary incontinence; VSGP: vertical supranuclear gaze palsy. *: VPS placed at 82 (no age at presentation given); ♣: Death at 77 (no age at presentation given); ♦: VPS placed at 66 (no age at presentation given); ♠: Death at 80 (no age at presentation given).

their presence in the setting of hydrocephalus tilts the diagnostic yield toward DLB; and 4) a "honeymoon" period may occur after shunting in patients with PSP but further progression would be expected thereafter. To the extent that transient symptomatic relief in the setting of a neurodegenerative disorder may be preferable to no relief at all, the approach to a hydrocephalic patient with "red flags" may still include fluid diversion, but patients and families need to be counseled about the anticipated short-term gains.

In sum, hydrocephalus in the setting of postural impairment and/or oculomotor abnormalities most probably represents PSP or DLB. Hallucinations may be the only early manifestation of the hydrocephalic presentation of DLB. An initial promising response to VPS placement does not exclude the possibility of an underlying neurodegenerative disease. Furthermore, a fully formed "classic" triad of gait impairment, urinary incontinence, and cognitive impairment appears to be more common in conditions other than NPH. The accumulating evidence suggests that early postural impairment, falls, oculomotor impairment, or hallucinations are inconsistent with the diagnosis of NPH regardless of ventricular size. Recognition of the hydrocephalic presentation of PSP and DLB can avoid unnecessary and potentially harmful shunting procedures.

Competing interests

Mr. Starr has nothing to disclose.

Dr. Hagen has nothing to disclose.

Dr. Espay is supported by the K23 career development award (NIMH, 1K23MH092735); has received grant support from CleveMed/Great Lakes Neurotechnologies, Davis Phinney Foundation, and Michael J Fox Foundation; personal compensation as a consultant/scientific advisory board member for Solvay/Abbott (now Abbvie), Chelsea Therapeutics, TEVA, Impax, Merz, Solstice Neurosciences, Eli Lilly, and USWorldMeds; and honoraria from Novartis, UCB, TEVA, the American Academy of Neurology, and the Movement Disorders Society. He serves as Associate Editor of Movement Disorders, Frontiers in Movement Disorders, and the Journal of Clinical Movement Disorders; and on the editorial boards of Parkinsonism and Related Disorders and The European Neurological Journal.

Authors' contributions

BS: Drafting of the manuscript, review of literature for important intellectual content. MH: Performed and reviewed of autopsy material, intellectual review of manuscript. AJE: acquisition of data, conception and design, interpretation of data, critically review the draft and subsequent versions for important intellectual content, provided final approval of the version to be published and agree to be accountable for all aspects of the work including accuracy and integrity of the data reported. All authors read and approved the final manuscript.

Acknowledgements

The authors acknowledge the Gardner Family Foundation for their support of the Brain Autopsy program at the University of Cincinnati.

Author details
[1]Gardner Family Center for Parkinson's Disease and Movement Disorders, Department of Neurology, University of Cincinnati, 260 Stetson St, Suite 2300, Cincinnati, OH 45267-0525, USA. [2]Department of Pathology, Division of Neuropathology, University of Cincinnati, Cincinnati, OH, USA.

References
1. Klassen BT, Ahlskog JE: **Normal pressure hydrocephalus: how often does the diagnosis hold water?** *Neurology* 2011, **77**(12):1119–1125.
2. Walchenbach R, Geiger E, Thomeer RT, Vanneste JA: **The value of temporary external lumbar CSF drainage in predicting the outcome of shunting on normal pressure hydrocephalus.** *J Neurol Neurosurg Psychiatry* 2002, **72**(4):503–506.
3. Hamilton R, Patel S, Lee EB, Jackson EM, Lopinto J, Arnold SE, Clark CM, Basil A, Shaw LM, Xie SX, Grady MS, Trojanowski JQ: **Lack of shunt response in suspected idiopathic normal pressure hydrocephalus with Alzheimer disease pathology.** *Ann Neurol* 2010, **68**(4):535–540.
4. Leinonen V, Koivisto AM, Savolainen S, Rummukainen J, Sutela A, Vanninen R, Jääskeläinen JE, Soininen H, Alafuzoff I: **Post-mortem findings in 10 patients with presumed normal-pressure hydrocephalus and review of the literature.** *Neuropathol Appl Neurobiol* 2012, **38**(1):72–86.
5. Cabral D, Beach TG, Vedders L, Sue LI, Jacobson S, Myers K, Sabbagh MN: **Frequency of Alzheimer's disease pathology at autopsy in patients with clinical normal pressure hydrocephalus.** *Alzheimers Dement* 2011, **7**(5):509–513.
6. Morariu MA: **Progressive supranuclear palsy and normal-pressure hydrocephalus.** *Neurology* 1979, **29**(11):1544–1546.
7. Alisky J: **Normal pressure hydrocephalus co-existing with a second dementia disorder.** *Neuropsychiatr Dis Treat* 2008, **4**(1):301–304.
8. Chakravarty A: **Unifying concept for Alzheimer's disease, vascular dementia and normal pressure hydrocephalus - a hypothesis.** *Med Hypotheses* 2004, **63**(5):827–833.
9. Silverberg GD, Mayo M, Saul T, Rubenstein E, McGuire D: **Alzheimer's disease, normal-pressure hydrocephalus, and senescent changes in CSF circulatory physiology: a hypothesis.** *Lancet Neurol* 2003, **2**(8):506–511.
10. Silverberg GD, Mayo M, Saul T, Fellmann J, Carvalho J, McGuire D: **Continuous CSF drainage in AD: results of a double-blind, randomized, placebo-controlled study.** *Neurology* 2008, **71**(3):202–209.
11. Magdalinou NK, Ling H, Smith JD, Schott JM, Watkins LD, Lees AJ: **Normal pressure hydrocephalus or progressive supranuclear palsy? A clinicopathological case series.** *J Neurol* 2013, **260**(4):1009–1013.
12. Curran T, Lang AE: **Parkinsonian syndromes associated with hydrocephalus: case reports, a review of the literature, and pathophysiological hypotheses.** *Mov Disord* 1994, **9**(5):508–520.
13. Burghaus L, Eggers C, Timmermann L, Fink GR, Diederich NJ: **Hallucinations in neurodegenerative diseases.** *CNS Neurosci Ther* 2012, **18**(2):149–159.

Multidisciplinary intensive rehabilitation treatment improves sleep quality in Parkinson's disease

Giuseppe Frazzitta[1,9*], Roberto Maestri[2], Davide Ferrazzoli[1], Giulio Riboldazzi[3], Rossana Bera[1], Cecilia Fontanesi[4,5], Roger P Rossi[6,7], Gianni Pezzoli[8] and Maria F Ghilardi[4,6*]

Abstract

Background: Sleep disturbances are among the most common non-motor symptoms of Parkinson's disease (PD), greatly interfering with daily activities and diminishing life quality. Pharmacological treatments have not been satisfactory because of side effects and interactions with anti-parkinsonian drugs. While studies have shown that regular exercise improves sleep quality in normal aging, there is no definitive evidence in PD.

Methods: In a retrospective study, we determined whether an intense physical and multidisciplinary exercise program improves sleep quality in a large group of patients with PD.
We analyzed the scores of PD Sleep Scale (PDSS), which was administered twice, 28 days apart, to two groups of patients with PD of comparable age, gender, disease duration and pharmacological treatment. The control group (49 patients) did not receive rehabilitation, The treated group (89 patients) underwent a 28-day multidisciplinary intensive rehabilitation program (three one-hour daily sessions comprising cardiovascular warm-up, relaxation, muscle-stretching, balance and gait training, occupational therapy to improve daily living activities).

Results: At enrolment, control and treated groups had similar UPDRS and PDSS scores. At re-test, 28 days later, UPDRS and total PDSS scores improved in the treated (p < 0.0001) but not in the control group. In particular, the treated group showed significant improvement in PDSS scores for sleep quality, motor symptoms and daytime somnolence. The control group did not show improvement for any item.

Conclusions: These results suggest that multidisciplinary intensive rehabilitation treatment may have a positive impact on many aspects of sleep in PD.

Keywords: PDSS, Rehabilitation, Plasticity, Sleep quality

Background

Sleep disturbances are among the most common non-motor symptoms of Parkinson's disease (PD). Their prevalence ranges from 40% to 90%, depending upon the type of study, and they include insomnia, excessive daytime sleepiness, REM sleep behavior disorder, restless legs and sleep apnea [1,2]. Sleep problems greatly interfere with daily activities and diminish the quality of life of the patients and their caregivers. Unfortunately, these symptoms can be associated with the use of dopaminergic

* Correspondence: frazzittag62@gmail.com; lice.mg79@gmail.com
[1]Department of Parkinson Disease Rehabilitation, Moriggia-Pelascini Hospital, Gravedona ed Uniti, Fondazione Europea Ricerca Biomedica FERB, "S.Isidoro" Hospital, Trescore Balneario, Italy
[4]Department of Physiol. Pharmacol. & Neuroscience, CUNY Medical School, Harris Hall 08, CCNY, 160 Convent Ave, New York, NY 10031, USA
Full list of author information is available at the end of the article

medications [3], and the pharmacological treatments have not produced satisfactory results [4,5]. Similarly, alternative approaches, such as repetitive transcranial magnetic stimulation, have been proven ineffectual [6].

In physiological aging, sleep complaints have been addressed mostly pharmacologically, but also with alternative or complementary strategies such as exercise: studies in normally aging subjects have indeed shown that sleep quality improves following regular exercises of moderate intensity [7,8]. There are increasing evidence that physical exercise of different sort and intensity can produce clinical benefits and might improve the general life quality of patients with PD [9,10]. Only few studies show a possible benefit of physical exercise on sleep in PD. *Nascimento et al.* demonstrated that a multimodal exercise program seem to be a feasible and effective alternative to decrease sleep-related disorders in people with PD and Alzheimer's disease [11]. However, this exercise program is not specific for PD, no objective measures (i.e. physical performance test) were included, and the used scale for the assessment of sleep-related disorder (Mini-Sleep Questionnarie) [12] is not properly suitable for PD. Recently, *Wassom DJ et al.* determined the impact of a six-week Qigong exercise intervention as a potential complementary therapy in the management of sleep-related symptoms in PD. Following Qigong, subjects showed improvement in some aspects of sleep quality [13]. However this is a very small (seven patients) and uncontrolled study. Other promising indications come from a study showing that scores improved in several areas related to quality of life, including sleep, following a twelve-week exercise program [14]. However, also this study was uncontrolled and, most importantly, it used a non-PD specific scale (the Nottingham Health Profile) [15], in which sleep quality, one of six items, was tested with questions that did not address the specific problems of PD.

PD Sleep Scale (PDSS) [16] is a visual analogue scale with 15 questions related to sleep problems that are commonly associated with PD, such as REM behavior disorders and nocturnal motor symptoms. In the last ten years, PDSS has been developed, tested and used in patients with PD in different types of studies [6,17,18]. Importantly, PDSS has good test–retest reliability and it has been validated in different populations of PD patients, including an Italian population [17].

It has been demonstrated that the physical treatments specifically made for PD should be multidisciplinary and have certain characteristics of intensity in order to be effective [9,10].

In this retrospective study, we examined PDSS scores to verify the effects of a four-week multidisciplinary intensive rehabilitation program on the sleep quality in a large group of patients with PD.

Methods

Patients

We retrospectively analyzed data from our prospectively collected database of patients with PD. We studied 138 patients (61 men, mean age ± SD: 69.1 ± 7.4 years) belonging to two groups: *Group 1-* patients who underwent multidisciplinary intensive rehabilitation treatment (MIRT, 89 patients); Group 2- patients who were kept on pharmacological therapy only (Controls, 49 patients).

All patients had a diagnosis of "clinically probable" idiopathic PD [19]; Hoehn-Yahr stage 2 or 3; Mini-Mental State Examination score > 26; subjective complaints of sleep disturbances; ability to walk without physical assistance; ability to perceive visual and auditory cues. Also, they did not have any other neurological conditions, postural hypotension, cardiovascular disorders, musculoskeletal

disorders, vestibular dysfunction limiting locomotion or balance. All patients had scores less than 8 at the Hamilton Depression scale.

This is a retrospective study based on our prospectively collected institutional database.

The Local Ethics Committee of Ospedale Moriggia-Pelascini approved the study. All patients provided written consent to the scientific treatment of their data in an anonymous form at the time of the assessment.

MIRT protocol

MIRT had been described in detail in previous papers [10,20-22]. It is specifically designed for PD. Briefly, it consisted of a 4-week physical therapy that entailed three daily sessions, five days a week, in a hospital setting. The duration of each session, including recovery periods, was about one hour. The first session comprised cardiovascular warm-up activities, relaxation, muscle-stretching (scapular, hip flexor, hamstring and gastrocnemius muscles), exercises to improve the range of motion of spinal, pelvic and scapular joints, exercises to improve the functionality of the abdominal muscles, and postural changes in the supine position. The second session included exercises to improve balance and gait using a stabilometric platform with visual cues (patients had to follow a circular pathway on a screen by using a cursor sensitive to their feet movements on the platform) and treadmill plus (treadmill training with both visual and auditory cues) [23]. All the exercise on the treadmill were aerobic with a hearth rate reserve 60% to 70% and a maximum speed of treadmill scrolling of 3.5 km/h. The last was a session of occupational therapy to improve autonomy in day living activities: transferring from sitting to standing, rolling from supine to sitting position and viceversa, dressing, use of tools, exercises to improve hand functionality and visuo-motor skills. The rehabilitation program, considering individually each patient, could also include: speech therapy, hydrotherapy (for severe disorders of balance and posture), and robotic-assisted walking training for specific gait disorders (i.e. freezing of gait).

Outcome measures

In both groups, we analyzed UPDRS III and II scores measured at enrolment and 28 days later, always at 10 AM, by the same neurologist, expert in movement disorders and blind with respect to the study design. Although UPDRS is a scale with some limitations (i.e. the low emphasis on the non-motor features of PD), we used this scale to establish the effect of MIRT on activities of daily life and on motor clinical aspects of the disease. These data were important in order to evaluate the correlations between the motor performance and the sleep parameters. Sleep complaints were assessed with an Italian translation of the PDSS [17]. Chaudhuri et al.

showed that the PDSS is easy to use and is a reliable instrument for measuring sleep disturbances in PD [16]. Each of the items or questions was scored on a scale between 0 (always suffer from the disorder) and 10 (never suffers the disorder). The PDSS items were also grouped into sub-domains or categories of sleep-related disorders; sleep quality (items 1–3), nocturnal restlessness (item 4 and 5), nocturnal distressing dreams and hallucinations (item 6 and 7), nocturia (item 8), nocturnal motor off and sensory symptoms (items 9–13), and daytime somnolence (item 14 and 15). Classification of patients with nocturnal symptoms was based on a pre-specified cutoff score of less than or equal to 100; single items with a score below 8 were considered as "sleep disturbances" [16,24].

Statistical analysis

Descriptive statistics are reported as mean ± SD. Shapiro–Wilk statistic was used to assess the normality of the distribution of all variables. To ascertain whether MIRT improved sleep quality, we used a mixed model ANOVA with Group (MIRT; Control) as between factor and Time (baseline, 28 days later) as within factor, and post-hoc tests. Correlations between PDSS, clinical and demographic data were assessed by the Pearson R coefficient. A p-value < 0.05 was considered statistically significant.

Results

PDSS at enrolment: characteristics of sleep in PD

Analyses on the combined group of 138 patients (MIRT: 89; Controls: 49) showed that, at enrolment, disease duration was 9.3 years (±3.3, SD); levodopa equivalent medication 611.5 mg (±341.8), Hoehn & Yahr stage 2.61 (±0.48), UPDRS II scores 11.4 (±5.5) and UPDRS III scores 14.87 (±7.1). On average, the total score of PDSS was 109.03 (±23.77) with 32% of the patients (44 in total, 36 in group 1 and 8 in group 2) having a total PDSS less or equal to 100. Table 1 reports average scores and percentages of patients with abnormal scores (<8) for each PDSS item. In general, these results were similar to the ones reported previously in different PD studies [16-18,24], with item 8 (nocturia) having the lowest scores and the greatest percentage of patients with abnormal scores.

We then correlated the global PDSS scores with the clinical and demographic data. Briefly, PDSS scores showed significant inverse correlation with UPDRS II scores (r = −0.29, p = 0.0005) and with the amount of levodopa equivalent therapy (r = −0.24, p = 0.005). No significant correlation was found between PDSS scores and age, gender, disease duration and UPDRS III scores.

Between-group comparisons at enrolment revealed no significant differences for disease duration (9.1 ± 3.6 vs. 9.7 ± 2.7 years, p = 0.32); levodopa equivalent medication (581.1 ± 351.7 vs. 666.8 ± 319.3 mg, p = 0.2), Hoehn &

Table 1 Average scores (±SD) and percentage of patients with abnormal scores (<8)

Item	Mean Score ± SD	Abnormal Score (%)
1	6.5 ± 2.6	57.2
2	6.6 ± 3.3	50.7
3	6.0 ± 3.2	65.2
4	7.3 ± 3.3	37.7
5	7.3 ± 3.1	42.8
6	8.4 ± 2.4	21.7
7	9.6 ± 1.3	5.1
8	4.2 ± 3.1	83.3
9	7.1 ± 3.4	39.9
10	7.6 ± 2.7	40.6
11	7.2 ± 2.9	47.8
12	7.3 ± 3.3	37.0
13	8.0 ± 2.9	27.5
14	7.2 ± 3.0	42.8
15	8.7 ± 1.9	26.1

Yahr stage (2.61 ± 0.52 vs. 2.61 ± 0.44, p = 0.999) and UPDRS III scores (14.33 ± 5.97 vs. 15.86 ± 8.76, p = 0.23).

The mean ± SD and the percentage of patients with abnormal scores (<8) for of each of the PDSS items are reported for each group in Figure 1 and Table 2. Briefly, at enrolment, there was no significant difference between the total scores (106.67 ± 27.29 vs. 113.3 ± 14.79, p = 0.12). However, we found between-group differences for some items: restlessness (item 4, MIRT < Controls, p = 0.013), nocturia (item 8, MIRT > Controls, p = 0.009), incontinence (item 9, MIRT < Controls, p = 0.01), numbness during sleep (item 10, MIRT < Controls, p = 0.04), pain at awakening (item 12, MIRT < Controls, p = 0.04), tiredness in the morning (item 14, MIRT < Controls, p = 0.0008), daytime sleepiness (item 15, MIRT > Controls, p = 0.05). Nevertheless, the scores' profiles of the two groups were similar, with item 8 (nocturia) having the lowest scores and item 7 (hallucinations) the greatest scores (Figure 1).

MIRT improves UPDRS scores and sleep quality

In both groups, pharmacological therapy did not change during the twenty-eight day period and it was the same at both testing times, thus ruling out a possible effects related to drug changes. Twenty-eight days after the baseline, UPDRS scores significantly decreased in the MIRT group (UPDRS III: 14.33 ± 5.97 vs. 8.34 ± 5.36 p < 0.0001; UPDRS II: 11.29 ± 4.88 vs. 6.63 ± 3.96, p < 0.0001), while they did not change in the controls (UPDRS III: 15.8 ± 8.76 vs. 15.65 ± 8.48, p = 0.23; UPDRS II: 11.69 ± 5.36 vs. 11.49 ± 6.44, p = 0.42).

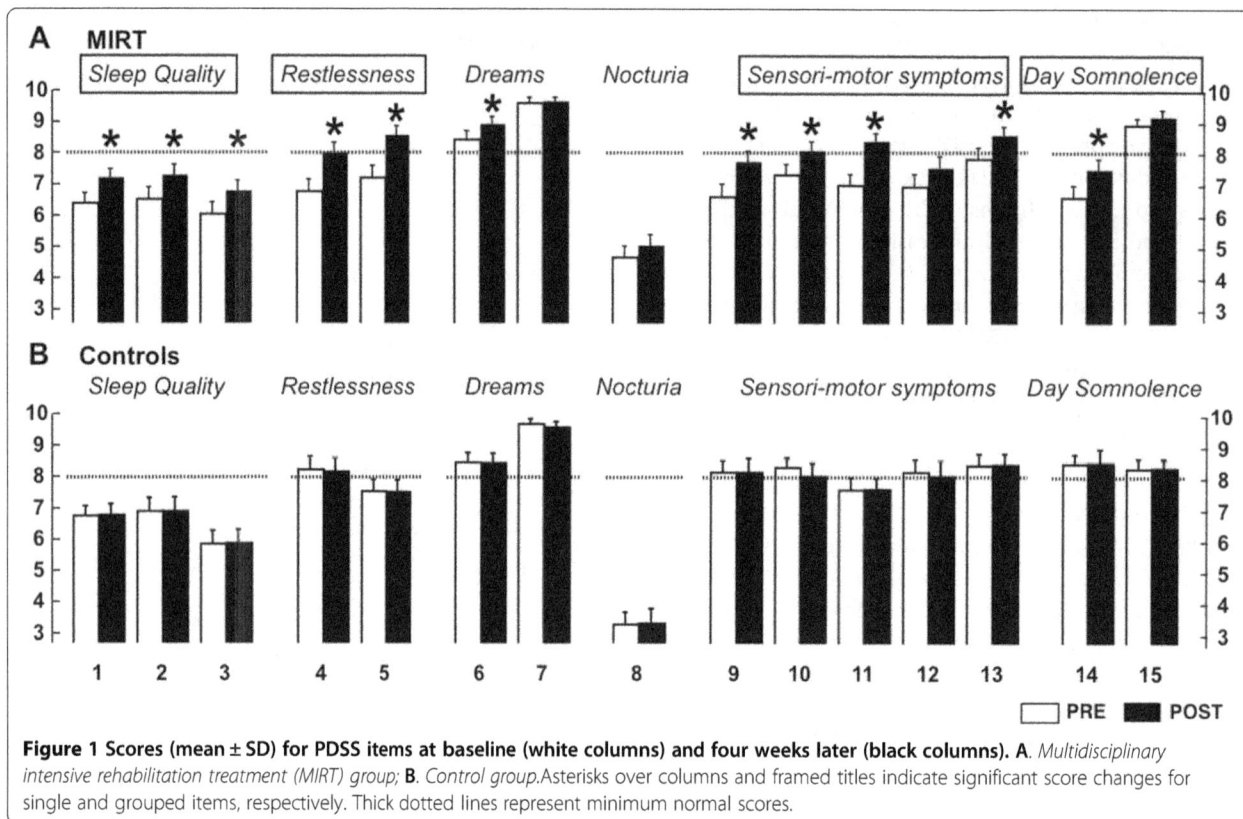

Figure 1 Scores (mean ± SD) for PDSS items at baseline (white columns) and four weeks later (black columns). **A**. *Multidisciplinary intensive rehabilitation treatment (MIRT) group;* **B**. *Control group.*Asterisks over columns and framed titles indicate significant score changes for single and grouped items, respectively. Thick dotted lines represent minimum normal scores.

An ANOVA on the total PDSS scores revealed a significant interaction between Groups and Time (Group: $F_{(1,136)} = 0.025$, $p = 0.88$; Time: $F_{(1,136)} = 18.22$; $p < 0.0001$; TimeXGroup: $F_{(1,1)} = 21.40$; $p < 0.0001$), suggesting a significant change in the MIRT group only. On

Table 2 Percentage of patients with abnormal scores (<8)

	Group 1			Group 2		
Item	PRE	POST	Difference	PRE	POST	Difference
1	55.06	49.44	5.62	61.22	61.22	0
2	50.56	40.45	10.11	51.02	48.98	2.04
3	62.92	53.93	8.99	69.39	67.35	2.04
4	43.82	28.09	15.73	26.53	28.57	−2.04
5	39.33	22.47	16.85	48.98	48.98	0
6	22.47	20.22	2.25	20.41	20.41	0
7	5.62	6.74	−1.12	4.08	4.08	0
8	75.28	71.91	3.37	97.96	97.96	0
9	44.94	37.08	7.87	30.61	30.61	0
10	40.45	31.46	8.99	40.82	44.90	−4.08
11	47.19	22.47	**24.72**	48.98	48.98	0
12	40.45	31.46	8.99	30.61	32.65	−2.04
13	30.34	24.72	5.62	22.45	24.49	−2.04
14	51.69	35.96	15.73	26.53	26.53	0
15	20.22	13.48	6.74	36.73	36.73	0

average, in the MIRT group, PDSS scores increased from 106.67 (±27.29) to 118.4 (±20.27; $p < 0.0001$), while they slightly decreased in the controls (from 113.3 ± 14.79 to 112.84 ± 14.78; $p = 0.03$). Also, as shown in Table 2 for each item, the percentage of patients with abnormal scores decreased in MIRT group and remained the same in the controls. In Figure 1, we report the scores of each item, separately and grouped by category, for the two groups at the two time points. Analysis of individual scores revealed that, in MIRT group, significant improvement occurred for almost all the items, with the exclusion of: items 7 (distressing hallucinations during the night) and 15 (daytime sleepiness), which had already average scores close to 10 before treatment; items 8 (nocturia) and 12 (painful posture in the morning), which showed only trends to improvement. In the controls, no statistical changes were noted, with the exception of a mild worsening for item 7 (from 9.63 ± 0.97 to 9.53 ± 1.0, $p = 0.024$). Thus, in summary, improvement in MIRT group was significant for the sensori-motor symptoms and restlessness (Group: $F_{(1, 138)} = 1.63$, $p = 0.2$; Time: $F_{(1, 138)} = 4.14$; $p = 0.04$; TimeXGroup: $F_{(1,1)} = 5.93$; $p = 0.0031$; post-hoc: MIRT: $p < 0.0001$, controls: $p = 0.24$); the quality of sleep items (Group: $F_{(1, 138)} = 0.22$, $p = 0.64$; Time: $F_{(1, 138)} = 9.17$; $p = 0.0029$; TimeXGroup: $F_{(1,1)} = 8.49$; $p = 0.0042$; post-hoc: MIRT: $p < 0.0001$, controls: $p = 0.32$); daytime somnolence (Group: $F_{(1, 138)} = 0.85$, $p = 0.36$;

Time: $F(1, 138) = 4.3$; $p = 0.04$; TimeXGroup: $F(1,1) = 3.8$; $p = 0.049$; post-hoc: MIRT: $p < 0.0088$; controls: $p = 0.32$).

We then verified whether the improvement in the general quality of sleep in the MIRT group was triggered by improvement in other categories or items: there were no significant correlations between improvements in any of the items or category and the quality of sleep. Nevertheless, we found significant correlations between improvements in nocturnal sensory-motor symptoms and daytime somnolence ($r = 0.39$; $p = 0.001$) as well as between restlessness (item 4 and 5) and distressing hallucinations during the night ($r = 0.38$; $p = 0.001$).

Finally, we found significant correlations in MIRT group between the changes in the PDSS total scores and in the UPDRS III and II scores (PDSS and UPDRS III: $r = 0.26$ $p = 0.009$; PDSS and UPDRS II: $r = 0.35$, $p = 0.005$). When we verified these correlations for each of the PDSS categories (Table 3), we found that sleep quality significantly correlated with the changes in UPDRS total and UPDRS II scores, as well as with the performance on the 6-minute walking time test. Improvement in the sensory-motor nocturnal symptoms instead significantly correlated with PDDS changes, while decrease in restlessness correlated with improvement in the total UPDRS scores.

While the total scores and the PDSS general profiles were similar in the two groups at baseline, there were significant between-group differences for some of the PDSS items. Since the control group had greater scores closer to the normal range, although unlikely, over time improvement in this group could have been prevented by a ceiling effect. Thus, we selected a subgroup of controls with abnormal PDSS scores (<8) in at least one item at baseline and matched them with subjects of MIRT group by PDSS scores, UPDRS scores, age, and levodopa equivalents. This procedure left us with 30 subjects per group. ANOVAs comparing the effect of exercise and group revealed results similar to those obtained with the entire groups: for the total PDSS scores we found a significant interaction between Groups and Time (Group: $F(1, 58) = 3.6$, $p = 0.064$; Time: $F(1, 58) = 36.3$; $p < 0.0001$; TimeXGroup: $F(1,1) = 41.8$; $p < 0.0001$), showing again a significant score improvement in the

Table 3 Correlations between improvements in PDSS category and clinical scores (r values)

	Sleep quality	Day sleepiness	Motor & Sensory	Psychosis	Restlessness
UPDRSTot	0.32*	0.08	0.20	0.05	0.29*
UPDRS_III	0.11	−0.07	0.01	−0.06	0.11
UPDRS_II	0.28*	0.07	0.14	0.07	0.21
PDDS	0.07	0.09	0.35*	0.10	0.21
sixMWT	−0.26*	0.04	−0.17	−0.16	−0.11

*Significant correlation between improvements in PDSS category and clinical scores (r values).

MIRT group only. These results further suggest that absence of improvement in the control group is not due to a "ceiling" effect.

Discussion and conclusions

The main result of this study is that a four-week intensive rehabilitation treatment in patients with PD has a positive effect on the sleep quality measured with PDSS, a scale that specifically addresses the sleep complaints of this disease. Second, the significant correlation between the improvements in UPDRS II and PDSS scores confirms that sleep plays an important role in improving autonomy in daily living activities and quality of life in patients with PD. Third, the finding of a significant inverse correlation between levodopa equivalents and PDSS scores suggests that increase of dopaminergic therapy has a negative impact on the quality of sleep of patients with PD. Altogether, these results suggest that sleep is an important factor in determining quality and autonomy in daily living activities in PD and that increasing levodopa levels might have a negative effect on sleep quality. Our data coincide with those recently appeared in recent studies showing that dopaminergic treatment decreases subjective and objective indices of sleep quality [25]. For instance, dopaminergic medication is thought to have a desynchronizing effect on sleep architecture that causes disruption of sleep continuity leading to excessive daytime sleepiness and "sleep attacks" [26]. Finally, these results confirm previous findings about the profile of the PDSS scores [15] in a different Italian population and suggest that PDSS yields highly reproducible results at one-month retest in the control group.

MIRT has a positive effect on sleep quality and on nocturnal motor symptoms

As in previous studies [10,20,22], UPDRS II and III scores significantly decreased after MIRT, while they did not change in the control group after a similar time interval. The novel finding is that the scores of PDSS, a scale geared to measure sleep problems that are specific to PD, also improved following MIRT. The most significant effects were seen in the general quality of sleep, nocturnal motor symptoms and daytime somnolence.

A few papers have already reported that exercise has a positive effect on the general quality of sleep in elderly normal subjects [7,8]. This is the first study in a large PD population showing that, besides improving the general quality of sleep, exercise decreases the severity of the nocturnal symptoms that are typical of this disease. Although improvements in those two categories could be related, as the general quality of sleep might benefit from decreased severity of nocturnal parkinsonian symptoms, we did not find any significant correlation between them. Nocturnal motor and sensory-related symptoms such as restlessness, off periods, numbness, tingling and cramps, are characteristically found in a majority of patients with PD and are responsible for frequent arousals and disruption of sleep. The origins of the specific nocturnal symptoms as well as of problems falling asleep and maintaining sleep are still obscure, mostly because the effects of multiple factors with a possible causal role cannot be disentangled. In fact, on one side, the disease is accompanied by the degeneration of the brainstem regulatory centers of sleep and wakefulness; on the other, dopaminergic treatment contributes to exacerbating sleep problems. What could be the mechanisms behind this exercise-related improvement?

It is possible that the general improvement in several aspects of motor performance, measured with the UPDRS III scores, might lead to a reduction of nocturnal hypokinesia resulting in both an enhancement of sleep quality and a reduction of sensory-motor nocturnal symptoms. However, although nocturnal hypokinesia might be a major determinant of sleep quality [27], we did not find significant correlations between improvements in PDSS and UPDRS III scores. We instead found significant correlations between improvements in the scores of PDSS and UPDRS II, which reflect autonomy in daily living activities. Although we cannot establish direct causality between sleep improvement and quality of daytime life, undoubtedly, exercise improves the quality of both sleep and daytime life, with a significant gain in personal autonomy.

Therefore, we found that MIRT significantly improved the sleep quality of Parkinsonian patients. Although further studies are needed, these results strongly suggest that exercise should be included in the management of sleep disturbances in PD.

The effects of MIRT on sleep might be linked to enhanced brain plasticity

A rather speculative interpretation of the mechanisms of MIRT effects on sleep quality might come from a recently formulated hypothesis, the synaptic homeostasis hypothesis [28], that provides a crucial link between plasticity-related phenomena and sleep. Briefly, this hypothesis states that during wake, activity induces long term potentiation (LTP)-related processes resulting in synaptic strength increases, which, in turn, promote sleep and, in particular, slow wave activity, the most restorative part of sleep. The function of slow wave activity is to renormalize, off-line, the synaptic weight and to restore the proper function, counteracting all costs of wake, both at cellular, system, and behavioral levels. Thus, more efficient are the LTP-related phenomena and the synapses strengthening during the day, greater is the slow wave activity during sleep. Indeed, exercise enhances the mechanisms related to brain plasticity, with positive effects on dopaminergic and

glutamatergic neurotransmission [29], striatal upregulation of brain-derived neurotrophic factor (BDNF) and glial cell line-derived neurotrophic factor in rat models of PD [30], hippocampal neurogenesis in normal mice [31], increased levels of peripheral BDNF in the elderly [32] and in patients in the early PD stages [33].

In patients with PD, electrophysiological and behavioral induction of LTP-like phenomena in the cortex seems impaired, with decreased potentiation phenomena [34-36] and decreased retention of new skills [30,37,38]. In addition, slow wave activity during sleep is reduced in patients with PD [26]. We thus might speculate that exercise, by enhancing LTP-related phenomena and promoting plasticity during wakefulness, might trigger a more restorative sleep. Indeed, prospective studies are needed to verify this hypothesis and to determine whether exercise produces improvements in LTP-related mechanisms and whether this improvement induces, in turn, changes in the sleep electroencephalography.

Study limitations

This study was based on retrospective analysis of a prospectively collected data-base. Even though this study design might constitute a potential limitation, we think that our results would not change significantly in a controlled study since data collection procedures were carefully designed and all relevant information were recorded on a structured protocol.

Although in this study was demonstrated a significant inverse correlation between levodopa equivalents and PDSS scores, the confounding effects of PD medications on sleep has not been completely addressed. Sleep disturbances in PD are dose related [39]: low-dose dopamine agonists have been associated with insomnia, whereas higher doses can lead to excessive daytime sleepiness. While initially associated with dopamine agonists, these symptoms can be induced by levodopa as well [3].

Limitations also include the different environmental conditions for the two groups. In fact, patients in the MIRT group were hospitalized for the entire 28-day period, while the controls were not. However, while hospitalization generally worsens sleep, in our study we have found an improving in sleep quality at the end of MIRT.

Another limitation arises from the difficulty to discern the effects related to the generic exercise and those directly attributable to MIRT. It is common opinion that better results in Parkinsonian patients have achieved using training program with a high training intensity, "beyond what they may self-select" [40], and with a multidisciplinary approach [41]. The aim of the study was to evaluate the efficacy of MIRT in Parkinsonian patients in comparison to patients treated only with drugs. The next step will be planning a study with a comparison between two different rehabilitation treatments.

A last criticism is the possible placebo effect of rehabilitation. The strength of expectation of clinical improvement during a rehabilitation or pharmacological treatment influences *per se* the release of dopamine [42]. This is another aspect that has to be clarified in a future study comparing two different rehabilitation treatments and providing for a follow-up period.

Abbreviations
PD: Parkinson's disease; PDSS: PD sleep scale; MIRT: Multidisciplinary intensive rehabilitation treatment; UPDRS: Unified Parkinson's disease rating scale; LTP: Long term potentiation; BDNF: Brain-derived neurotrophic factor.

Competing interests
The authors declare that they have no competing interests.

Authors' contributions
GF: Research project: A. Conception, B. Organization, C. Execution; Statistical Analysis: A. Design, B. Execution, C. Review and Critique; Manuscript: A. Writing of the first draft, B. Review and Critique. RM: Research project: B. Organization, C. Execution; Statistical Analysis: A. Design, B. Execution, C. Review and Critique; Manuscript: B. Review and Critique. GR: Research project: B. Organization, C. Execution; Manuscript: A. Writing of the first draft, B. Review and Critique. DF: Research project: B. Organization, C. Execution; Manuscript: A. Writing of the first draft, B. Review and Critique. RB: Research project: B. Organization, C. Execution; Manuscript: A. Writing of the first draft, B. Review and Critique. CF: Statistical Analysis: B. Execution, C. Review and Critique; Manuscript: A. Writing of the first draft, B. Review and Critique. RPR: Research project: A. Conception, B. Organization, Statistical Analysis: C. Review and Critique; Manuscript: A. Writing of the first draft, B. Review and Critique. GP: Research project: A. Conception, B. Organization, C. Execution; Statistical Analysis: A. Design, B. Execution, C. Review and Critique; Manuscript: A. Writing of the first draft, B. Review and Critique. MFG: Research project: A. Conception, B. Organization, C. Execution; Statistical Analysis: A. Design, B. Execution, C. Review and Critique; Manuscript: A. Writing of the first draft, B. Review and Critique. All authors read and approved the final manuscript.

Authors' information
Cecilia Fontanesi:
Employment: CCNY
Grants: CUNY Science Scholarship
M. Felice Ghilardi:
Consultancies: New York University
Employment: CUNY
Grants: NPF, McDonnell Foundation, NIH

Funding
This work was supported by grants from the National Parkinson Foundation (MFG), the National Institutes of Health Grant NS-054864 (MFG).

Author details
[1]Department of Parkinson Disease Rehabilitation, Moriggia-Pelascini Hospital, Gravedona ed Uniti, Fondazione Europea Ricerca Biomedica FERB, "S.Isidoro" Hospital, Trescore Balneario, Italy. [2]Department of Biomedical Engineering, Scientific Institute of Montescano, S. Maugeri Foundation IRCCS, Montescano, Italy. [3]Center for Parkinson's Disease, Macchi Foundation, Varese and Department of Rehabilitation, "Le Terrazze" Hospital, Cunardo, Italy. [4]Department of Physiol. Pharmacol. & Neuroscience, CUNY Medical School, Harris Hall 08, CCNY, 160 Convent Ave, New York, NY 10031, USA. [5]The Graduate Center, Biology - Neuroscience PhD Program, CUNY, New York, NY, USA. [6]Department of Physical Medicine & Rehabilitation, JFK Johnson Rehabilitation Institute, Edison, NJ, USA. [7]NYU Movement Disorder Center, New York University, New York, NY, USA. [8]Parkinson Institute, Istituti Clinici di Perfezionamento, Milano, Italy. [9]Department of Parkinson Rehabilitation, Ospedale Moriggia Pelascini, Via Pelascini 3, Gravedona ed Uniti, Como 22015, Italy.

References
1. Barone P, Antonini A, Colosimo C, Marconi R, Morgante L, Avarello TP, et al. The PRIAMO study: A multicenter assessment of nonmotor symptoms and their impact on quality of life in Parkinson's disease. Mov Disord. 2009;15:1641–9.
2. Kumar S, Bhatia M, Behari M. Sleep disorders in Parkinson's disease. Mov Disord. 2002;17:775–81.
3. Park A, Stacy M. Dopamine-induced nonmotor symptoms of Parkinson's disease. Parkinsons Dis. 2011;2011:485063.
4. Budur K, Rodriguez C, Foldvary-Schaefer N. Advances in treating insomnia. Cleve Clin J Med. 2007;74:251–2. 5–8, 61–2 passim.
5. Paus S, Brecht HM, Koster J, Seeger G, Klockgether T, Wullner U. Sleep attacks, daytime sleepiness, and dopamine agonists in Parkinson's disease. Mov Disord. 2003;18:659–67.
6. Arias P, Vivas J, Grieve KL, Cudeiro J. Double-blind, randomized, placebo controlled trial on the effect of 10 days low-frequency rTMS over the vertex on sleep in Parkinson's disease. Sleep Med. 2010;11:759–65.
7. King AC, Oman RF, Brassington GS, Bliwise DL, Haskell WL. Moderate-intensity exercise and self-rated quality of sleep in older adults. A randomized controlled trial. JAMA. 1997;277:32–7.
8. Santos RV, Viana VA, Boscolo RA, Marques VG, Santana MG, Lira FS, et al. Moderate exercise training modulates cytokine profile and sleep in elderly people. Cytokine. 2012;60:731–5.
9. Ellis T, Katz DI, White DK, DePiero TJ, Hohler AD, Saint-Hilaire M. Effectiveness of an inpatient multidisciplinary rehabilitation program for people with Parkinson disease. Phys Ther. 2008;88:812–9.
10. Frazzitta G, Bertotti G, Riboldazzi G, Turla M, Uccellini D, Boveri N, et al. Effectiveness of intensive inpatient rehabilitation treatment on disease progression in parkinsonian patients: a randomized controlled trial with 1-year follow-up. Neurorehabil Neural Repair. 2012;26:144–50.
11. Nascimento CM, Ayan C, Cancela JM, Gobbi LT, Gobbi S, Stella F. Effect of a multimodal exercise program on sleep disturbances and instrumental activities of daily living performance on Parkinson's and Alzheimer's disease patients. Geriatr Gerontol Int. 2014;14:259–66.
12. Gorenstein C. Reliability of a sleep self-evaluation questionnaire. AMB Rev Assoc Med Bras. 1983;29:155–7.
13. Wassom DJ, Lyons KE, Pahwa R, Liu W. Qigong exercise may improve sleep quality and gait performance in Parkinson's disease: a pilot study. Int J Neurosci 2014, Oct 22. [Epub ahead of print]. doi:10.3109/00207454.2014.966820.
14. Rodrigues De Paula F, Teixeira Salmela LF, Coelho De Morais Faria CD, Rocha De Brito P, Cardoso F. Impact of an exercise program on physical, emotional, and social aspects of quality of life of individuals with Parkinson's disease. Mov Disord. 2006;21:1073–7.
15. Hunt SM, McKenna SP, McEwen J, Backett EM, Williams J, Papp E. A quantitative approach to perceived health status: a validation study. J Epidemiol Community Health. 1980;34:281–6.
16. Chaudhuri KR, Pal S, DiMarco A, Whately-Smith C, Bridgman K, Mathew R, et al. The Parkinson's disease sleep scale: a new instrument for assessing sleep and nocturnal disability in Parkinson's disease. J Neurol Neurosurg Psychiatry. 2002;73:629–35.
17. Pellecchia MT, Antonini A, Bonuccelli U, Fabbrini G, Ferini Strambi L, Stocchi F, et al. Observational study of sleep-related disorders in Italian patients with Parkinson's disease: usefulness of the Italian version of Parkinson's disease sleep scale. Neurol Sci. 2012;33:689–94.
18. Trenkwalder C, Kies B, Rudzinska M, Fine J, Nikl J, Honczarenko K, et al. Rotigotine effects on early morning motor function and sleep in Parkinson's disease: a double-blind, randomized, placebo-controlled study (RECOVER). Mov Disord. 2011;26:90–9.
19. Gelb DJ, Oliver E, Gilman S. Diagnostic criteria for Parkinson disease. Arch Neurol. 1999;56:33–9.
20. Frazzitta G, Morelli M, Bertotti G, Felicetti G, Pezzoli G, and Maestri R. Intensive Rehabilitation Treatment in Parkinsonian Patients with Dyskinesias: A Preliminary Study with 6-Month Follow-up. Parkinson's Disease 2012, (2012). Article ID 910454, 4 pages. doi:10.1155/2012/910454
21. Frazzitta G, Bertotti G, Uccellini D, Boveri N, Rovescala R, Pezzoli G, Maestri R. Short- and Long-Term Efficacy of Intensive Rehabilitation Treatment on Balance and Gait in Parkinsonian Patients: A Preliminary Study with a 1-Year Follow-up. Parkinson's Disease 2013, (2013) Article ID 583278, 5 pages. doi:10.1155/2013/583278.
22. Frazzitta G, Maestri R, Bertotti G, Riboldazzi G, Boveri N, Perini M, Uccellini D, Turla M, Comi C, Pezzoli G, Ghilardi MF. Intensive Rehabilitation Treatment

in Early Parkinson's Disease: A Randomized Pilot Study With a 2-Year Follow-Up. Neurorehabilitation and Neural Repair 2014, 2014.

23. Frazzitta G, Maestri R, Uccellini D, Bertotti G, Abelli P. Rehabilitation treatment of gait in patients with Parkinson's disease with freezing: a comparison between two physical therapy protocols using visual and auditory cues with or without treadmill training. Mov Disord. 2009;24:1139–43.

24. Chaudhuri RK, Martinez-Martin P, Rolfe KA, Cooper J, Rockett CB, Giorgi L, et al. Improvements in nocturnal symptoms with ropinirole prolonged release in patients with advanced Parkinson's disease. Eur J Neurol. 2012;19:105–13.

25. Chahine LM, Daley J, Horn S, Duda JE, Colcher A, Hurtig H, et al. Association between dopaminergic medications and nocturnal sleep in early-stage Parkinson's disease. Parkinsonism Relat Disord. 2013;19:859–63.

26. Brunner H, Wetter TC, Hogl B, Yassouridis A, Trenkwalder C, Friess E. Microstructure of the non-rapid eye movement sleep electroencephalogram in patients with newly diagnosed Parkinson's disease: effects of dopaminergic treatment. Mov Disord. 2002;17:928–33.

27. Louter M, Munneke M, Bloem BR, Overeem S. Nocturnal hypokinesia and sleep quality in Parkinson's disease. J Am Geriatr Soc. 2012;60:1104–8.

28. Tononi G, Cirelli C. Sleep and the price of plasticity: from synaptic and cellular homeostasis to memory consolidation and integration. Neuron. 2014;81:12–34.

29. Petzinger GM, Fisher BE, Van Leeuwen JE, Vukovic M, Akopian G, Meshul CK, et al. Enhancing neuroplasticity in the basal ganglia: the role of exercise in Parkinson's disease. Mov Disord. 2010;1:S141–5.

30. Cotman CW, Berchtold NC, Christie LA. Exercise builds brain health: key roles of growth factor cascades and inflammation. Trends Neurosci. 2007;30:464–72.

31. van Praag H, Shubert T, Zhao C, Gage FH. Exercise enhances learning and hippocampal neurogenesis in aged mice. J Neurosci. 2005;25:8680–5.

32. Voss MW, Prakash RS, Erickson KI, Basak C, Chaddock L, Kim JS, et al. Plasticity of brain networks in a randomized intervention trial of exercise training in older adults. Front Aging Neurosci. 2010;2:32. 10.3389/fnagi.2010.00032.

33. Frazzitta G, Maestri R, Ghilardi MF, Riboldazzi G, Perini M, Bertotti G, et al. Intensive Rehabilitation Increases BDNF Serum Levels in Parkinsonian Patients: A Randomized Study. Neurorehabil Neural Repair. 2014;28:163–8.

34. Kishore A, Joseph T, Velayudhan B, Popa T, Meunier S. Early, severe and bilateral loss of LTP and LTD-like plasticity in motor cortex (M1) in de novo Parkinson's disease. Clin Neurophysiol. 2012;123:822–8.

35. Koch G. Do studies on cortical plasticity provide a rationale for using Non-invasive brain stimulation as a treatment for Parkinson's disease patients? Front Neurol. 2013;4:180.

36. Morgante F, Espay AJ, Gunraj C, Lang AE, Chen R. Motor cortex plasticity in Parkinson's disease and levodopa-induced dyskinesias. Brain. 2006;129:1059–69.

37. Bedard P, Sanes JN. Basal ganglia-dependent processes in recalling learned visual-motor adaptations. Exp Brain Res. 2011;209:385–93.

38. Marinelli L, Crupi D, Di Rocco A, Bove M, Eidelberg D, Abbruzzese G, et al. Learning and consolidation of visuo-motor adaptation in Parkinson's disease. Parkinsonism Relat Disord. 2009;15:6–11.

39. Verbaan D, van Rooden SM, Visser M, Marinus J, van Hilten JJ. Nighttime sleep problems and daytime sleepiness in Parkinson's disease. Mov Disord. 2008;23:35–41.

40. Hirsch MA, Farley BG. Exercise and neuroplasticity in persons living with Parkinson's disease. Eur J Phys Rehabil Med. 2009;45:215–29.

41. Post B, van der Eijk M, Munneke M, Bloem BR. Multidisciplinary care for Parkinson's disease: not if, but how! Pract Neurol. 2011;11:58–61.

42. Lidstone SC, Schulzer M, Dinelle K, Mak E, Sossi V, Ruth TJ, et al. Effects of expectation on placebo-induced dopamine release in Parkinson disease. Arch Gen Psychiatry. 2010;67:857–65.

3

Freezing of gait and white matter changes: a tract-based spatial statistics study

Kazumi Iseki[1,2,3,4*], Hidenao Fukuyama[1], Naoya Oishi[1], Hidekazu Tomimoto[5], Yoshinobu Otsuka[1], Manabu Nankaku[6], David Benninger[2], Mark Hallett[2] and Takashi Hanakawa[1,7,8]

Abstract

Background: We hypothesized that the integrity of white matter might be related to the severity of freezing of gait in age-related white matter changes.

Methods: Twenty subjects exhibiting excessive hyperintensities in the periventricular and deep white matter were recruited. The subjects underwent the Freezing of Gait Questionnaire, computerized gait analyses, and diffusion tensor magnetic resonance imaging. Images of axial, radial and mean diffusivity, and fractional anisotropy were calculated as indices of white matter integrity and analyzed with tract-based spatial statistics.

Results: The fractional anisotropy, mean, axial and radial diffusivity averaged across the whole white matter structure were all significantly correlated with Freezing of Gait Questionnaire scores. Regionally, a negative correlation between Freezing of Gait Questionnaire scores and fractional anisotropy was found in the left superior longitudinal fasciculus beneath the left premotor cortex, right corpus callosum, and left cerebral peduncle. The scores of the Freezing of Gait Questionnaire were positively correlated with mean diffusivity in the left corona radiata and right corpus callosum, and with both axial and radial diffusivity in the left corona radiata. The white matter integrity in these tracts (except the corpus callosum) showed no correlation with cognitive or other gait measures, supporting the specificity of those abnormalities to freezing of gait.

Conclusion: Divergent pathological lesions involved neural circuits composed of the cerebral cortex, basal ganglia and brainstem, suggesting that freezing of gait has a multifactorial nature.

Keywords: Age-related white matter change (ARWMC), Diffusion tensor imaging (DTI), Disconnection, Freezing of gait (FOG), Tract-based spatial statistics (TBSS), Vascular Parkinsonism

Background

Freezing of gait (FOG) is a characteristic symptom observed in some patients with gait disorders. FOG is defined as an "inability to generate effective stepping movement" [1]. It is often observed in patients with idiopathic Parkinson's disease (PD), and is even more prevalent in patients with atypical Parkinsonism (including vascular Parkinsonism) than in those with PD [2]. FOG can be seen in age-related white matter changes (ARWMC), which refer to the neuroradiological

* Correspondence: kazumi.iseki@gmail.com
[1]Human Brain Research Center, Kyoto University Graduate School of Medicine, 54 Kawahara-cho, Shogoin, Sakyo-ku, Kyoto 606-8507, Japan
[2]Human Motor Control Section, Medical Neurology Branch, National Institute of Neurological Disorders and Stroke, National Institutes of Health, Bethesda, MD, USA
Full list of author information is available at the end of the article

state of diffusely extended white matter lesions in elderly subjects [3-5].

The pathophysiology of FOG remains unclear [6]. The most reliable measure of the severity in FOG to date is the total score on the Freezing of Gait Questionnaire (FOGQ) [7]. Following recent development, white matter (WM) integrity can now be evaluated using diffusion tensor imaging (DTI). A directional bias of water diffusion can be quantified by measuring fractional anisotropy (FA), while mean diffusivity (MD) indicates the degree of diffusion [8].

Analysis of DTI can directly test whether the cortico-subcortical disconnection of WM tracts is responsible for gait disturbance as suggested by previous studies on gait disturbance in ARWMC [9,10]. Tract-based spatial statistics (TBSS) analysis of DTI data was recently developed as an automatic, hypothesis-free and precise method for the assessment of integrity of the WM [11]. Here we investigated the degree of integrity and directionality of the WM tracts in ARWMC patients, by means of TBSS analysis of DTI in combination with FOGQ scores.

Methods

Subjects

Twenty subjects with ARWMC were enrolled at the Neurology Clinic of Kyoto University Hospital. The inclusion criteria were: (1) aged between 65 and 84 years old, and (2) T_2-weighted magnetic resonance images (MRI) revealing both irregular periventricular hyperintensities extending into the deep WM (Fazekas' PVH 3) and confluent hyperintensities in the deep WM (Fazekas' DWMH 3), diffusely involving at least bilateral fronto-subcortical areas and not confined to a single vascular territory [12]. Exclusion criteria were: (1) a history of acute stroke in the previous 3 months, (2) neurological and neuroradiological findings or history of surgery which suggests complication of other neurological or orthopedic diseases affecting gait including possible idiopathic normal pressure hydrocephalus (NPH). Specifically, an experienced neurologist first selected subjects solely according to the neuroimaging findings in the neurology clinic. The subjects whose diagnoses were other than ARWMC were excluded afterwards according to the exclusion criteria. The research protocol was approved by the ethics committee of Kyoto University Graduate School and Faculty of Medicine, and written informed consent was obtained from each subject.

Assessment of FOGQ and gait performance

All subjects completed the FOGQ [7], and underwent neurological evaluation by a board-certified neurologist (K.I.). While subjects walked at their own pace repeatedly, the presence of FOG was checked, with special attention being paid to their gait initiation and turning. Moreover, they were assessed with a three-dimensional (3D) locomotion analysis system (GATAL-ITS-60, Sumitomo Metal Inc., Osaka, Japan). Velocity, cadence, stride length (SL), stride width (SW), gait cycle (GC), and the ratios of double support time per GC (DST/GC) were measured. The correlations between the gait-related parameters and the sum of FOGQ scores were tested (Spearman's test). Additionally, the total score of FOGQ was compared between the FOG positive and FOG negative groups as classified by the clinical observation (Mann–Whitney U test). Findings were considered significant at the level of $P < 0.05$.

Assessment of cognitive status

Mini-mental state examination (MMSE) scores were obtained. They were not intended to provide a precise evaluation of cognitive impairment, as our main focus was the analysis of FOG. We conducted Spearman's tests to test the correlations between FOGQ and MMSE scores. Findings were considered significant at the level of $P < 0.05$.

Image data acquisition

DTI, T_1 and T_2-weighted images were acquired with a 3-Tesla MRI scanner (Trio; Siemens, Erlangen, Germany). DTI data were obtained using a single-shot, spin-echo, echo-planar imaging sequence applying motion probing gradient pulses to 12 non-colinear axes with b = 700 s/mm^2. To enhance the signal-to-noise ratio, imaging was repeated four times.

A magnetization-prepared rapid gradient echo (MPRAGE) sequence was used for anatomical T_1-weighted volume data acquisition. T_2-weighted images were acquired with a turbo spin-echo sequence.

Data analysis

The DTI data were pre-processed using DTI-Fit software included in the Functional MRI of the Brain (FMRIB) Diffusion Toolbox (FDT) (FSL4.1, http://www.fmrib.ox.ac.uk/fsl). We computed FA images and diffusivity images representing axial diffusivity (AD, λ_1) and radial diffusivity (RD, $\lambda_2 + \lambda_3/2$) to the principal direction [13], and also mean diffusivity (MD). Representative T_2-weighted images demonstrating PVH and DWMH, and maps of diffusion measures, both of which were taken from the same subject are shown in Figure 1.

First, we tested the relationship between the FOGQ score and the global changes of the diffusion measures reflecting different aspects of WM integrity (global correlation analysis). We hypothesized that FA would be decreased in accord with the severity of FOG (reflected by greater FOGQ scores) and that there would be a negative correlation between FOGQ and FA. As for the parameters representing diffusivity, MD is thought to reflect overall WM disruption similarly to FA, while RD and AD are thought to be useful as an index of myelin integrity and axonal integrity, respectively [13-15]. The most commonly reported pattern in previous studies is an increase in RD, AD, and MD in accord with the severity of age-related white matter damage [16]. We hence hypothesized that those diffusivity measures would be increased in relation to the severity of FOG and that there would be a positive correlation between FOGQ score and the three diffusivity parameters (MD, RD and AD). The correlation of FOGQ scores with each of FA, MD, AD and RD in the mean WM skeleton was tested using Spearman's rank correlation.

To explore possible correlation between brain atrophy and FOGQ scores, the Structural Image Evaluation using Normalization of Atrophy (SIENAX) method [17] was then applied to the T_1-weighted image for each

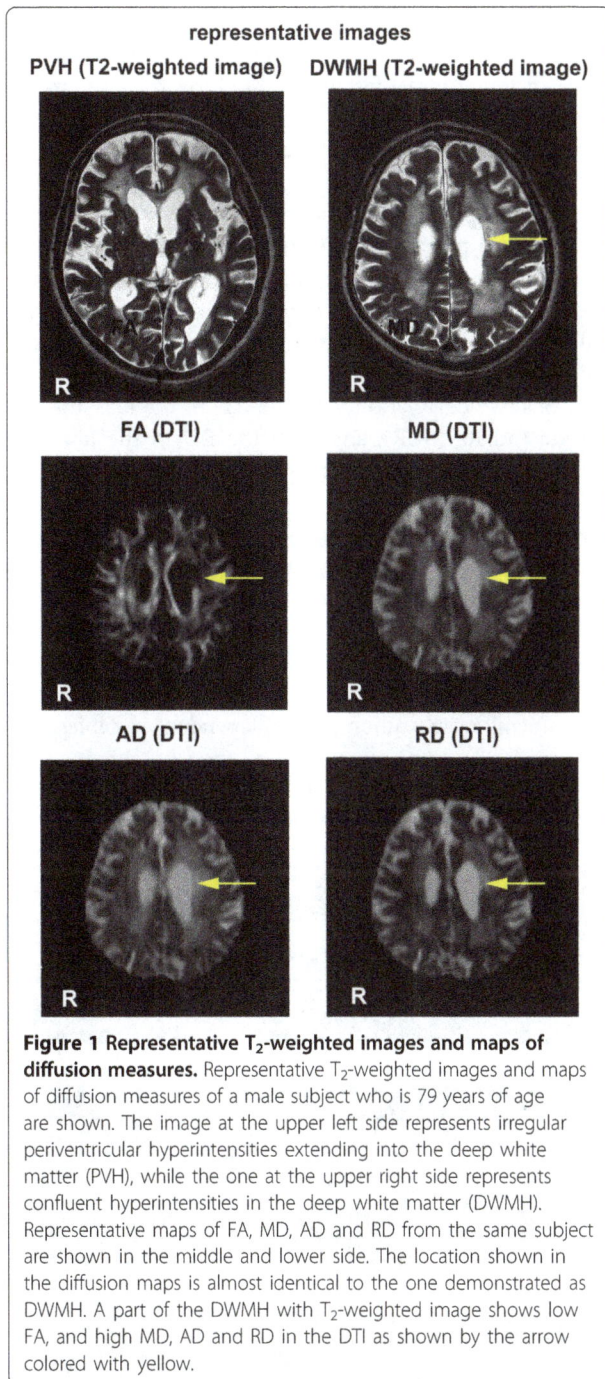

Figure 1 Representative T$_2$-weighted images and maps of diffusion measures. Representative T$_2$-weighted images and maps of diffusion measures of a male subject who is 79 years of age are shown. The image at the upper left side represents irregular periventricular hyperintensities extending into the deep white matter (PVH), while the one at the upper right side represents confluent hyperintensities in the deep white matter (DWMH). Representative maps of FA, MD, AD and RD from the same subject are shown in the middle and lower side. The location shown in the diffusion maps is almost identical to the one demonstrated as DWMH. A part of the DWMH with T$_2$-weighted image shows low FA, and high MD, AD and RD in the DTI as shown by the arrow colored with yellow.

subject to estimate the total, gray and white matter brain volumes.

Second, we tested regional correlations between the FOGQ score and the image representing each of the diffusion parameters (FA, MD, AD, and RD) on a voxel-by-voxel basis using the TBSS software. For the regional correlation analysis, we also speculated that the FOGQ score would be negatively correlated with FA values, and positively correlated with MD, AD and RD values.

Statistical inference was obtained using a non-parametric method called Threshold-Free Cluster Enhancement (TFCE) with 5,000 permutations [18]. Changes were considered significant at the level of $P < 0.05$, which was fully corrected for multiple comparisons. To test the specific relation of FOGQ scores with the diffusion measures identified in the regional correlation analysis, a confirmatory multiple linear regression analysis was applied. We computed the average value of FA, MD, AD and RD in each cluster, which showed significant regional correlation with FOGQ score as a sole dependent variable. The FOGQ scores, MMSE scores, walking velocity, cadence, SL, SW, GC and DST/GC were used as independent variables. Testing the multicollinearity that affects the result of the analysis is considered to be important when employing the multivariate analysis. Multicollinearity between these independent variables was tested by calculating the variance inflation factor (VIF), which is widely used for this purpose. If the VIF reveals specific variables to be unacceptable in the model, it is advised to exclude those specific variables. A well-accepted cutoff value of VIF is 10 [19,20]. The result was considered significant at the level of $P < 0.05$.

Results

Behavioral parameters

Clinical assessment of the subjects, including the FOGQ scores and the presence of FOG, is shown in Table 1. The FOGQ scores (mean ± S.D.; 4.2 ± 5.0) were significantly correlated with the DST/GC (0.31 ± 0.074, $r = 0.63$, $P = 0.003$), walking velocity (0.98 ± 0.30, $r = -0.79$, $P < 0.001$) and SL (0.96 ± 0.25, $r = -0.74$, $P < 0.001$) (Table 2). Furthermore, there was a significant difference in FOGQ scores between subjects who were judged to exhibit FOG (9.2 ± 5.7, n = 6) and those who were not (2.5 ± 2.7, n = 14) ($P = 0.003$, Mann–Whitney U test). In addition, the FOGQ and the MMSE scores (28 ± 1.4) also showed a significant correlation ($r = -0.62$, $P = 0.003$; Table 2).

Correlation of FOG with global changes in brain volumes and DTI measures

The assessment of brain atrophy with SIENAX failed to show a correlation between FOGQ scores and the volume of the total brain ($P = 0.59$), gray matter ($P = 0.68$) or white matter ($P = 0.10$). Nevertheless, when the diffusion measures averaged across the mean white matter skeleton were assessed, FOGQ scores showed a significant negative correlation with mean FA (0.38 ± 0.032 $r = -0.49$, $P = 0.026$), and a significant positive correlation with MD (0.99 ± 0.059 $r = 0.50$, $P = 0.022$), AD (1.4 ± 0.042, $r = 0.48$, $P = 0.029$) and RD (0.79 ± 0.069, $r = 0.48$, $P = 0.031$; Table 2).

Local correlation of DTI measures with FOGQ scores

In the TBSS analysis for the assessment of voxel-by-voxel local correlation, FA showed a significant negative

Table 1 Clinical assessment of the subjects

Subject	Velocity (m/s)	SL (m)	DST/GC	FOGQ	Presence of FOG
1	0.71	0.68	0.35	16	yes
2	0.58	0.8	0.33	6	yes
3	0.72	0.69	0.33	6	yes
4	0.54	0.59	0.46	17	yes
5	0.71	0.83	0.39	6	yes
6	0.62	1.2	0.46	4	yes
7	1.06	1.1	0.33	0	no
8	0.96	0.66	0.31	3	no
9	0.83	0.6	0.37	8	no
10	0.84	0.77	0.28	1	no
11	1.1	1.2	0.25	0	no
12	1.4	0.95	0.34	0	no
13	1.1	1	0.26	1	no
14	1.3	1.1	0.31	4	no
15	0.99	1.0	0.27	7	no
16	1.1	1.2	0.22	1	no
17	1.6	1.3	0.25	0	no
18	1.4	1.3	0.20	0	no
19	1.1	1.3	0.21	0	no
20	0.9	0.9	0.28	3	no

SL: stride length, SW: stride width, DST: double support time, GC: gait cycle, FOGQ: freezing of gait questionnaire, FOG: freezing of gait.
While subjects walked at their own pace repeatedly, the presence of FOG was checked, with special attention being paid to their gait initiation and turning.

Table 2 The behavioral and DTI measures, and their correlations with FOGQ scores

Correlation with FOGQ scores			
Parameters	Mean ± S.D.	r	P
DST/GC	0.31 ± 0.074	0.63	0.003*
Velocity	0.98 ± 0.30	−0.79	<0.001*
SL	0.96 ± 0.25	−0.74	<0.001*
MMSE score	28 ± 1.4	−0.62	0.003*
FA	0.38 ± 0.032	−0.49	0.026*
	(†0.45 ± 0.02)		
MD	0.99 ± 0.059	0.50	0.022*
	(†0.78 ± 0.03)		
AD	1.4 ± 0.042	0.48	0.029*
	(†1.18 ± 0.03)		
RD	0.79 ± 0.069	0.48	0.031*
	(†0.58 ± 0.04)		

For the DTI measures (FA, MD, AD and RD), values reported by Burzynska et al. using 63 healthy elderly subjects are shown in the parentheses as a reference. P-values considered to be significant are followed by an asterisk.
DST/GC: double support time/gait cycle, SL: stride length.

correlation with the FOGQ scores in three clusters (Figure 2 and Table 3). They were composed of the left superior longitudinal fasciculus (SLF) located close to the premotor area (PM) (Brodmann's area [BA] 6), the right corpus callosum (CC) nearby the anterior cingulate cortex (BA32), and the cerebral peduncle (CP) in the midbrain. A correlation analysis between the FOGQ scores and the MD revealed two significant WM clusters composed of the left posterior limb of the internal capsule (PLIC) located close to the putamen, and of the right cingulum close to the cingulate gyrus (BA24) (Figure 3 and Table 3). In addition, the FOGQ scores showed a significant positive correlation with the AD in the left superior corona radiata (SCR), and with the RD in the left SCR close to the putamen (Figure 3 and Table 3).

Multiple linear regression analysis

To test how much of the variability in the regional diffusion measures was explained by FOG when other parameters were considered, multiple linear regression analyses were performed on the data extracted from the clusters detected by local correlation analysis. In the test of multicollinearity among the independent variables, VIF

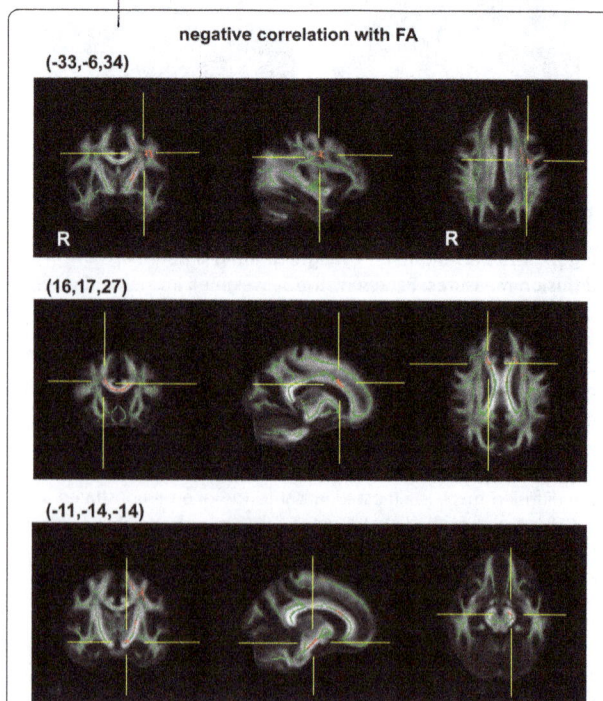

Figure 2 Correlation between the FOGQ and FA. The coordinates of detected regions within clusters that showed a significant correlation between the FOGQ and FA. The detected regions are colored with red and superimposed onto the white matter skeleton (green, thresholded at tract voxel FA >0.2) and the grayscale mean FA image of all the subjects. Note that the points of the crossed yellow lines represent the location with significant activation. See Tables 3 and 4 for details.

Table 3 The location of each area which showed local correlation between DTI measures and FOGQ scores

Diffusion measure	MNI coordinates			Cluster size	Side	Area	Nearest GM
	x	y	z				
FA	−33	−6	34	2060	left	SLF	precentral gyrus (BA6)
	16	17	27	732	right	CC	anterior cingulate (BA32)
	−11	−14	−14	196	left	CP	midbrain
MD	−23	−5	18	1037	left	PLIC	putamen
	6	18	19	178	right	cingulum	anterior cingulate (BA33)
AD	−26	−20	29	256	left	SCR	no GM found*
RD	−23	−5	19	173	left	SCR	putamen

SLF: superior longitudinal fasciculus, CC: corpus callosum, CP: cerebral peduncle, PLIC: posterior limb of the internal capsule, SCR: superior corona radiata, BA: Brodmann's area, GM: gray matter.
*No gray matter was found around the 11×11×11-mm^3 cube around this coordinate.

was less than 10 for the FOGQ score (2.8), MMSE score (3.7), SL (7.7), DSP (4.8), cadence (6.8) and SW (2.2) while it was more than 10 for the velocity (25) and GC (22). Since a well-accepted cutoff value of VIF is 10 [19,20], the walking velocity and GC were excluded from the

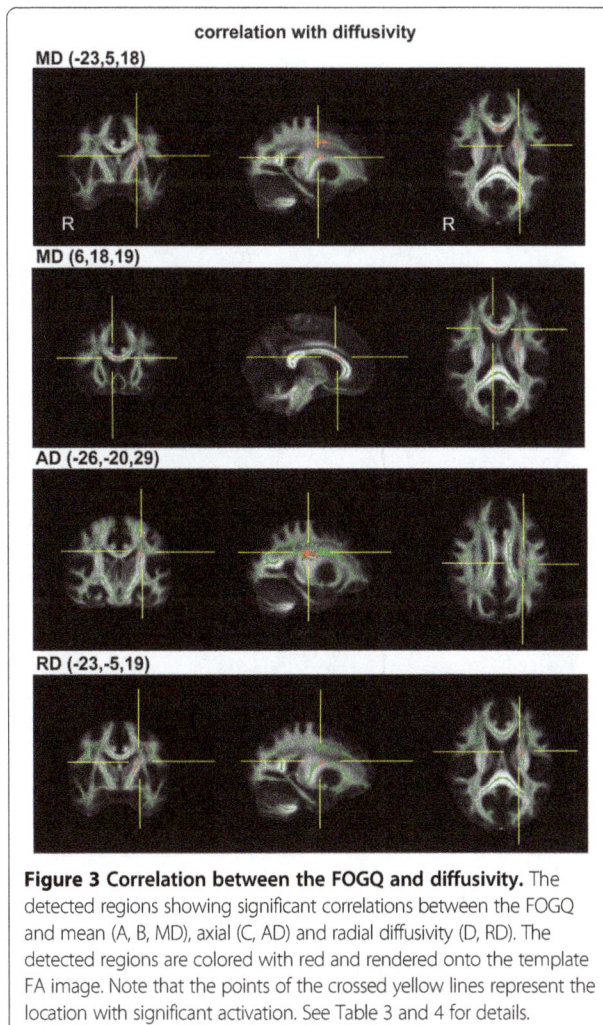

Figure 3 Correlation between the FOGQ and diffusivity. The detected regions showing significant correlations between the FOGQ and mean (A, B, MD), axial (C, AD) and radial diffusivity (D, RD). The detected regions are colored with red and rendered onto the template FA image. Note that the points of the crossed yellow lines represent the location with significant activation. See Table 3 and 4 for details.

independent variables. In this variable-reduced model, VIF was less than 3 for all the FOGQ (2.6), MMSE scores (1.8), SL (2.8), DSP (2.6), cadence (1.7) and SW (1.8). The adaptability of this reduced multi-regression model was significant for all dependent variables (P <0.05), supporting the appropriateness of the selected independent variables for predicting each dependent variable. In most of the WM regions, only the total FOGQ scores exhibited a significant association (P <0.05, Table 4). In the right CC, however, both the FOGQ score and the MMSE score exhibited significant associations.

Further, to test the effects of the velocity and GC that were excluded from the reduced multi-regression model, we replaced the FOGQ with the velocity or GC in another series of multiple regression analysis. When the velocity was used, the adaptability of the model was found to be non-significant in all WM clusters, except the right CC (F = 4.06, P = 0.016). In the right CC, only MMSE scores significantly explained the variance in the diffusion-derived variables (P = 0.045). When the GC was substituted for the FOGQ scores, the adaptability of the model was non-significant in all WM clusters, except for the right CC (F = 4.05, P = 0.016). Again in the right CC, only the MMSE scores revealed significant effects (P = 0.012).

This analysis suggested that DTI measures of the WM regions, except for the right CC, were specifically correlated with the FOGQ scores, but not with other cognitive or gait parameters.

Discussion
Assessment of FOG
The present study revealed a strong correlation between the FOGQ scores and the gait parameters from the computerized gait analysis. PD subjects with FOG have gait disturbance, which result in the abnormality of the gait parameters. For example, FOG affects GC which results in the increase of the stride-to-stride variability [21]. Furthermore, gradual reduction of stride length is associated with

Table 4 Multilinear regression analysis

Diffusion measure	Area	Variables	Coefficient	T	P
FA	left SLF	FOGQ	−0.81	−3.7	0.003*
		MMSE	0.43	2.0	0.067
		SL	−0.42	−1.8	0.092
		DST/GC	−0.30	−1.3	0.20
		Cad	−0.18	−0.99	0.34
		SW	0.14	0.76	0.46
FA	right CC	FOGQ	−0.57	−2.7	0.018*
		MMSE	0.60	3.4	0.005*
		SL	−0.27	−1.2	0.23
		DST/GC	0.02	0.093	0.93
		Cad	0.03	0.18	0.86
		SW	−0.18	−1.0	0.32
FA	left CP	FOGQ	−0.90	−4.28	<0.001*
		MMSE	0.45	2.0	0.071
		SL	−0.47	−2.2	0.063
		DST/GC	−0.08	−0.38	0.71
		Cad	−0.18	−1.1	0.30
		SW	−0.01	−0.06	0.95
MD	left PLIC	FOGQ	0.73	3.4	0.005*
		MMSE	−0.37	−2.1	0.07
		SL	0.15	0.64	0.53
		DST/GC	0.11	0.50	0.62
		Cad	0.16	0.92	0.38
		SW	0.03	0.18	0.86
MD	right cingulum	FOGQ	0.91	4.4	<0.001*
		MMSE	−0.26	−1.3	0.21
		SL	0.17	0.81	0.44
		DST/GC	0.11	0.55	0.59
		Cad	0.04	0.26	0.80
		SW	−0.37	−2.1	0.08
AD	left SCR	FOGQ	0.96	3.7	0.003*
		MMSE	0.05	0.22	0.83
		SL	0.21	0.76	0.46
		DST/GC	−0.17	−0.63	0.54
		Cad	−0.06	−0.3	0.77
		SW	0.14	0.65	0.53
RD	left SCR	FOGQ	0.69	2.7	0.019*
		MMSE	−0.08	−0.39	0.71
		SL	−0.06	−0.21	0.84
		DST/GC	0.12	0.48	0.64
		Cad	0.02	0.11	0.91
		SW	−0.07	−0.32	0.75

The table shows the results of multilinear regression analysis of all those six independent variables using average activation of each area in which significant local correlation between FOGQ and FA was found as a dependent variable. The significant *P*-values are noted by an asterisk.

FOGQ: Freezing of Gait Questionnaire, MMSE: Mini-Mental State Examination, SL: stride length, DST/GC: double support time/gait cycle, cad: cadence, SW: stride width.

FOG [22]. The result from the present study concurs with these findings, although we should be careful not to simply equate FOG and gait disturbance. That is, although most subjects with FOG show profound gait disturbance, some subjects with FOG may show normal gait parameters upon a gait analysis, reflecting fluctuating nature of FOG [6].

Nevertheless, the multiple regression analysis indicated that only the FOGQ score exhibited a significant effect as an independent variable explaining changes of the DTI measures in almost all the WM clusters detected in the local correlation analysis. The multiple regression analysis substituting the FOGQ scores for the walking velocity or GC failed to produce significant results in the model in most of the WM clusters. These results indicate that the diffusion measures in the WM clusters (except for CC) were strongly correlated with the severity of FOG specifically, not with cognitive decline or gait disturbance in general.

Interhemispheric connections

In the CC, FA exhibited a significant negative correlation with FOGQ and MMSE scores. WM integrity of the CC is significantly correlated with quantitative measures of gait in the elderly population [9]. It has been suggested that the CC may transfer sensory information necessary for gait planning interhemispherically [23]. Moreover, a recent study demonstrated that perceptual judgment of an upcoming doorway is more strongly affected in patients with FOG than those without [24]. These findings suggest that CC may affect the ability of gait planning according to sensory information in the environment which might be related to FOG.

Corticofugal and thalamocortical fibers

The present study revealed a negative correlation between FOGQ scores and FA in the ventromedial part of the CP at the midbrain level. The CP includes the corticofugal tract, which connects the brainstem and the spinal cord with cortical motor areas including the primary motor cortex, supplementary motor area (SMA) and PM [25]. The CP may also include the fibers projecting to the pedunculopontine nucleus (PPN) and/or the mesencephalic locomotor region (MLR). The neural circuits connecting the PPN, basal ganglia, motor cortex and limbic system are hypothesized to be responsible for FOG [26]. Moreover, recent study revealed that the PD patients with FOG showed more increase of brain activity in the PPN/MLR during imagery of walking compared with those without FOG [27]. Taken together, the disruption of the projecting fibers to PPN/MLR at the level of CP appears to be responsible for FOG.

There was a positive correlation between MD in the PLIC and FOGQ scores. Damage to the PLIC encompassing parts of the corticofugal tracts could result in poor motor outcomes [28]. In infants with low birth weight, reduced FA in the PLIC has been shown to be correlated with the severity of gait deficits in the future [29].

Both AD and RD were significantly correlated with the FOGQ scores in the left SCR. Hence, the damage to both myelin and axons might contribute to the WM damage seen here. Damage of the thalamocortical sensory tracts at the SCR can cause both sensory deficits and gait disturbance [30]. Considering that FOG can be ameliorated or exacerbated by sensory stimuli [31], sensorimotor networks are likely to be involved.

Fronto-parietal connections and cingulum

It has been suggested that FOG may result from dysfunction of the PM-parietal circuits [32]. Consistent with this view, we found a significant negative correlation between FA and FOGQ scores in the SLF close to the PM. The SLF is likely to contribute to visuospatial processing [33] which might be related to FOG.

The cingulum collects projections from the cingulate cortex and extends into the temporal or frontal lobe [34]. In the present study, MD in the cingulum exhibited a positive correlation with FOGQ, consistent with the hypothesis that a local network in SMA and adjacent cingulate cortex might be responsible for FOG [35]. The cingulate regions are activated during gait movement [10,36] and are also thought to be involved in the planning of gait [37,38]. The cingulum bundle participates in the limbic circuit, which is thought to be involved in FOG together with the motor and cognitive circuits in patients with PD [26]. Based on these considerations, the present findings in the cingulum might reflect not only the motor but also the emotional aspects of FOG.

Brain volume, global diffusion measures and FOG

Previous studies indicate that gray matter atrophy is related to gait impairment [39], as well as the volume of WM lesions [40]. However, our analysis failed to reveal a significant correlation between WM atrophy and FOGQ, whereas all of the diffusion measures were significantly correlated with FOGQ. Thus, it appears that the diffusion measures were more sensitive than WM atrophy in patients with ARWMC.

We did not take the WM lesion volume into account in the TBSS analysis since we focused on the integrity of the white matter. However, we could not exclude a possibility that such WM volume changes might affect the TBSS results.

Proposed mechanisms underlying FOG

The present findings raise the question of how the WM abnormalities identified above (CC, PLIC, SCR, CP, and SLF) might explain FOG. Youn et al. [41] performed a region-of-interest (ROI) analysis on DTI data and found that the FA values of the bilateral PPN, bilateral PM, right orbitofrontal area and left SMA were lower in the ARWMC patients with FOG compared to those without. Their finding partly concurs the present result, which showed that the FA in the SLF close to the PM, and also in the CP close to the midbrain PPN, was correlated with FOG. The areas detected slightly differed probably because of the difference in the methodology, especially the spatial normalization procedure (TBSS versus ROI analysis). The present result suggests that multiple neural substrates related to the control of walking may be involved in FOG in consistent with the study by Youn et al. [41]. This notion favors the view that FOG is likely to be a clinical condition resulting from multiple pathophysiological issues involving one or more nodes of the neural network regulating walking behavior. Since visual stimuli or some other extra cues can help or exacerbate FOG [31], the phenomenon might emerge when extra demands for sensory, cognitive, or emotional processing overburden the damaged neural substrates.

Limitations of this study

We enrolled patients who were regularly visiting a neurology outpatient clinic. Thus, the population might be different from those who were diagnosed as having ARWMC in radiology departments or in general elderly population. Therefore, a further study will be required to test if the present finding can be generalized to those population.

In the present study, we focused on the relationship between WM abnormality and FOG. We employed a relatively small number of subjects to perform a comprehensive investigation. Since there is no established objective measure of FOG, we avoided classifying subjects with FOG and those without, and used FOGQ as a parameter for a correlation analysis instead. Because of this strategy, we have included the subjects who did not clearly present FOG, which is often invisible at the physician's room. To reduce ambiguity regarding the subject selection, we did our best to discriminate FOG and general gait disturbance in the multiple regression analysis, but it would still be difficult to discuss the mechanisms of FOG completely segregated from those of gait disturbance in general.

In the present study, we used the T_2-weighted images only for the purpose of subject recruitment, but did not analyze these non-quantitative data. We reviewed the individual T_2-weighted images of each subject, and visually investigated if the regions detected in the DTI analysis corresponded to ARWMC regions in the T_2-weighted images. In most of the subjects, ARWMC were present in all the detected regions except for the CP. This result is reasonable since we tested the correlation between the FOGQ scores and the diffusion parameters, which

should reflect different aspects of anatomical structure seen in the T_2-weighted images. For example, as minor reduction of white matter integrity resulting from remote ischemic lesions would be captured by DTI, but not necessarily by T_2-weighted images. Future research comparing DTI and quantitative T_2-weighted images is awaited. We discussed FOG mainly in relation to the underlying pathophysiology of FOG in PD. The symptoms of FOG seem very similar across different diseases such as PD and other types of Parkinsonism. However, it remains unclear whether the mechanisms underlying FOG are shared across related diseases. Therefore, caution must be exercised in generalizing the mechanisms of FOG suggested here. Future studies are necessary to compare the mechanisms of FOG across different diseases.

Conclusion

While disconnections in the brain have previously been suggested as a cause of FOG, few studies have directly addressed this issue. To our knowledge, the present study provides the first experimental evidence that FOG is related to WM disruption, with the current results revealing that WM damage in the SLF, CC, PLIC, cingulum, CR and CP was correlated with FOG.

Abbreviations
ARWMC: Age related white matter change; FA: Fractional anisotropy; FOG: Freezing of gait; PD: Parkinson's disease.

Competing interests
The authors declare that they have no competing interests.

Authors' contributions
KI designed and conducted the study, collected data, drafted and revised the paper. He also has full access to all the data. He is a guarantor. HF designed and supervised the study, and revised the paper with intellectual suggestions. NO conducted analyses and revised the paper with intellectual suggestions. HT recruited the subjects, served for the interpretation of the data, and revised the manuscript with intellectual suggestions. YO recruited the subjects, served for the interpretation of the data, and revised the manuscript with intellectual suggestions. MN served for the interpretation of the data, and revised the manuscript with intellectual suggestions. DB served for the interpretation of the data, and revised the manuscript with intellectual suggestions. MH served for the interpretation of the data, and revised the manuscript with intellectual suggestions. TH designed and supervised the study, and revised the manuscript with intellectual suggestions. All the authors listed approved for the present paper to be published.

Funding
The research was partly supported by grants from KAKENHI (24500573) and the Sumitomo Life Social Welfare Services Foundation to K.I., and by grants from Japanese Society in the Promotion of Science (21613004) and Global COE Program to N.O., and by grants from KAKENHI (26120008) and Development of BMI Technologies for Clinical Application carried out under the Strategic Research Program for Brain Sciences to T.H. The NINDS Intramural Program provided additional support.

Author details
[1]Human Brain Research Center, Kyoto University Graduate School of Medicine, 54 Kawahara-cho, Shogoin, Sakyo-ku, Kyoto 606-8507, Japan. [2]Human Motor Control Section, Medical Neurology Branch, National Institute of Neurological Disorders and Stroke, National Institutes of Health, Bethesda, MD, USA. [3]Department of Behavioral Neurology and Cognitive Neuroscience, Tohoku University, Graduate School of Medicine, Sendai, Miyagi, Japan.

[4]Department of Neurology, Sakakibara-Hakuho Hospital, Tsu, Mie, Japan.
[5]Department of Neurology, Mie University, Graduate School of Medicine, Tsu, Mie, Japan. [6]Department of Physical Therapy, Kyoto University Hospital, Kyoto, Japan. [7]Department of Advanced Neuroimaging, Integrative Brain Imaging Center, National Center of Neurology and Psychiatry, Kodaira, Japan. [8]PRESTO, JST, Kawaguchi, Saitama, Japan.

References

1. Giladi N, Nieuwboer A: **Understanding and treating freezing of gait in parkinsonism, proposed working definition, and setting the stage.** *Mov Disord* 2008, **23**(Suppl 2):S423–S425.

2. Factor SA: **The clinical spectrum of freezing of gait in atypical parkinsonism.** *Mov Disord* 2008, **23**(Suppl 2):S431–S438.

3. de Leeuw FE, de Groot JC, Achten E, Oudkerk M, Ramos LM, Heijboer R, Hofman A, Jolles J, van Gijn J, Breteler MM: **Prevalence of cerebral white matter lesions in elderly people: a population based magnetic resonance imaging study: the Rotterdam Scan Study.** *J Neurol Neurosurg Psychiatry* 2001, **70**:9–14.

4. Hachinski VC, Potter P, Merskey H: **Leuko-araiosis.** *Arch Neurol* 1987, **44**:21–23.

5. Inzitari M, Pozzi C, Rinaldi LA, Masotti G, Marchionni N, Di Bari M: **Cognitive and functional impairment in hypertensive brain microangiopathy.** *J Neurol Sci* 2007, **257**:166–173.

6. Nutt JG, Bloem BR, Giladi N, Hallett M, Horak FB, Nieuwboer A: **Freezing of gait: moving forward on a mysterious clinical phenomenon.** *Lancet Neurol* 2011, **10**:734–744.

7. Giladi N, Shabtai H, Simon ES, Biran S, Tal J, Korczyn AD: **Construction of freezing of gait questionnaire for patients with Parkinsonism.** *Parkinsonism Relat Disord* 2000, **6**:165–170.

8. Charlton RA, Barrick TR, McIntyre DJ, Shen Y, O'Sullivan M, Howe FA, Clark CA, Morris RG, Markus HS: **White matter damage on diffusion tensor imaging correlates with age-related cognitive decline.** *Neurology* 2006, **66**:217–222.

9. Bhadelia RA, Price LL, Tedesco KL, Scott T, Qiu WQ, Patz S, Folstein M, Rosenberg I, Caplan LR, Bergethon P: **Diffusion tensor imaging, white matter lesions, the corpus callosum, and gait in the elderly.** *Stroke* 2009, **40**:3816–3820.

10. Iseki K, Hanakawa T, Hashikawa K, Tomimoto H, Nankaku M, Yamauchi H, Hallett M, Fukuyama H: **Gait disturbance associated with white matter changes: a gait analysis and blood flow study.** *Neuroimage* 2010, **49**:1659–1666.

11. Smith SM, Jenkinson M, Johansen-Berg H, Rueckert D, Nichols TE, Mackay CE, Watkins KE, Ciccarelli O, Cader MZ, Matthews PM, Behrens TE: **Tract-based spatial statistics: voxelwise analysis of multi-subject diffusion data.** *Neuroimage* 2006, **31**:1487–1505.

12. Fazekas F, Chawluk JB, Alavi A, Hurtig HI, Zimmerman RA: **MR signal abnormalities at 1.5 T in Alzheimer's dementia and normal aging.** *AJR Am J Roentgenol* 1987, **149**:351–356.

13. Song SK, Sun SW, Ramsbottom MJ, Chang C, Russell J, Cross AH: **Dysmyelination revealed through MRI as increased radial (but unchanged axial) diffusion of water.** *Neuroimage* 2002, **17**:1429–1436.

14. Budde MD, Kim JH, Liang HF, Schmidt RE, Russell JH, Cross AH, Song SK: **Toward accurate diagnosis of white matter pathology using diffusion tensor imaging.** *Magn Reson Med* 2007, **57**:688–695.

15. Song SK, Sun SW, Ju WK, Lin SJ, Cross AH, Neufeld AH: **Diffusion tensor imaging detects and differentiates axon and myelin degeneration in mouse optic nerve after retinal ischemia.** *Neuroimage* 2003, **20**:1714–1722.

16. Bennett IJ, Madden DJ, Vaidya CJ, Howard DV, Howard JH Jr: **Age-related differences in multiple measures of white matter integrity: A diffusion tensor imaging study of healthy aging.** *Hum Brain Mapp* 2010, **31**:378–390.

17. Smith SM, Zhang Y, Jenkinson M, Chen J, Matthews PM, Federico A, De Stefano N: **Accurate, robust, and automated longitudinal and cross-sectional brain change analysis.** *Neuroimage* 2002, **17**:479–489.

18. Smith SM, Nichols TE: **Threshold-free cluster enhancement: addressing problems of smoothing, threshold dependence and localisation in cluster inference.** *Neuroimage* 2009, **44**:83–98.

19. Chatterjee S, Hadi A: In *Regression Analysis by Examples.* 4th edition. Edited by Balding DJ. New York: John Wiley & Sons; 2006.

20. Freund R, Wilson W, Ping S: **Regression analysis.** In *Statistical Modeling of a Response Variable.* Edited by Singer T. San Diego: Academic; 2006.

21. Hausdorff JM, Schaafsma JD, Balash Y, Bartels AL, Gurevich T, Giladi N: **Impaired regulation of stride variability in Parkinson's disease subjects with freezing of gait.** *Exp Brain Res* 2003, **149**:187–194.

22. Chee R, Murphy A, Danoudis M, Georgiou-Karistianis N, Iansek R: **Gait freezing in Parkinson's disease and the stride length sequence effect interaction.** *Brain* 2009, **132**:2151–2160.

23. Park HJ, Kim JJ, Lee SK, Seok JH, Chun J, Kim DI, Lee JD: **Corpus callosal connection mapping using cortical gray matter parcellation and DT-MRI.** *Hum Brain Mapp* 2008, **29**:503–516.

24. Almeida QJ, Lebold CA: **Freezing of gait in Parkinson's disease: a perceptual cause for a motor impairment?** *J Neurol Neurosurg Psychiatry* 2010, **81**:513–518.

25. Newton JM, Ward NS, Parker GJ, Deichmann R, Alexander DC, Friston KJ, Frackowiak RS: **Non-invasive mapping of corticofugal fibres from multiple motor areas–relevance to stroke recovery.** *Brain* 2006, **129**:1844–1858.

26. Lewis SJ, Barker RA: **A pathophysiological model of freezing of gait in Parkinson's disease.** *Parkinsonism Relat Disord* 2009, **15**:333–338.

27. Snijders AH, Leunissen I, Bakker M, Overeem S, Helmich RC, Bloem BR, Toni I: **Gait-related cerebral alterations in patients with Parkinson's disease with freezing of gait.** *Brain* 2011, **134**:59–72.

28. Jang SH: **A review of corticospinal tract location at corona radiata and posterior limb of the internal capsule in human brain.** *NeuroRehabilitation* 2009, **24**:279–283.

29. Rose J, Mirmiran M, Butler EE, Lin CY, Barnes PD, Kermoian R, Stevenson DK: **Neonatal microstructural development of the internal capsule on diffusion tensor imaging correlates with severity of gait and motor deficits.** *Dev Med Child Neurol* 2007, **49**:745–750.

30. Shinoura N, Suzuki Y, Yoshida M, Yamada R, Tabei Y, Saito K, Yagi K: **Assessment of the corona radiata sensory tract using awake surgery and tractography.** *J Clin Neurosci* 2009, **16**:764–770.

31. Hallett M: **The intrinsic and extrinsic aspects of freezing of gait.** *Mov Disord* 2008, **23**(Suppl 2):S439–S443.

32. Bartels AL, Leenders KL: **Brain imaging in patients with freezing of gait.** *Mov Disord* 2008, **23**(Suppl 2):S461–S467.

33. Hoeft F, Barnea-Goraly N, Haas BW, Golarai G, Ng D, Mills D, Korenberg J, Bellugi U, Galaburda A, Reiss AL: **More is not always better: increased fractional anisotropy of superior longitudinal fasciculus associated with poor visuospatial abilities in Williams syndrome.** *J Neurosci* 2007, **27**:11960–11965.

34. Schmahmann JD, Pandya DN, Wang R, Dai G, D'Arceuil HE, de Crespigny AJ, Wedeen VJ: **Association fibre pathways of the brain: parallel observations from diffusion spectrum imaging and autoradiography.** *Brain* 2007, **130**:630–653.

35. Hashimoto T: **Speculation on the responsible sites and pathophysiology of freezing of gait.** *Parkinsonism Relat Disord* 2006, **12**:S55–S62.

36. Hanakawa T, Fukuyama H, Katsumi Y, Honda M, Shibasaki H: **Enhanced lateral premotor activity during paradoxical gait in Parkinson's disease.** *Ann Neurol* 1999, **45**:329–336.

37. Dobkin BH, Firestine A, West M, Saremi K, Woods R: **Ankle dorsiflexion as an fMRI paradigm to assay motor control for walking during rehabilitation.** *Neuroimage* 2004, **23**:370–381.

38. Iseki K, Hanakawa T, Shinozaki J, Nankaku M, Fukuyama H: **Neural mechanisms involved in mental imagery and observation of gait.** *Neuroimage* 2008, **41**:1021–1031.

39. Rosano C, Sigurdsson S, Siggeirsdottir K, Phillips CL, Garcia M, Jonsson PV, Eiriksdottir G, Newman AB, Harris TB, van Buchem MA, Gudnason V, Launer LJ: **Magnetization transfer imaging, white matter hyperintensities, brain atrophy and slower gait in older men and women.** *Neurobiol Aging* 2010, **31**:1197–1204.

40. Soumare A, Elbaz A, Zhu Y, Maillard P, Crivello F, Tavernier B, Dufouil C, Mazoyer B, Tzourio C: **White matter lesions volume and motor performances in the elderly.** *Ann Neurol* 2009, **65**:706–715.

41. Youn J, Cho JW, Lee WY, Kim GM, Kim ST, Kim HT: **Diffusion tensor imaging of freezing of gait in patients with white matter changes.** *Mov Disord* 2012, **27**:760–764.

4

Isolated vocal tremor as a focal phenotype of essential tremor

Amar Patel* and Steven J Frucht

Abstract

Background: Essential tremor (ET) is a common condition associated with significant physical and psychosocial disability. "Classic" ET is a clinical syndrome of action tremor in the upper limbs and less commonly the head, jaw, voice, trunk, or lower limbs. Current diagnostic criteria for ET exclude isolated vocal tremor (IVT). Failure to recognize IVT as a form of ET may contribute to misdiagnosis and missed opportunities for treatment.

Methods: We conducted a retrospective review of cases referred for voice disturbance. Patients with a primary diagnosis of vocal tremor were included while those with a diagnosis of spasmodic dysphonia where excluded.

Results: 19 cases of vocal tremor were identified, of which 17 patients (89%) were female. The average age of vocal symptom onset was 64 (SD 8.0) and patients had been symptomatic an average of 6 years (SD 4) at their initial visit. 8 patients had IVT while 11 also had evidence of subtle head or limb tremor. 8 patients (42%) had a family history of ET, with vocal tremor specifically identified in 5 of those cases (26%). 11 patients (58%) noted transient tremor improvement after alcohol consumption. Primidone and propranolol were the most common medications prescribed to these patients prior to consultation. 7 patients were given a trial of 1 gm of sodium oxybate in the office as part of a clinical trial, with at least mild improvement in vocal tremor noted by qualitative assessment.

Conclusions: ET may present as vocal tremor with little or no associated limb tremor. It may be a more common manifestation of ET in women. A family history of tremor and improvement in tremor after consuming alcohol can often be elicited on history. We propose that IVT may be part of the spectrum of ET.

Keywords: Vocal tremor, Isolated vocal tremor, Essential tremor, Pharyngeal tremor, Sodium oxybate

Background

Essential tremor (ET) is the most common pathological cause of tremor, defined as a rhythmic, oscillatory movement of a body part about an axis. ET is the most common movement disorder in the general population and of those presenting for neurological evaluation [1]. Many cases of ET are familial, with anywhere from 17% to 100% cited in various studies, and inherited most likely in an autosomal dominant fashion with variable penetrance [2,3]. The tremor of ET occurs during voluntary movement, posture and action [4]. ET has been defined by the Movement Disorder Society Consensus Statement on Tremor as a "bilateral, largely symmetric postural or kinetic tremor involving hands and forearms that is visible and persistent" [5]. These criteria were based on Tremor Investigation Group guidelines which also included duration of illness as a major criterion [6]. Other causes of tremor, e.g. dystonia, must be excluded, and although traditionally vocal tremor is recognized as a feature of ET in anywhere from 10 to 25% of cases, isolated vocal tremor (IVT), defined as tremor of the voice in the absence of other observable tremor, does not meet current criteria for ET [7]. Voice tremor has thus classically been considered a secondary feature of ET which does not occur without upper limb tremor.

Here we describe a series of cases in which tremor of the phonatory apparatus is the sole or predominant manifestation of ET. We also compare the current series to previously described essential voice tremor populations. We propose that the phenomenologic characteristics of isolated vocal tremor (IVT) are consistent with its inclusion as a focal form of ET; and where both vocal and limb

* Correspondence: amar.patel@mountsinai.org
Department of Neurology, Icahn School of Medicine at Mount Sinai, 5 E 98th Street, New York, NY 10029, USA

tremor occur, the former need not be a secondary feature of the latter, but rather the primary concern of the patient.

Methods

We conducted a retrospective review of the medical records of patients referred to the senior author for voice disturbance over a ten-year period. Patients with a diagnosis of vocal tremor were included, while those with a diagnosis of spasmodic dysphonia where excluded. The study was approved by the Institutional Review Board of Mount Sinai School of Medicine. Written informed consent was obtained for the use of video examinations. A waiver of consent for review of medical records was granted by the IRB.

Results

19 patients with a primary diagnosis of vocal tremor were evaluated between 2003 and 2013 (Table 1). 17 patients (89%) were female. The average age of onset of vocal difficulty was 64 (SD 8.0). Patients had been symptomatic an average of 6 years (SD 4) upon their initial consultation. 8 patients (42%) had a family history of ET, with vocal tremor specifically identified in 5 of those cases (26%). 11 patients (58%) noted transient tremor improvement after alcohol consumption; the remaining patients did not drink alcohol. On examination, 17 patients (89%) had a visible tremor of the pharyngeal musculature when speaking. Sustained vowel (A and E) phonation most reliably brought out the rhythmic oscillations of voice intensity at a frequency of approximately 4–8 Hz. Supplementary patient videos show this in greater detail for a sample of the patients described in this case series [see Additional file 1: Videos S1 and S2 and Additional file 2: Video S3]. All 9 patients who were referred for or had prior videostroboscopic evaluation of the vocal cords had visual confirmation of vocal tremor. 6 patients (32%) were noted to have very slight head tremor while 3 patients (16%) had very mild action tremor of the upper extremities. Two patients had both mild head and limb tremor. Of these 11 patients with vocal tremor plus tremor elsewhere, 4 had videostroboscopic evaluation of the vocal cords that was more consistent with vocal tremor rather than spasmodic dysphonia. Rest tremor of the upper limbs was present in only one patient, and none had signs of rigidity or bradykinesia to support a diagnosis of parkinsonism. No patient had sought medical treatment of their head or limb tremor prior to consultation for their voice tremor. Primidone and propranolol were the most common medications prescribed to these patients prior to consultation. 7 patients were treated with 1 gm of the alcohol analogue sodium oxybate after their consultation as part of a separate IRB-approved clinical trial. All 7 patients were observed to have at least mild improvement in vocal tremor, as noted by a reduction in the amplitude of the tremor without a change in its

frequency. Patients were subsequently followed for as little as 6 months and as long as 10 years without the development of dystonia or parkinsonism.

Discussion

The present case series provides some comparisons and contrasts with previously reported populations of voice tremor (Table 2). In agreement with previous reports is the finding that voice tremor is a condition of the elderly. The largest study population of voice tremor patients included only two cases of voice tremor presenting in the second and third decade of life [8]. This matches the association of another "midline" symptom, head tremor, with older age independent of duration of tremor [9]. Although epidemiological studies of ET find an equal gender distribution [10], voice tremor seems to affect more women, who represent approximately 80% of the patients identified in the literature. This corresponds with a similar gender bias in head tremor [9], suggesting that older age and female gender are defining characteristics of midline ET symptoms. Given the relatively small number of patients in some of these case series selection bias is possible, and a population-based study of essential voice tremor would be needed to more definitively address the question. Rates of familial voice tremor appear to be similar to those of familial limb tremor, although the heterogeneity of inheritance rates and patterns in the latter make this comparison less useful clinically [2].

A significant proportion of patients in the present case series reported transient tremor improvement after drinking alcohol, at rates similar to other studies of voice tremor. In fact, all alcohol "non-responders" were unaware of their response due to reported abstention from alcohol. This would suggest that an even greater percentage of voice tremor cases would respond if challenged with alcohol and objectively measured. Such a high percentage of voice tremor response to alcohol is in line with reported rates of response of limb tremor in those patients aware of the effect of alcohol on tremor [18]. Given the robust response to alcohol, it is not surprising that all patients treated with sodium oxybate had at least a mild reported improvement in voice tremor. Sodium oxybate is the salt form of γ-hydroxybutyric acid. Mice deficient in $GABA_a$ receptor have an ET-like tremor that improves with ethanol, suggesting a GABAergic mechanism in ET [19]. A previous open-label, single-blinded trial of sodium oxybate with medically refractory ET showed a dose-dependent improvement in tremor ratings [20]. Three of the patients in the current case series who responded to sodium oxybate had previously had no response to primidone and propranolol. Proper diagnosis of voice tremor can thus lead to alternative medication strategies for this often refractory condition.

Table 1 Case series

Case	Gender	Age of onset	Duration (years)	Family history	Alcohol response	Medications	Head tremor	Kinetic arm tremor	Rest tremor	Video-stroboscopy	Visible palatal or pharyngeal muscle tremor	Response to 1 gm sodium oxybate
1	F	56	4	No	Unaware	Primidone (mild response, side effects)	No	No	No	Yes	Yes	N/A
2	F	71	3	No	Yes	None	Slight	Slight	No	Yes	Not commented upon	N/A
3	F	64	2	Vocal tremor (Mother)	Unaware	None	Slight	No	No	No	Yes	N/A
4	F	70	10	No	Unaware	Lorazepam (slight improvement)	Slight	No	No	No	Yes	N/A
5	F	69	2	No	Unaware	Atenolol (No response)	Slight	No	No	Yes	Yes	N/A
6	F	87	1	No	Unaware	Lorazepam (No Response)	Slight	No	No	No	Yes	N/A
7	F	54	15	Parkinson	Yes	None	No	Slight	No	No	Yes	Mild improvement
8	F	69	3	Action tremor (Mother), Vocal tremor (Sister)	Yes	Mirapex (No response); Primidone (No Response)	No	Slight	No	Yes	Not Commented Upon	Mild improvement
9	F	56	5	Vocal tremor (Mother, Sister)	Yes	Propranolol (No Response)	No	No	No	Yes	Yes	Mild improvement
10	F	64	6	No	Unaware	Propranolol (No Response)	No	No	No	Yes	Yes	Mild improvement
11	M	72	15	No	Yes	None	Slight	No	No	No	Yes	Mild improvement
12	F	63	2	Action tremor (Father)	Yes	Primidone (Unknown Response)	No	No	No	No	Yes	N/A
13	F	66	3	Vocal tremor (Mother)	Unaware	Primidone (Mild improvement, Yes side effects)	No	Slight	No	No	Yes	N/A
14	F	45	20	Action tremor (Father, Son)	Yes	Primidone (Moderate improvement)	Slight	No	Slight	No	Yes	N/A
15	F	70	2	No	Unaware	None	No	No	No	No	Yes	N/A
16	F	81	3	No	Yes	Primidone (Moderate improvement)	No	No	No	No	Yes	N/A
17	M	56	6	Tremor (Father, Paternal Aunt/Uncle/Grandmother)	Yes	Propranolol (Mild improvement)	No	No	No	Yes	Yes	Mild improvement
18	F	65	9	No	Yes	Propranolol, Primidone (Mild improvement)	Slight	Slight	No	Yes	Yes	Mild improvement
19	F	45	2	Action tremor (Father), Vocal tremor (Paternal Aunt)	Yes	Propranolol (Moderate improvement)	No	No	No	Yes	Yes	N/A

Table 2 Vocal tremor case series comparative analysis

Study	Year	No. of cases	Mean age	Mean duration of symptoms (years)	Female (%)	Family history (%)	Isolated vocal tremor (%)	Alcohol response (%)
Brown et al. [11]	1963	31			55	52	19	
Koller et al. [12]	1985	7	64	16	14	57	14	
Busenbark et al. [13]	1996	9	73	32	89			
Hertegard et al. [14]	2000	15	73		87			
Warrick et al. [15]	2000	10	64	12	80	20		40
Adler et al. [16]	2004	13	73		85	38	54	
Bove et al. [17]	2006	20	66	8	55	45		45
Sulica and Louis [8]	2010	34	70	7	93	38	56	27
Patel and Frucht	2014	19	64	6	89	42	42	58

Our case series supports the findings of more recent studies of voice tremor which suggest that voice tremor can occur in isolation or with limb tremor of little or no consequence. Sulica and Louis determined that 56% of patients in their voice tremor study had arm tremor within the range observed in similarly matched aged controls, as determined by the WHIGET scale [8]. Our retrospective review found a similar percentage of patients without clinically significant limb tremor through a qualitative assessment. In our series, the 8 patients with IVT and 11 patients with vocal tremor plus head/limb tremor showed similar characteristics of age, gender, and alcohol responsivity. The historical categorization of voice tremor as a secondary feature of ET thus likely contributes to the under-recognition of essential voice tremor in clinical practice. Further longitudinal studies are needed to determine if these IVT patients develop tremor elsewhere or better resemble classic ET patients over time.

At the same time, it is important to recognize that inclusion of IVT in groups of ET patients may not be helpful when investigating the etiology and pathogenesis of ET. Indeed, emerging understanding of the broad heterogeneity of ET, which IVT adds to, suggests that ET may be a family of disorders rather than a single entity. This has significant research implications for correctly identifying disease risk factors, prognostic markers, and future clinical trial design which may be specific to the "type" of ET studied [21].

Limitations of our retrospective review include the lack of electrophysiologic characterization of voice and limb tremor. Similarly, not all patients had videostroboscopic evaluation. Mild cases of adductor spasmodic dysphonia may be misdiagnosed as essential voice tremor. Without electromyographic evaluation of the vocal cords or limbs, subtle dystonic tremor which appears regular can mimic essential tremor on qualitative evaluation [22]. However, the similar age of onset, rates of familial tremor, lack of other dystonic features (phoneme-specific voice breaks, sensory geste antagoniste), and robust alcohol response in our cases compared with known ET characteristics all suggest that misdiagnosis in these cases was less likely. Further confounding this distinction between dystonia and ET is the possibility that involuntary movements like dystonia may co-occur in long-standing "pure" ET patients; raising the question as to whether such patients have two diseases or a secondary feature of a singular condition [23]. Indeed, patient 1 in Additional file 1: Video S1 has a slight head tilt during singing and a co-occuring cervical dystonia may not be excluded by exam alone.

Conclusions

This retrospective review adds to the growing understanding of essential voice tremor as part of the heterogeneous presentation of ET. Recognition of IVT occurring in the absence of "classic" ET features may aid in improving diagnosis and identifying new therapeutics for this functionally disabling and often medically refractory condition.

Abbreviations
IVT: Isolated vocal tremor; ET: Essential tremor.

Competing interests
The authors declare that they have no competing interests.

Authors' contributions
AP participated in study design and drafting the manuscript. SF conceived of the study, participated in its design and helped to revise the manuscript. Both authors read and approved the final manuscript.

References

1. Louis ED. Essential tremor. Lancet Neurol. 2005;4(2):100–10.
2. Jimenez-Jimenez FJ, Alonso-Navarro H, Garcia-Martin E, Lorenzo-Betancor O, Pastor P, Agundez JA. Update on genetics of essential tremor. Acta Neurol Scand. 2013;128(6):359–71.
3. Louis ED, Ottman R. How familial is familial tremor? The genetic epidemiology of essential tremor. Neurology. 1996;46(5):1200–5.
4. Elble RJ. Diagnostic criteria for essential tremor and differential diagnosis. Neurology. 2000;54(11 Suppl 4):S2–6.
5. Deuschl G, Bain P, Brin M. Consensus statement of the movement disorder society on tremor. Mov Disord. 1998;13 Suppl 3:2–23.
6. Findley LJ, Koller WC. Definitions and behavioral classifications. In: Findley LJ, Koller W, editors. Handbook of tremor disorders. New York: Marcel Dekker; 1995. p. 1–5.
7. Jankovic J. Essential tremor: clinical characteristics. Neurology. 2000;54(11 Suppl 4):S21–5.
8. Sulica L, Louis ED. Clinical characteristics of essential voice tremor: a study of 34 cases. Laryngoscope. 2010;120(3):516–28.
9. Louis ED. When do essential tremor patients develop head tremor? Influences of age and duration and evidence of a biological clock. Neuroepidemiology. 2013;41(2):110–5.
10. Romero JP, Benito-Leon J, Bermejo-Pareja F. The NEDICES study: recent advances in the understanding of the epidemiology of essential tremor. Tremor Other Hyperkinet Mov. 2012;2:tre-02-70-346-2. Epub 2012 Jun 15.
11. Brown JR, Simonson J. Organic voice tremor: a tremor of phonation. Neurology. 1963;13:520–5.
12. Koller W, Graner D, Mlcoch A. Essential voice tremor: treatment with propranolol. Neurology. 1985;35(1):106–8.
13. Busenbark K, Ramig L, Dromey C, Koller WC. Methazolamide for essential voice tremor. Neurology. 1996;47(5):1331–2.
14. Hertegard S, Granqvist S, Lindestad PA. Botulinum toxin injections for essential voice tremor. Ann Otol Rhinol Laryngol. 2000;109(2):204–9.
15. Warrick P, Dromey C, Irish JC, Durkin L, Pakiam A, Lang A. Botulinum toxin for essential tremor of the voice with multiple anatomical sites of tremor: a crossover design study of unilateral versus bilateral injection. Laryngoscope. 2000;110(8):1366–74.
16. Adler CH, Bansberg SF, Hentz JG, Ramig LO, Buder EH, Witt K, et al. Botulinum toxin type A for treating voice tremor. Arch Neurol. 2004;61(9):1416–20.
17. Bove M, Daamen N, Rosen C, Wang CC, Sulica L, Gartner-Schmidt J. Development and validation of the vocal tremor scoring system. Laryngoscope. 2006;116(9):1662–7.
18. Koller WC, Busenbark K, Miner K. The relationship of essential tremor to other movement disorders: report on 678 patients. Ann Neurol. 1994;35(6):717–23.
19. Kralic JE, Criswell HE, Osterman JL, O'Buckley TK, Wilkie ME, Matthews DB, et al. Genetic essential tremor in gamma-aminobutyric acidA receptor alpha1 subunit knockout mice. J Clin Invest. 2005;115(3):774–9.
20. Frucht SJ, Houghton WC, Bordelon Y, Greene PE, Louis ED. A single-blind, open-label trial of sodium oxybate for myoclonus and essential tremor. Neurology. 2005;65(12):1967–9.
21. Louis ED. 'Essential tremor' or 'the essential tremors': is this one disease or a family of diseases? Neuroepidemiology. 2014;42:81–9.
22. Elble RJ. Defining dystonic tremor. Curr Neuropharmacol. 2013;11(1):48–52.
23. Louis ED, Hernandez N, Alcalay RN, Tirri DJ, Ottman R, Clark LN. Prevalence and features of unreported dystonia in a family study of "pure" essential tremor. Parkinsonism Relat Disord. 2013;19(3):359–62.

5

Effect of prior exposure to dopamine agonists on treatment with gabapentin enacarbil in adults with moderate-to-severe primary restless legs syndrome: pooled analyses from 3 randomized trials

William G Ondo[1*], Neal Hermanowicz[2], Diego García Borreguero[3], Mark J Jaros[4], Richard Kim[5] and Gwendoline Shang[5]

Abstract

Background: Dopamine agonists (DAs) are a first-line therapy for moderate-to-severe restless legs syndrome (RLS), but these treatments may lead to complications, such as augmentation and impulse control disorders, requiring switching to another therapeutic class. Here we assess efficacy and tolerability of gabapentin enacarbil (GEn) in adults with moderate-to-severe primary RLS, with or without prior DA exposure.

Methods: Data from 3 trials were pooled. Patients were identified as DA-naive or DA-exposed, based on prior treatment with ropinirole, pramipexole, rotigotine, or pergolide mesylate, and the dopamine precursor levodopa. Details on prior treatment duration and dose were unavailable. Patients with a history of augmentation were excluded. Within DA-naive/DA-exposed patients we investigated the co-primary end points from the pivotal trials: mean change from baseline to week 12 in International RLS (IRLS) Rating Scale total score and proportion of responders ("much"/"very much" improved) on the investigator-rated Clinical Global Impression–Improvement (CGI-I) scale. Safety was also assessed.

Results: 671 patients were randomized (DA-naive: placebo, n = 194; GEn 600 mg, n = 131; GEn 1200 mg, n = 214; DA-exposed: placebo, n = 50; GEn 600 mg, n = 30; GEn 1200 mg, n = 52). Across treatment arms, no significant differences between DA-naive and DA-exposed subgroups in IRLS Rating Scale total score change from baseline at any visit were seen, except week 1 in the placebo group (−6.1 DA-naive vs −3.4 DA-exposed, $P = .020$). No significant differences in the odds of CGI-I response at week 12 between DA-naive vs DA-exposed patients in any treatment group were seen; however, with placebo there was a nonsignificant trend toward fewer responders among DA-exposed (34.0%) vs DA-naive (44.3%) patients. Both GEn doses significantly improved the IRLS Rating Scale total score change from baseline and CGI-I response vs placebo, regardless of prior DA exposure. The most common treatment-emergent adverse events were dizziness and somnolence.

Conclusions: Prior DA exposure had no significant effect on efficacy or tolerability of GEn (600 or 1200 mg) in this pooled analysis of adults with moderate-to-severe primary RLS. These data support the use of GEn in DA-exposed and DA-naive patients.

Keywords: Restless legs syndrome, Gabapentin enacarbil, Dopamine agonist, International restless legs syndrome rating scale, Clinical global impression–improvement, Augmentation

* Correspondence: William.Ondo@uth.tmc.edu
[1]University of Texas Health Science Center at Houston, 6410 Fannin Street, Suite 1010, Houston, TX 77030, USA
Full list of author information is available at the end of the article

Background

Restless legs syndrome (RLS), also known as Willis-Ekbom disease, is a common neurological disorder characterized by an urge to move the legs. This urge is frequently accompanied by unpleasant sensations in the legs, worsens in the evening and at rest, and is transiently improved with activity [1,2]. Patients with RLS experience significant impairments in sleep, daytime or social functioning, and overall quality of life [3,4].

Over the past decade, dopamine agonists (DAs) have been used as first-line therapy for patients with moderate-to-severe primary RLS [5]. Three DAs—ropinirole, pramipexole, and rotigotine—have been approved by the US Food and Drug Administration (FDA) for the treatment of moderate-to-severe primary RLS [2]. Though initially effective, the benefit of treatment with DAs may lessen over time owing to a variety of factors which may include augmentation, tolerance, or dopaminergic downregulation. In particular, augmentation leads to a paradoxical scenario involving a worsening and earlier phase shift of RLS symptoms during treatment [6,7]. Some RLS patients who are treated with DAs may also develop impulse control disorders [2,8]. These developments may warrant switching to an alternate class of drugs when these side effects develop.

Gabapentin enacarbil (GEn), an agent in the alpha-2-delta ligand class of drugs, is an actively transported prodrug of gabapentin. GEn is approved by the FDA at a dose of 600 mg once daily for the treatment of moderate-to-severe primary RLS in adults. GEn is also approved for the management of postherpetic neuralgia in adults (600 mg twice daily) [9] and remains the only FDA-approved non-DA alternative for the treatment of moderate-to-severe primary RLS. In 3 randomized, double-blind, placebo-controlled studies in adult patients with moderate-to-severe primary RLS (XP052/XP053/XP081), GEn (600 mg and 1200 mg) significantly improved RLS symptoms compared with placebo, as assessed by the mean change from baseline in International RLS (IRLS) Rating Scale total score and the proportion of responders on the investigator-rated Clinical Global Impression–Improvement (CGI-I) scale at week 12. In all 3 studies, the most commonly reported adverse events were somnolence and dizziness [10-12].

When physicians consider how to treat patients with RLS, the potential effect of prior DA exposure on the efficacy of the new agent could be a factor. The effect of starting alternative agents, such as GEn, following exposure to DAs has not yet been examined. To investigate the effect of prior DA exposure on response to GEn treatment in adult patients with moderate-to-severe primary RLS, we compared outcomes for patients with and without prior DA exposure using pooled data from the XP052, XP053, and XP081 studies.

Methods

Study design and patients

The study designs and patient populations of the 3 primary studies (XP052, XP053, and XP081) have been published previously (ClinicalTrials.gov NCT00298623, NCT00365352, and NCT01332305) [10-12]. These were phase 2 or 3, double-blind, 12-week, placebo-controlled trials in adults with moderate-to-severe primary RLS, as defined by the IRLS Study Group diagnostic criteria [13].

For this analysis, data were pooled for each treatment from the XP052 (GEn 1200 mg and placebo) and XP053 (GEn 600 mg, GEn 1200 mg, and placebo) studies. Patients were grouped based on previous DA treatment status. Considering that augmentation was an exclusion criterion from study participation, the rate of any preceding augmentation was not rigorously assessed and thus remains unknown. In addition, the extent of treatment duration and dose of prior DA therapy were also not available. All subjects provided written informed consent prior to study participation. The primary studies were conducted in accordance with good clinical practice guidelines and the Declaration of Helsinki.

Co-primary end points from the pivotal trials, and investigated in the present analysis, were mean change in IRLS Rating Scale total score from baseline to week 12 [14], and the proportion of responders ("much" or "very much" improved) on the investigator-rated CGI-I scale [15] at week 12 for GEn 600 mg and GEn 1200 mg compared with placebo. Safety outcomes included treatment-emergent adverse events (TEAEs) and serious AEs.

Statistical analyses

Efficacy analyses were performed on the modified intent-to-treat population (all patients in the safety population with a baseline and ≥1 post-baseline IRLS Rating Scale total score). Missing data were imputed using the last observation carried forward for analyses of the investigator-rated CGI-I data, and a mixed-effect model for repeated measures (MMRM) with observed cases (no imputation) was used for analysis of the IRLS Rating Scale total score. The main comparisons for all efficacy analyses were within treatments across DA status (by visit for IRLS Rating Scale total score).

For the change from baseline IRLS Rating Scale total scores, the effects of prior DA exposure were analyzed using MMRM with an unstructured covariance matrix, including fixed effects for treatment, visit, treatment-by-visit interaction, baseline IRLS Rating Scale total score, DA history (yes/no), DA history-by-treatment interaction, DA history-by-visit interaction, and DA history-by-treatment-by-visit interaction. For the percentage of CGI-I responders, the effect of prior DA exposure was analyzed using a logistic regression model with the following factors: treatment, DA history (yes/no), and DA history-by-treatment interaction.

Results

Patients

In this pooled analysis, 19.7% (132/671) of patients had been previously exposed to DAs. Ropinirole was the most frequently reported prior DA across the 3 treatment arms (Table 1). In general, a greater proportion of DA-exposed patients had severe RLS at baseline compared with DA-naive patients (IRLS Rating Scale total score ≥24; 59.9% vs 42.7%). In the DA-naive group, 16.7% (90/539) of patients received non-DA prior treatment for RLS. Although not FDA-approved for the treatment of primary moderate-to-severe primary RLS, these non-DA prior treatments included gabapentin, non-steroidal anti-inflammatory drugs, sleep aids, clonazapam, tramadol, cyclobenzaprine, and quinine (Table 1). The mean duration of RLS symptoms

was 12.5 to 13.9 years in the DA-naive group and 16.1 to 17.9 years in the DA-exposed group. Of the DA-naive patients, 82.0% (159/194) in the placebo group, 84.7% (111/131) in the GEn 600-mg group, and 86.0% (184/214) in the GEn 1200-mg group completed their respective study. Among the DA-exposed patients, 82.0% (41/50) in the placebo group, 90.0% (27/30) in the GEn 600-mg group, and 86.5% (45/52) in the GEn 1200-mg group completed their respective study (Table 1).

End points

At week 12, prior DA exposure had no effect on the change in IRLS Rating Scale total score from baseline in the placebo (treatment difference between DA-naive and DA-exposed patients: −0.6 [1.3], $P = .673$), GEn 600-mg (treatment difference: −0.5 [1.6], $P = .762$), or GEn 1200-mg (treatment difference: 0.1 [1.3], $P = .964$) groups (Figure 1). With the exception of week 1 in the placebo group, there were no statistically significant differences in

Table 1 Baseline characteristics of DA-naive and DA-exposed patients (mITT population)

Characteristic	DA-naive (n = 539)			DA-exposed (n = 132)		
	Placebo (n = 194)	GEn 600 mg (n = 131)	GEn 1200 mg (n = 214)	Placebo (n = 50)	GEn 600 mg (n = 30)	GEn 1200 mg (n = 52)
Age at screening, mean years (SD)	48.9 (12.78)	47.2 (12.85)	49.8 (11.99)	50.5 (10.33)	52.4 (11.26)	54.2 (14.40)
Sex, n (%)						
Female	122 (63)	75 (57)	122 (57)	29 (58)	21 (70)	31 (60)
Male	72 (37)	56 (43)	92 (43)	21 (42)	9 (30)	21 (40)
Race, n (%)						
White/Caucasian	186 (96)	123 (94)	206 (96)	48 (96)	29 (97)	50 (96)
Mean baseline IRLS Rating Scale total score, points (SD)	22.5 (4.76)	23.2 (4.98)	22.9 (5.07)	25.2 (4.72)	24.0 (5.34)	24.6 (5.28)
Mean IRLS Rating Scale total score, n (%)						
<24 at baseline	116 (60)	67 (51)	126 (59)	18 (36)	14 (47)	21 (40)
≥24 at baseline	78 (40)	64 (49)	88 (41)	32 (64)	16 (53)	31 (60)
Duration of RLS symptoms, years						
Mean (SD)	13.1 (12.29)	12.5 (12.82)	13.9 (13.33)	17.0 (15.13)	17.9 (12.09)	16.1 (16.80)
Prior RLS treatment, n (%)						
Yes[a]	39 (20)[c]	20 (15)[c]	31 (14)[c]	50 (100)	30 (100)	52 (100)
Prior dopamine agonist treatment, n (%)						
Ropinirole	N/A	N/A	N/A	39 (78)	26 (87)	38 (73)
Pramipexole	N/A	N/A	N/A	9 (18)	5 (17)	10 (19)
Levodopa-carbidopa[b]	N/A	N/A	N/A	7 (14)	2 (7)	4 (8)
Rotigotine	N/A	N/A	N/A	2 (4)	2 (7)	2 (4)
Pergolide mesylate	N/A	N/A	N/A	1 (2)	0	0
Levodopa[b]	N/A	N/A	N/A	0	0	1 (2)

[a]Includes patients whose treatment terminated prior to the month before the start of study drug, and those who received treatment within the month of the start of study drug or within the previous month. [b]Classified as dopaminergic agents. Patients with a past history of treatment with levodopa-carbidopa and levodopa were included in the DA-exposed group. [c]Examples of non-DA prior treatment include: gabapentin, non-steroidal anti-inflammatory drugs, zolpidem, diphenhydramine HCL, clonazepam, diazepam, trazodone, tramadol, propoxyphene, cyclobenzaprine, and quinine. Please note, these treatments are not FDA approved treatments for primary moderate-to-severe RLS and list is not inclusive of all prior treatments reported.

DA, dopamine agonist; GEn, gabapentin enacarbil; IRLS, International Restless Legs Syndrome; mITT, modified intent-to-treat; N/A, not available; RLS, restless legs syndrome; SD, standard deviation.

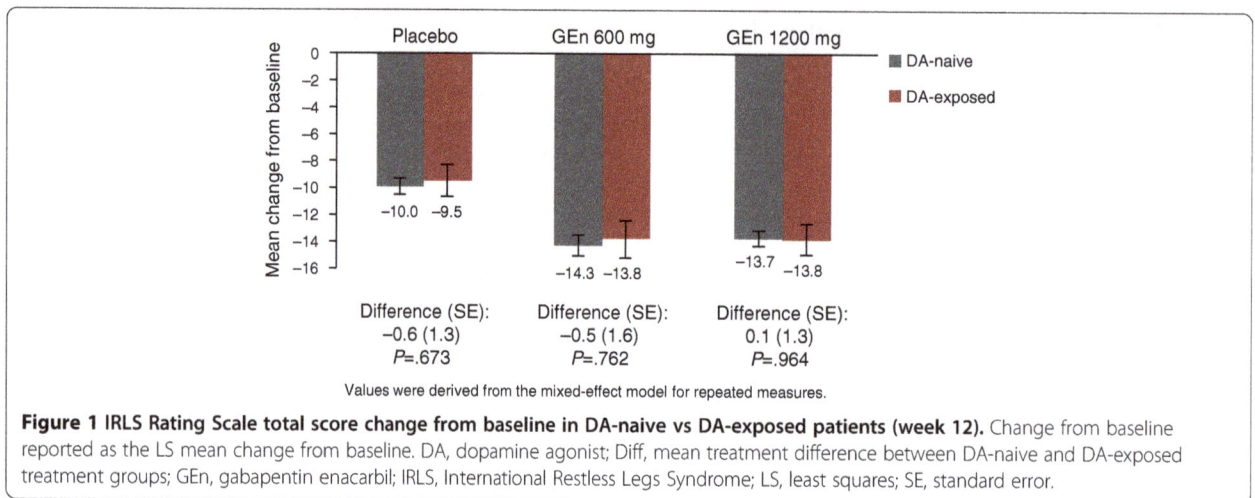

Figure 1 IRLS Rating Scale total score change from baseline in DA-naive vs DA-exposed patients (week 12). Change from baseline reported as the LS mean change from baseline. DA, dopamine agonist; Diff, mean treatment difference between DA-naive and DA-exposed treatment groups; GEn, gabapentin enacarbil; IRLS, International Restless Legs Syndrome; LS, least squares; SE, standard error.

change in IRLS Rating Scale total score from baseline between the DA-naive vs DA-exposed patients in any treatment arm at any of the visits (Figure 2). At week 1, the change from baseline in the IRLS Rating Scale was greater in the DA-naive patients compared with the DA-exposed patients treated with placebo (−6.1 vs −3.4, P = .020).

There were also no significant differences in the odds of being a CGI-I responder between the DA-naive vs DA-exposed patients in any of the treatment groups at week 12 (Figure 3), although the DA-exposed placebo group showed a nonsignificant trend toward fewer responders compared with the DA-naive placebo group (34.0% vs 44.3%, respectively).

Regardless of whether they had prior DA exposure, patients showed significant improvements in IRLS Rating Scale total score change from baseline with both GEn doses compared with placebo at most time points (Figure 2). Significantly more patients receiving GEn (600 mg or 1200 mg) were CGI-I responders compared with patients receiving placebo in both DA-naive and DA-exposed groups (Figure 3).

Tolerability
The TEAE profile was similar between DA-exposed and DA-naive patients. The most commonly reported TEAEs in the safety population were somnolence and dizziness (Table 2). Thirty-eight patients (7%) in the DA-naive group (GEn 600 mg, n = 10; GEn 1200 mg, n = 18; placebo, n = 10) and 6 patients (5%) in the DA-exposed group (GEn 600 mg, n = 1; GEn 1200 mg, n = 5; placebo, n = 0) discontinued treatment because of an AE. The majority of AEs were rated as mild or moderate in intensity. A total of 6 patients reported serious AEs: cellulitis (DA-naive, GEn 600 mg), worsened peripheral arterial disease (DA-naive, placebo), worsening cholelithiasis (DA-naive, GEn 1200 mg), cholelithiasis (DA-exposed, placebo), appendicitis (DA-exposed, placebo), and herniated

disc (DA-exposed, GEn 600 mg). None of these events were considered treatment-related, and 5 of the 6 patients recovered (the outcome of 1 patient with worsened peripheral arterial disease was unknown).

Discussion
In this pooled analysis of 671 adult patients with moderate-to-severe RLS, previous exposure to DAs did not significantly alter the efficacy and TEAE profile of GEn (600 mg or 1200 mg) given once daily compared with placebo. There were no significant differences in the change in IRLS Rating Scale total score (looking at change from baseline both at week 12 and by visit) or in the investigator-rated CGI-I responder status between the DA-naive and DA-exposed patients in any of the treatment groups. Although these findings are preliminary, it is worth noting that the limitations of these analyses include the fact that information on prior DA treatment duration and dose were not available nor was the rate of augmentation rigorously assessed, particularly because patients with symptom augmentation were excluded from the trial. Regardless of prior DA exposure, both GEn doses significantly improved change from baseline in IRLS Rating Scale total score and CGI-I response compared with placebo. The TEAE profile was similar between DA-naive and DA-exposed patients, with somnolence and dizziness being the most commonly reported TEAEs. The TEAEs reported in this study are consistent with those of the primary analyses [10-12] and with the overall safety profile of GEn [9].

Although DAs are the most commonly prescribed agents for the treatment of RLS [5,7], there is mounting concern about AEs associated with treatment with DA, particularly augmentation and impulse control disorders [16]. Augmentation involves an increase in the duration (earlier onset), anatomy, and intensity of RLS symptoms. Further, the incidence and severity of augmentation

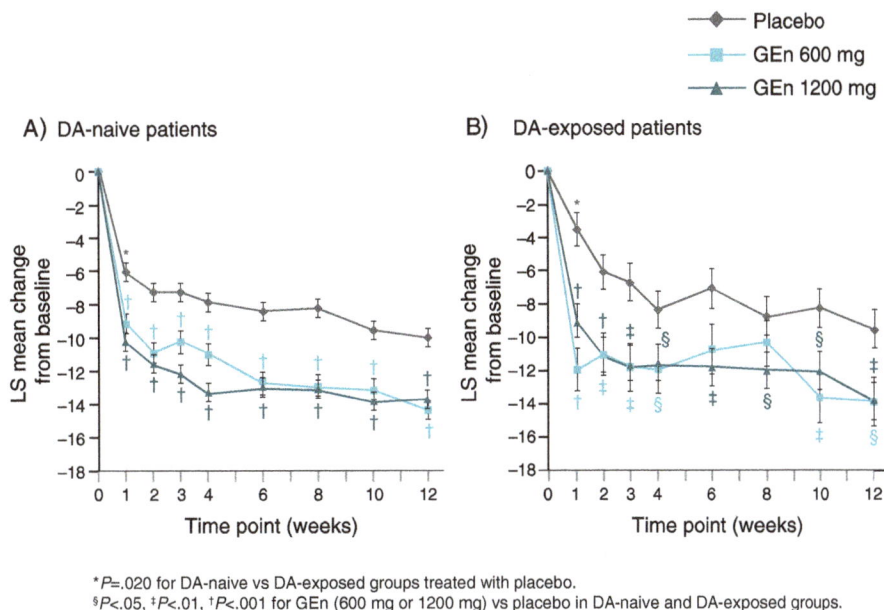

*P=.020 for DA-naive vs DA-exposed groups treated with placebo.
§P<.05, ‡P<.01, †P<.001 for GEn (600 mg or 1200 mg) vs placebo in DA-naive and DA-exposed groups.

Figure 2 **IRLS Rating Scale total score changes from baseline by visit in DA-naive (A) and DA-exposed (B) patients.** MMRM analysis. Change from baseline reported as the LS mean change from baseline. Within the placebo group, there were no statistically significant differences in change in IRLS Rating Scale total score from baseline between the DA-naive vs DA-exposed patients in any treatment arm at any of the visits, except at week 1. Within the GEn 600-mg and GEn 1200-mg groups, there were no statistically significant differences in change in IRLS Rating Scale total score from baseline between the DA-naive vs DA-exposed patients in any treatment arm at any of the visits. DA, dopamine agonist; GEn, gabapentin enacarbil; IRLS, International Restless Legs Scale; LS, least squares; MMRM, mixed-effect model for repeated measures; W, week.

increases linearly with the duration of DA treatment and usually resolves over weeks once DA treatment is discontinued [6]. This period, however, can be complicated by severe RLS symptoms, which are not always resolved by switching from one DA to another [17,18]. These are important points to note when considering treatment with DAs, as the dose and duration of prior DA exposure are related to the likelihood of augmentation, and augmentation is associated with a decrease in the response to subsequent DA treatment [16]. A retrospective

analysis found that DAs are also associated with impulse control disorders including pathological gambling, compulsive shopping, and hypersexuality [19]. These data show the need for more prominent warnings for DAs as part of their prescribing information.

To our knowledge, the effect of starting non-DA treatments after a short washout period has not been studied in adequately controlled clinical trials, although a case report detailed that the alpha-2-delta ligand pregabalin improved RLS symptoms in a patient previously treated

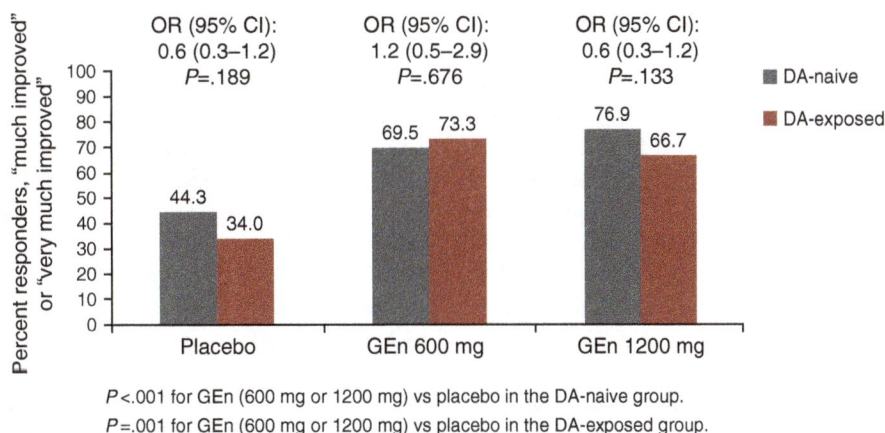

P<.001 for GEn (600 mg or 1200 mg) vs placebo in the DA-naive group.
P=.001 for GEn (600 mg or 1200 mg) vs placebo in the DA-exposed group.

Figure 3 **Percentage of responders on the investigator-rated CGI-I in DA-naive vs DA-exposed patients (week 12).** Response on the CGI-I was defined as "much" or "very much" improved at week 12. CGI-I, Clinical Global Impression–Improvement; CI, confidence interval; DA, dopamine agonist; GEn, gabapentin enacarbil; OR, odds ratio.

Table 2 Most frequent TEAEs in ≥5% of the safety population of any treatment groups[a]

Adverse event, n (%)	DA-naive			DA-exposed		
	Placebo (n = 195)	GEn 600 mg (n = 133)	GEn 1200 mg (n = 217)	Placebo (n = 50)	GEn 600 mg (n = 30)	GEn 1200 mg (n = 52)
Any event	149 (76)	105 (79)	187 (86)	34 (68)	27 (90)	40 (77)
Somnolence	12 (6)	25 (19)	54 (25)	0	7 (23)	7 (14)
Dizziness	9 (5)	20 (15)	44 (20)	2 (4)	2 (7)	15 (29)
Headache	22 (11)	12 (9)	36 (17)	5 (10)	7 (23)	4 (8)
Nasopharyngitis	10 (5)	13 (10)	17 (8)	6 (12)	1 (3)	4 (8)
Nausea	8 (4)	5 (4)	15 (7)	4 (8)	4 (13)	4 (8)
Fatigue	10 (5)	5 (4)	15 (7)	1 (2)	3 (10)	3 (6)
Diarrhea	10 (5)	3 (2)	7 (3)	2 (4)	3 (10)	3 (6)
Upper respiratory tract infection	7 (4)	6 (5)	5 (2)	2 (4)	3 (10)	1 (2)
Dry mouth	4 (2)	4 (3)	11 (5)	1 (2)	1 (3)	1 (2)
Constipation	6 (3)	0	7 (3)	2 (4)	3 (10)	3 (6)
Insomnia	6 (3)	7 (5)	4 (2)	1 (2)	1 (3)	2 (4)
Irritability	3 (2)	2 (2)	8 (4)	0	4 (13)	3 (6)
Back pain	6 (3)	4 (3)	6 (3)	1 (2)	2 (7)	1 (2)
Sinusitis	5 (3)	2 (2)	6 (3)	1 (2)	3 (10)	1 (2)
Increased weight	3 (2)	2 (2)	7 (3)	2 (4)	2 (7)	2 (4)

[a]Additional AEs reported in ≥5% of the safety population (at an overall frequency lower than those shown in the table) were: flatulence, contusion, abnormal coordination, toothache, increased appetite, urinary tract infection, depression, viral gastroenteritis, neck pain.
DA, dopamine agonist; GEn, gabapentin enacarbil; TEAE, treatment-emergent adverse events.

with the DA pramipexole [20]. According to recent guidelines, patients who experience augmentation due to DAs may benefit from alternative treatments, including alpha-2-delta ligands such as GEn [4], but no studies have investigated this. Our analysis suggests that GEn can be used to effectively treat RLS symptoms in patients with or without prior DA treatment, after a short washout period.

RLS studies can also be complicated by a robust placebo response, and prior DA treatment status has been shown to affect placebo response in patients with RLS [21,22]. In a meta-analysis of double-blind, randomized, placebo-controlled studies of patients with RLS, the placebo effect was particularly large for the primary outcome measure (IRLS Rating Scale) but less so for scales of daytime functioning [21]. Our analysis also found a treatment difference in the change in IRLS Rating Scale total score from baseline between DA-naive and DA-exposed populations within the placebo group at week 1. A blunted short-term placebo response resulting from prior DA treatment could be a possible explanation for these data.

Our analysis is limited to the data available from the individual trials. In particular, data on prior DA exposure is limited to the type of DA used, and the washout period following DA treatment was ≥2 weeks. As noted previously, information is not available to describe

the duration, dosage, and other details of previous dopaminergic treatment, leaving an important gap. As the severity and duration of RLS symptoms were greater in the DA-exposed group than in the DA-naive group, one might expect the DA-exposed group to have less of a response to GEn treatment; however, this was not the case. Although DA treatment ended at least 2 weeks before study initiation, the exact washout period following DA treatment was also unknown, raising the question of potential additive effects of DA treatment in the DA-exposed group. In addition to these limitations, the sample size of the DA-naive group was considerably larger than the DA-exposed group, and there were fewer patients with severe RLS in the DA-naive group than in the DA-exposed group, as one might expect. This was not a formal meta-analysis; therefore, the scope of this pooled analysis was limited to the GEn doses, treatment duration, and patient populations assessed in the XP052, XP053, and XP081 trials. Despite these limitations, the question whether previous exposure to a DA affects the efficacy of an alternate agent after changing treatment remains important clinically, and further studies that address these limitations properly are necessary. In particular, it would be worthwhile to examine prospectively whether earlier vs more delayed treatment with a non-DA medication, such as GEn, may lead to differential treatment effects in patients with RLS.

Conclusions

In summary, limited, prior exposure to DA had no significant effects on the efficacy or tolerability of GEn (600 mg or 1200 mg) once daily in this pooled analysis of adult patients with moderate-to-severe primary RLS. These preliminary data might support the use of GEn in non-augmented patients who were previously treated with DA after a ≥2-week washout period, as well as in those who are DA-naive.

Abbreviations

CGI-I: Clinical Global Impression–Improvement; DA: Dopamine agonist; FDA: United States Food and Drug Administration; GEn: Gabapentin enacarbil; IRLS: International Restless Legs Syndrome; mITT: Modified intent-to-treat; MMRM: Mixed-effect model for repeated measures; RLS: Restless legs syndrome; TEAE: Treatment-emergent adverse event.

Competing interests

WO served as a speaker for UCB Pharma, Lundbeck, Merz, and TEVA and received grant support from US World Meds, UCB Pharma, and Ipsen. NH served as a consultant for Allergan, Amgen, GlaxoSmithKline, Lundbeck, Teva, UCB Pharma, and US Worldmeds, and received research support from Allergan, Biotie, Chelsea Therapeutics, Merck, Pfizer, and Teva. DGB served as a consultant for UCB, XenoPort Inc., Impax Pharmaceuticals, and Otsuka. MJ is a consultant to XenoPort, Inc. RK and GS are employees of and own stock in XenoPort, Inc.

Authors' contributions

WO participated in the interpretation of data and critical revision of the draft for important intellectual content. NH participated in the interpretation of data and critical revision of the draft for important intellectual content. DGB participated in the interpretation of data and critical revision of the draft for important intellectual content. MJ performed the analyses and helped to draft the manuscript. RK participated in the analysis and interpretation of data and critical revision of the draft for important intellectual content. GS participated in the analysis and interpretation of data and helped draft the manuscript. All authors have made substantial contributions to this work in accordance with authorship criteria and have provided final approval of the submitted version of this manuscript.

Acknowledgments

These studies and this analysis were conducted by XenoPort, Inc., Santa Clara, CA. Medical writing support was provided by Sachi Yim and Meredith Kalish from CodonMedical, a division of KnowledgePoint360 (an Ashfield Company), and was funded by XenoPort, Inc.

Author details

[1]University of Texas Health Science Center at Houston, 6410 Fannin Street, Suite 1010, Houston, TX 77030, USA. [2]University of California Irvine Movement Disorders Program, 100 Irvine Hall, Irvine, CA 92697, USA. [3]Sleep Research Institute, Alberto Alcocer 19, 28036 Madrid, Spain. [4]Summit Analytical, LLC, 2422 Stout Street, Denver, CO 80205, USA. [5]XenoPort, Inc., 3410 Central Expressway, Santa Clara, CA 95051, USA.

References

1. Allen RP, Picchietti DL, Garcia-Borreguero D, Ondo WG, Walters AS, Winkelman JW, et al. Restless legs syndrome/Willis-Ekbom disease diagnostic criteria: updated International Restless Legs Syndrome Study Group (IRLSSG) consensus criteria - history, rationale, description, and significance. Sleep Med. 2014;15:860–73.
2. Garcia-Borreguero D, Kohnen R, Silber MH, Winkelman JW, Earley CJ, Högl B, et al. The long-term treatment of restless legs syndrome/Willis-Ekbom disease: evidence based guidelines and clinical consensus best practice guidance: a report from the International Restless Legs Syndrome Study Group. Sleep Med. 2013;14:675–84.
3. Allen RP, Walters AS, Montplaisir J, Hening W, Myers A, Bell TJ, et al. Restless legs syndrome prevalence and impact: REST general population study. Arch Intern Med. 2005;165:1286–92.
4. Garcia-Borreguero D, Stillman P, Benes H, Buschmann H, Chaudhuri KR, Gonzalez Rodriguez VM, et al. Algorithms for the diagnosis and treatment of restless legs syndrome in primary care. BMC Neurol. 2011;11:28.
5. Buchfuhrer MJ. Strategies for the treatment of restless legs syndrome. Neurotherapeutics. 2012;9:776–90.
6. Garcia-Borreguero D, Allen RP, Kohnen R, Högl B, Trenkwalder C, Oertel W, et al. Diagnostic standards for dopaminergic augmentation of restless legs syndrome: report from a World Association of Sleep Medicine-International Restless Legs Syndrome Study Group consensus conference at the Max Planck Institute. Sleep Med. 2007;8:520–30.
7. Ondo W, Romanyshyn J, Vuong KD, Lai D. Long-term treatment of restless legs syndrome with dopamine agonists. Arch Neurol. 2004;61:1393–7.
8. Cornelius JR, Tippmann-Peikert M, Slocumb NL, Frerichs CF, Silber MH. Impulse control disorders with the use of dopaminergic agents in restless legs syndrome: a case–control study. Sleep. 2010;33:81–7.
9. HORIZANT® [package insert]. Santa Clara, CA: XenoPort Inc., 2013. Available at: http://www.horizant.com/assets/docs/Horizant_PrescribingInformation.pdf.
10. Kushida CA, Becker PM, Ellenbogen AL, Canafax DM, Barrett RW, XP052 Study Group. Randomized, double-blind, placebo-controlled study of XP13512/GSK1838262 in patients with RLS. Neurology. 2009;72:439–46.
11. Lee DO, Ziman RB, Perkins AT, Poceta JS, Walters AS, Barrett RW, et al. A randomized, double-blind, placebo-controlled study to assess the efficacy and tolerability of gabapentin enacarbil in subjects with restless legs syndrome. J Clin Sleep Med. 2011;7:282–92.
12. Lal R, Ellenbogen A, Chen D, Zomorodi K, Atluri H, Luo W, et al. A randomized, double-blind, placebo-controlled, dose–response study to assess the pharmacokinetics, efficacy, and safety of gabapentin enacarbil in subjects with restless legs syndrome. Clin Neuropharmacol. 2012;35:165–73.
13. Allen RP, Picchietti D, Hening WA, Trenkwalder C, Walters AS, Montplaisi J, et al. Restless legs syndrome: diagnostic criteria, special considerations, and epidemiology. A report from the restless legs syndrome diagnosis and epidemiology workshop at the National Institutes of Health. Sleep Med. 2003;4:101–19.
14. Walters AS, LeBrocq C, Dhar A, Hening W, Rosen R, Allen RP, et al. Validation of the International Restless Legs Syndrome Study Group rating scale for restless legs syndrome. Sleep Med. 2003;4:121–32.
15. Busner J, Targum SD. The clinical global impressions scale: applying a research tool in clinical practice. Psychiatry (Edgmont). 2007;4:28–37.
16. Allen RP, Ondo WG, Ball E, Calloway MO, Manjunath R, Higbie RL, et al. Restless legs syndrome (RLS) augmentation associated with dopamine agonist and levodopa usage in a community sample. Sleep Med. 2011;12:431–9.
17. Nirenberg MJ. Dopamine agonist withdrawal syndrome: implications for patient care. Drugs Aging. 2013;30:587–92.
18. García-Borreguero D, Allen RP, Benes H, Earley C, Happe S, Högl B, et al. Augmentation as a treatment complication of restless legs syndrome: concept and management. Mov Disord. 2007;22 suppl 18:S476–84.
19. Moore TJ, Glenmullen J, Mattison DR. Reports of pathological gambling, hypersexuality, and compulsive shopping associated with dopamine receptor agonist drugs. JAMA Intern Med. 2014;174:1930–3.
20. Silber MH. Sleep-related movement disorder. Continuum (Minneap Minn). 2013;19:170–84.
21. Fulda S, Wetter TC. Where dopamine meets opioids: a meta-analysis of the placebo effect in restless legs syndrome treatment studies. Brain. 2008;131:902–17.
22. Ondo WG, Hossain MM, Gordon MF, Reess J. Predictors of placebo response in restless legs syndrome studies. Neurology. 2013;81:193–4.

6

Epidemiology and treatment of 23 musicians with task specific tremor

André Lee[*], Shinichi Furuya and Eckart Altenmüller

Abstract

Background: Task specific tremors in musicians have been mainly described as primary bowing tremor in string instrumentalists in relatively small sample sizes. Our aim was to describe epidemiology, risk factors, phenomenology and treatment options of this disorder in 23 musicians of different instruments.

Methods: We included 23 professional musicians (4 female, 19 male; mean age 51.5 ± 11.4 years) with a TSTM. During anamnesis, clinical examination, by mail or via telephone patients were asked for epidemiological, phenomenological information, risk factors and treatments. We then compared our findings to primary writing tremor, the most common task specific tremor.

Results: Age at onset of the TST was 44.6 ± 13.6 years and tremor appeared 35.1 ± 13.5 years after beginning to play the instrument. The majority of patients were string instrumentalists, followed by woodwind instrumentalists. Other instrumentalists were a guitarist, pianist and percussionist respectively. In contrast to primary writing tremor, we also found proximal muscles of the upper extremity involved in tremor. A positive family history was found in Prior trauma was more common than in primary writing tremor. Treatment with a positive effect on tremor were in order of efficacy: Botulinumtoxin, Primidone, Propranolol, Trihexyphenidyl. No patient had undergone deep brain stimulation.

Conclusion: Task specific tremor in musicians is a heterogeneous disorder with a male gender predominance that shares many commonalities with PWT. The onset age as well as the time between starting to play the instrument and tremor onset has a wide range. Because previous trauma and overuse appear to be risk factors, preventive measures against playing related injuries are necessary. There appears to be a genetic predisposition for TST. No single beneficial medication exists and treatment of patients remains highly individual. It should be discussed, whether deep brain stimulation should be offered not only to patients that do not respond to any other medication but early in the course of the disease.

Keywords: Dystonia, Essential tremor, Movement disorders, Botulinum toxin, Deep brain stimulation

Background

Task specific tremor in musicians (TSTM) is a highly disabling disorder that occurs only or mainly while playing the instrument and has primarily been described in string instrumentalists as primary bowing tremor (PBT) [1-3]. The most common form of a task specific tremor is primary writing tremor (PWT), first described by Rothwell in 1979 [4]. Two forms can be distinguished: type A tremor (task specific) and type B (position specific) [5]. While there are many studies on epidemiology, pathophysiology and treatment of PWT [5-20] only a few studies are available for TSTM [1-3,21]. Thus the sample sizes described so far are small, allowing only for limited conclusions e.g. with regard to risk factors or treatment. The aim of this paper therefore was to describe epidemiological data and treatment in 23 musicians with TSTM at a variety of instruments and compare the findings to PBT and PWT.

Methods

The study was approved by the local ethics committee and written informed consent was obtained from all participants.

* Correspondence: andre.lee@hmtm-hannover.de

Inistitute of Music Physiology and Musicians' Medicine, Hannover University of Music, Drama and Media, Hannover, Germany

We included 23 professional musicians (4 female, 19 male; mean age 51.5 ± 11.4 years) with a TSTM who were seen at our outpatient clinic. Four violinists with PBT described previously were included. During anamnesis, by mail or via telephone the following information were asked for: Age, age when starting to play the instrument and age at onset of tremor; time between starting to play the instrument and tremor onset; previous trauma; whether the professional position as before tremor was still upheld (e.g. an orchestra musician was still playing in an orchestra); responsiveness to alcohol; family history for movement disorders. Tremor frequency; side of tremor; spreading of tremor to other tasks; treatments and their efficacy. In order to distinguish between kinetic tremor and postural tremor at the instrument, the former and latter was considered type A and B tremor, respectively. However we are aware that this distinction may be debatable (Table 1). Tremor was quantified with electromyogram and accelerometer in 22 patients and the mean frequency is given for those participants. Details will be reported elsewhere.

To assess the gender distribution we applied two χ^2-tests: The first assuming no gender predominance and a second one assuming a gender predominance as in musician's dystonia [22] (f:m =1:4), if the first should reveal a significant difference.

Results
Epidemiology
Mean ± standard deviation (SD) of age of our patients was 51.5 ± 11.4 years. Tremor duration was 7.0 ± 5.1 years. Patients started their instrument at an age of 9.4 ± 3.2 years. Age at onset of the TST was 44.6 ± 13.6 years and duration between starting to play the instrument and tremor onset was 35.1 ± 13.5 years (Figure 1). Of our patients, sixteen were string instrumentalists (69.6%), four were woodwind instrumentalists (17.4%) one was a guitarist, pianist and percussionist respectively (each 4.3%). Nine patients (39%) reported a trauma or injury prior to onset of tremor: three had an overuse injury of the respective arm after intensively practicing and playing the instrument, one had an injury of the middle and ring finger and one had a fracture of the radius and ulna. Three patients had shoulder related problems: One had surgery of the shoulder, one surgery of the rotator cuff and one a pain syndrome. Nine patients (39%) had a positive family history for tremor: Two (9%) had relatives with Parkinson's disease, of which one had another relative with a tremor disorder. One patient (4%) had a relative with writer's cramp, four (17%) had a relative with essential tremor and one (4%) had a relative with an unknown tremor disorder. In eight of the patients (35%) a first-degree relative and in four (17%) a second-degree relative was affected. Three patients (13%) had two affected relatives. Three of the four

relatives with essential tremor were first-degree relatives (parents) and one was a second degree relative (grandparents). Two patients did not recall which kind of tremor disorder their relatives were suffering from. In one patient, a first degree relative (father) was suffering from writer's cramp. One patient had a dystonia before onset of TSTM, however at clinical examination no dystonic posturing was visible, and only tremor was discernible.

Phenomenology
Tremor frequency was 6.5 ± 0.9 Hz. Ten patients (43%) were diagnosed as type B tremor. Fifteen patients (65.2%) had a wrist tremor, three (13.0%) had a forearm pronation supination tremor, four (17.4%) had an elbow tremor and one (4.3%) had a shoulder tremor. In eight patients (35%) tremor was at the left upper extremity. Seventeen patients (74%) were orchestra musicians (including big band), two (9%) were students, two (9%) were teachers, one (4%) was self-employed and one (4%) was retired. In all patients, tremor started while playing the instrument and remained unilateral. None of the patients developed rest tremor and no other posture than for playing the instrument was affected. In eleven patients (48%) tremor has spread to other activities. In one patient tremor spread first to shaving, in another to an instrument that was not affected at first, in two tremor appeared when holding a pen, in five when filling a glass with water, one patient had difficulties holding the telephone or typing on a computer keyboard, one had tremor when playing table-tennis. Spreading of tremor occurred between 1 and 6 years after tremor during playing the instrument. Tremor was alcohol responsive in six patients (33% of 18 patients, five patients did not drink any alcohol). In none of those patients did alcohol lead to a complete remission of tremor, therefore its effect was not rated as sufficient by any of the patients. All opposed taking alcohol before concerts. None of those patients reported a dose response curve to alcohol; however, none had consciously assessed a possible dose–response. Likewise none of those patients reported a rebound effect.

Treatment
Propranolol was taken in dosages between 5–80 mg/day by 15 patients, of whom 9 had an improvement of tremor (60%); Trihexyphenidyl was taken by 10 patients at a dosage of 6 mg/day of whom 2 reported an improvement (20%); four patients took Primidone at 60 mg/day, of whom 3 had an improvement of tremor (75%); Madopar® at a dosage of 62,5 mg/day and Escitalopram at a dosage of 10 mg/day were taken by three patients respectively without effect; Gabapentin at a dosage of 2.4 g/day, Venlafaxin at a dosage of 150 mg/day, Topiramat at a dosage of 200 mg/day and Lorazepam at a dosage of 1 mg/day was each taken by one patient without effect. Five patients were treated with injections of Botulinumtoxin

Table 1 Patients' characteristics of all 23 patients with a task specific tremor at the instrument

	Gender	Age (yrs)	Instrument	Age when starting to play the instrument (yrs)	Age at onset of TST (yrs)	Time until TST onset since beginning to play (yrs)	TST duration (yrs)	Tremor location	Type A tremor
Pat. 1	Male	40	Sax	12	27	15	13	Wrist	l
Pat. 2	Male	62	Violin	8	46	38	16	Wrist	r
Pat. 3	Male	54	Violin	12	43	31	11	Wrist	r
Pat. 4	Male	48	Violin	4	40	36	8	Wrist	r
Pat. 5	Female	50	Violin	13	43	30	7	Wrist	r
Pat. 6	Female	24	Violin	5	10	5	14	Wrist	r
Pat. 7	Male	59	Violin	7	58	51	1	Wrist	r
Pat. 8	Male	62	Violin	7	59	52	3	Wrist	r
Pat. 9	Male	54	Violin	10	44	34	10	Wrist	r
Pat. 10	Male	54	Guitar	11	45	34	9	Pron/Sup	r
Pat. 11	Female	58	Cello	7	56	49	2	Pron/Sup	l
Pat. 12	Male	63	Cello	9	61	52	2	Pron/Sup	l
Pat. 13	Male	56	Sax	10	47	37	9	Wrist	l
Pat. 14	Female	55	Oboe	15	50	35	5	Elbow	r
Pat. 15	Male	57	Violin	10	40	30	17	Shoulder	r
Pat. 16	Male	63	Viola	6	62	56	1	Elbow	l
Pat. 17	Male	23	Piano	6	19	13	4	Wrist	l
Pat. 18	Male	38	Cello	5	28	23	10	Wrist	r
Pat. 19	Male	58	Violin	9	57	48	1	Wrist	l
Pat. 20	Male	55	Violin	12	54	42	1	Wrist	l
Pat. 21	Male	59	Violin	12	49	37	10	Elbow	r
Pat. 22	Male	55	Oboe	13	54	41	1	Elbow	l
Pat. 23	Male	38	Percussion	14	33	19	5	Wrist	l

Table 1 Patients' characteristics of all 23 patients with a task specific tremor at the instrument (*Continued*)

	Type B tremor	Spreading of tremor	Previous trauma	Medication	Botulinum toxin	Ethanol responsive	Family history for movement disorders	DBS	Tremor frequency (Hz)	Still plays in the orchestra
Pat. 1	n	y	y (overuse)	Thx	y	n	n	n	7.3	n
Pat. 2	n	y	y (car accident)	Prop, Thx, Gabap,Topi, Prim	y	y	y (WC)	n	6.4	y
Pat. 3	n	y	n	Prim, Prop	n	y	y (tremor)	n	4.9	y
Pat. 4	n	y	n	Prim, Prop	y	y	n	n	6.8	y
Pat. 5	y	n	y (overuse)	Prop, Thx	n	n	n	n	6.4	y
Pat. 6	n	n	n	Thx, Mad, Cip, Prop	n	?	n	n	6.8	Student
Pat. 7	n	n	y (finger injury)	Thx	n	n	n	n	8.3	y
Pat. 8	n	y	y (overuse)	Prop, Thx	n	?	n	n	7.1	y
Pat. 9	y	n	n	Prop	n	n	y (tremor, PD)	n	4.6	y
Pat. 10	y	y	n	Thx	n	y	n	n	6.8	Teacher
Pat. 11	n	n	y (fracture radius + ulna)	Prop	n	?	n	n	6.1	y
Pat. 12	n	n	n	none	n	n	n	n	5.1	Retired
Pat. 13	n	y	n	Prop	y	y	n	n	6.4	y (Big Band)
Pat. 14	n	y	n	Prop, Prim	y	n	n	n	6.4	y
Pat. 15	y	n	y (surgery shoulder)	Vfx, Mtz, Loraz, Thx	n	?	n	n	6.6	y
Pat. 16	y	y	n	Prop, Mad	n	n	n	n	6.4	y
Pat. 17	n	n	n	Prop	n	n	n	n	6.4	Student
Pat. 18	y	n	n*	Thx, Cip, Mad	n	n	y	n	6.8	y
Pat. 19	y	n	y (surgery rotaor cuff)	Bromazepam	n	n	y (ET)	n	7.6	y
Pat. 20	y	n	y (pain shoulder)	Prop	n	y	y (ET)	n	6.1	y
Pat. 21	y	n	n	-	n	?	y (ET)	n	7.8	Teacher
Pat. 22	y	y	n	Prop	n	n	y (ET)	n	6.1	Self employed
Pat. 23	n	y	n	Cip, Prop	n	n	y (PD)	n	-	y

*This patient had a dystonia that improved before tremor occured. *Abbreviations:* *yrs* years, *Pat.* patient, *DBS* deep brain stimulation, *r* right, *l* left, *y* yes, *n* no, *Prop* propranolol, *Thx* Trihexyphenidyl, *Gabap* Gabapentin, *Topi* topiramat, *Prim* primidone, *Mad* madopar, *Cip* cipralex, *Vfx* venlafaxin, *Loraz* lorazepam, *WC* writer's cramp, *PD* Parkinson's Disease, *ET* essential tremor.

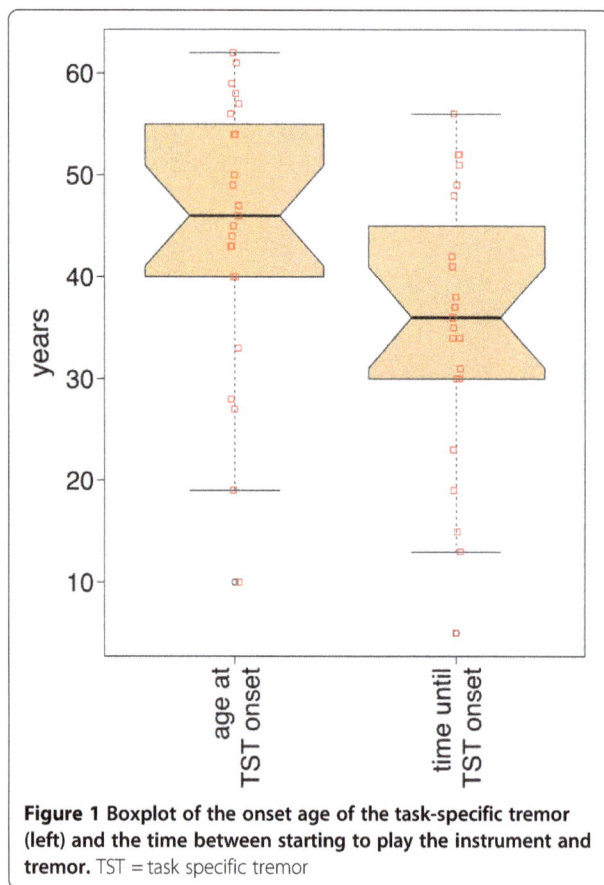

Figure 1 Boxplot of the onset age of the task-specific tremor (left) and the time between starting to play the instrument and tremor. TST = task specific tremor

with amounts of 10–117.5 Units or 5–23.4 Units/muscle, where the amount of muscles varied between two and six. No adverse events were reported under this treatment. Four of these patients reported an improvement of tremor (80%). Treatment and response to treatment are given in Table 2 and Figure 2.

Gender distribution

χ^2-test assuming an equal gender distribution (f:m =1:1) demonstrated that χ^2 = 9.8, df =1, and p =0.002. χ^2-test assuming a gender distribution as in musicians dystonia (f:m =1:4) showed χ^2 = 0.1, df =1, p =0.8.

A summary of epidemiology, phenomenology and treatment in this study, in PBT and in PWT is given in Table 3.

Discussion

Tremor frequency corresponds to what has been found in PWT [5,6,8,12]. The main differences to PWT are firstly that we found an involvement of proximal muscles, which to our knowledge has not been reported in PWT. The necessity to hold the entire arm against gravity while playing the instruments in contrast to writing may be an explanation for this phenomenon. Secondly type B tremor occurs more often in TSTM than in PWT [5-8,12,14,19]. This is interesting because it supports the notion that the tonic nature of playing the affected instruments as mentioned above seems to play a role in TSTM. No difference to PWT [5-8,12,14,19] was found with regard to alcohol responsiveness, although a wide range between 0% [14] and 75% [6] exists in PWT (Table 3). Spreading of tremor to other tasks as we found in TSTM is a phenomenon described in TST and a strict task-specificity was questioned recently [5,19,23]. An evolution of the disorder over time [19] was discussed that may apply to TSTM, as well.

The mean onset age of TSTM is 43.5 years and does not differ to PBT [1,2] and is only marginally lower than in PWT [5-8,12,14,19] (Table 3). The high standard deviation in PBT [2] and in PWT [5-8,12,14,19] reflects the great range of the age at tremor onset (Table 3). Tremor appeared on average 35 years after starting to exert the triggering task, an information to our knowledge not reported in PWT. However there is a wide range of 5 years to more than 50 years. Mean tremor-affected duration of our patients was 7.6 ± 5.2 years. In this context it is noteworthy that only one of the musicians playing in an ensemble had to stop playing because of tremor and all musicians who are primarily teaching continue to exert their profession. One musician was retired (Table 3). This is an important finding, since for most musicians tremor poses a serious threat to their professional career. Which treatments are available that may allow patients to continue performing (Table 3)? Botulinum-toxin-injection with a response rate of 80% was the most effective treatment. High response rates have been reported in PWT [5,14,15], where it was fond to be the second-best rated treatment after deep brain stimulation [19]. The most effective oral medication was Primidone with a response rate of 75%. Propranolol was the most often prescribed

Table 2 Medications prescribed

	Prop	Thx	Prim	Madop	Gabap	Cip	Ven	Topi	Loraz	Btx*
Number of patients	15	10	4	3	1	3	1	1	1	5
Improvement	9	2	3	0	0	0	0	0	1	4
No improvement	6	8	1	3	1	3	1	1	0	1
Dosage	5-80 mg	6 mg	60 mg	62.5 mg	2.4 g	10 mg	150 mg	200 mg	1 mg	5-23.4/muscle

*Units of Dysport® were converted intor units of Botox® with the factor 3:1. Thx = Trihexyphendyl; Gabap = Gabapentine; Madop = Madopar; Prop = Propranolol; Prim = Primidone; Cip = Citalopram; Ven = Venlafaxin; Topi = Topiramate; Loraz = Lorazepam; Btx = Botulinumtoxin; resp = responder; non-resp = non-responder.

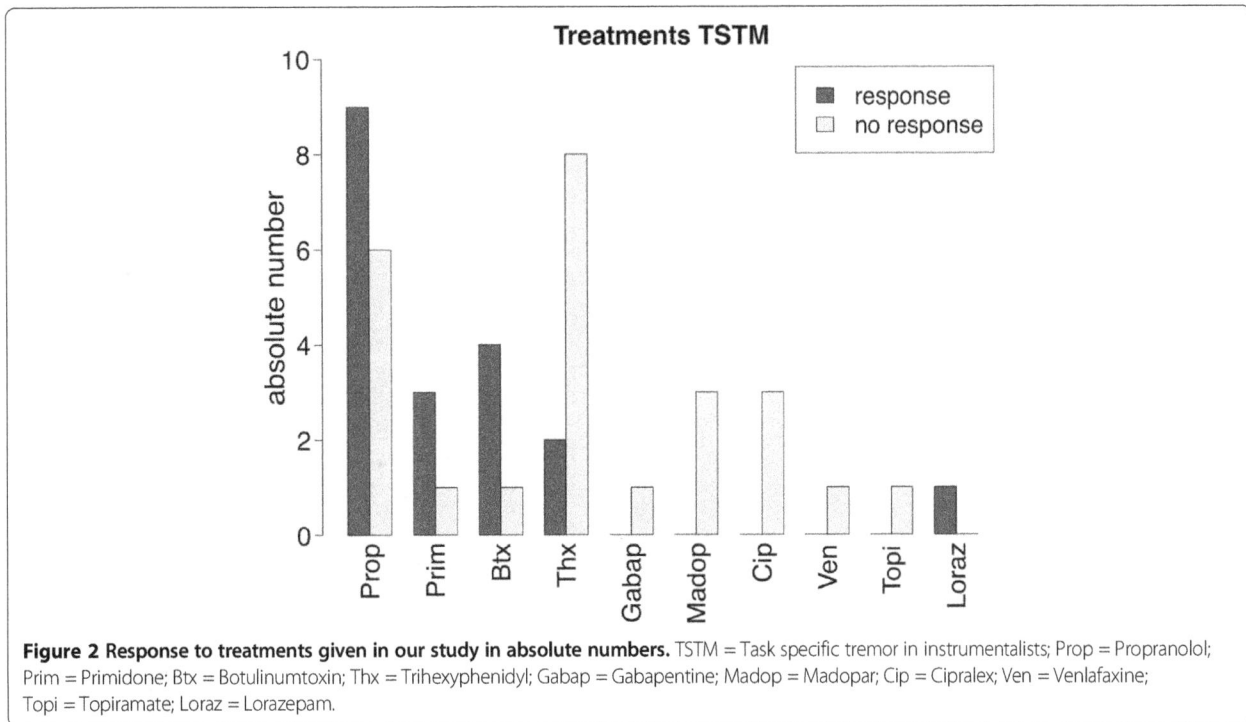

Figure 2 Response to treatments given in our study in absolute numbers. TSTM = Task specific tremor in instrumentalists; Prop = Propranolol; Prim = Primidone; Btx = Botulinumtoxin; Thx = Trihexyphenidyl; Gabap = Gabapentine; Madop = Madopar; Cip = Cipralex; Ven = Venlafaxine; Topi = Topiramate; Loraz = Lorazepam.

treatment and beneficial for 60% of our patients, although, as in PWT [6-8] improvement was not related to the dosage: one patient reported an improvement under 5 mg whereas 80 mg did not have any effect in another patient. As in PWT [5,7,8,14], Trihexyphenidyl was beneficial for only 20% of the patients, although one patient had an almost complete remission. The effect of Lorazepam, taken by one patient was due to reduction of stress caused by the tremor. None of the other medications had any effect. Treatment in PWT and PBT are given in Table 2.

None of our patients has undergone DBS so far, although two had considered it. The main concern is the lack of experience with DBS in musicians as well as high expectations of a complete remission. Therefore a recent case report of an oboist with TST is of interest, where a marked improvement through bilateral stimulation of the ventralis intermedius nucleus was reported [24]. In PWT several reports of successful treatment with DBS of the thalamus exist [9,11,17].

The response to Primidone and Propranolol is suggestive of essential tremor and it remains under debate whether task-specific tremors are a form of essential tremor, of focal dystonia or an entity of its own [7,18,23,25].

The high prevalence of string and woodwind instrumentalists has been reported before in a study by Lederman [21]. It has to be noted, however, that in the study by Lederman tremors other than TST were included. It is of interest that in the present study that includes only patients with TSTM, tremor is much more common in instrumentalists requiring steady (tonic) postural

muscular activity (holding the bow, the oboe etc.) as in instrumentalists mainly relying on phasic and ballistic movements such as pianists and percussionists. This of course may be related to the professional consequences, in that postural tremor reduces perceived sound quality to a much higher degree as compared to tremor in phasic movements.

A recent study of five string instrumentalists with PBT consisted of three female and two male participants suggesting an female gender predominance [2], however, due to the small sample size general conclusions were difficult. Our test for gender distribution suggests a male gender predominance in TSTM that does not differ to musician's dystonia [22] or PWT.

Of our patients, 39% reported a trauma of the affected limb prior to tremor onset, which is known from PWT, albeit at a lower prevalence (19% [5] and 30% [6]), however, we are aware that this question is subject to recall bias. Whether traumata are related to the development of TST, however, cannot be concluded from our data alone. One patient had a dystonia that had markedly improved before developing tremor and during examination at the instrument no dystonic posturing was visible and only tremor was evident. This is interesting, because dystonia preceding PWT was described by Bain et al. [5] and likewise tremor preceding dystonia has been described before [26]. A positive family history as risk factor was found in PBT [2] as well as in PWT, although in PWT, two studies reported no family history in ten [6] or five [14] patients respectively (Table 3).

Table 3 Summary of epidemiology, phenomenology and treatment in this study, in primary bowing tremor (PBT) and primary writing tremor (PWT)

	Mean age at onset (yrs)	SD of onset age (yrs)	Sample size	Alcohol responsive	Antichol	Dosage per day	Prop	Dosage per day	Prim	Dosage per day	BTX	Type B	Dosage per day	Family history	Trauma	Tremor frequency (Hz)	Ratio f:m
TST in musicians																	
This paper	51.5	11.4	n = 23	6/18 (33%)	2/10 (20%)	6 mg	9/15 (60%)	5-80 mg	3/4 (75%)	60 mg	4/5 (80%)	10 (43%)	5-23.4 U/m	9 (39%)	9 (39%)	6.5 (+− 0.9)	4:19
PBT																	
Lederman [2]	41	23.2	n = 5	1/1 (100%)	0/1	6 mg	1/1 (100%)	20 mg	-	-	-	2 (40%)	-	2 (40%)	-	-	3:02
PWT																	
Rosenbaum & Jankovic [7]	50.5	14.8	n = 10	2/4 (50%)	4/5 (80%)	-	4/4 (100%)	-	-	-	-	3 (30%)	-	3 (30%)	-	-	3:07
Bain et al. [5]	50.1	range (16–76)	n = 21	7/17 (41%)	4/12 (33%)	-	4/12 (33%)	120-240 mg+	3/4 (75%)	62.5-125 mg	2/2 (100%)	10 (48%)	33 U/m	7 (33%)	4 (19%)	5.5 (4.1-7.3)	1:20
Kachi et al. [6]	40.8	18.1	n = 10*	3/4 (75%)	-	-	10/11 (91%)#	-	-	-	-	3 (30%)	-	0	3 (30%)	5-Jun	2:08
Elble et al. [8]	37	13.9	n = 5	1/4 (25%)	1/3 (33%)##	12-15 mg++	0/3 (0%)	240 mg	0/2 (0%)	750 mg	-	2 (40%)	-	1 (20%)	-	5-Jul	1:04
Modugno et al. [12]	51.7	16.2	n = 7	-	-	-	-	-	-	-	-	1 (14%)	-	3 (43%)	-	5-Jul	1:06
Ondo & Satija [19]	47.2	18	n = 56	-	-	-	31**	-	18**	-	17**	11 (20%)	-	27 (48%)	-	-	41:15:00
Papapetropoulos & Singer [14]	48.4	15.5	n = 5	0/5	1/2 (50%)	6 mg	-	-	-	-	4/4 (100%)	2 (40%)	10-12.5 U/m	0	-	-	2:03

*One patient had golfing tremor; # in five patients propranolol was administered intravenously and not orally, of whom 4 responded; +only orally administered propranolol; ##2xtrihexyphenidyl, 1xbenztropine (no effect); ++dosage only for trihexyphenidyl; **only the number of treated patients was reported with a mean rating of success; ## not including the range given by Bain et al. *Abbreviations: TST* Task-specific tremor, *PBT* Primary bowing tremor, *PWT* Primary writing tremor, *yrs* years, *SD* standard deviation, *Type B* type B task-specific tremor, *Antichol* anticholinergic medication, *Prop* propranolol, *Prim* primidone, *f* female, *m* male, *appr* approximately.
For the treatment and alcohol responsiveness, the numerator indicates positive response to the respective medication/alcohol whereas the denominator indicates the number of patients treated with the respective medicament/alcohol in the respective study.

Conclusion

To our knowledge, this is the largest sample of TSTM described in detail so far. It is a heterogeneous disorder that shares many commonalities with PWT. It occurs mainly between the age of 30 and 55, appears between 21 and 48 years after starting to play the instrument and has a male gender predominance. It may spread to other tasks. Because previous trauma may precede TSTM, it is important to raise awareness for preventive measures against playing related injuries as e.g. overuse. There appears to be a genetic predisposition for TST. A variety of treatment options exist, of which most beneficial are Botulinumtoxin, Propranolol, and Primidone. Since no single beneficial medication exists, treatment of patients remains highly individual. Given the positive results of DBS in PWT and the positive case report of an oboist with TSTM, it should be discussed, whether this should be offered not only to patients that do not respond to any other medication but early in the course of the disease. However, further studies are necessary to address this question.

Competing interests
The authors declare that they have no competing interests.

Authors' contribution
AL: Conception and design of the study, acquisition, analysis and interpretation of data. Drafting of the manuscript. Final approval. Agrees to be accountable for all aspects of the work in ensuring that questions related to the accuracy or integrity of any part of the work are appropriately investigated and resolved. SF: Analysis and interpretation of data. Revision of manuscript for important intellectual content. Final approval. Agrees to be accountable for all aspects of the work in ensuring that questions related to the accuracy or integrity of any part of the work are appropriately investigated and resolved. EA: Conception and design of the study, interpretation of data. Revision of manuscript for important intellectual content. Final approval. Agrees to be accountable for all aspects of the work in ensuring that questions related to the accuracy or integrity of any part of the work are appropriately investigated and resolved. All authors read and approved the final manuscript.

Acknowledgements
Funding for AL and EA: Hannover University of Music, Drama and Media.

References
1. Lee A, Chadde M, Altenmüller E, Schoonderwaldt E: **Characteristics of task-specific tremor in string instrument players.** *Tremor Hyperkinetic Mov N Y N* 2013. in press.
2. Lederman RJ: **Primary bowing tremor: a task-specific movement disorder of string instrumentalists.** *Med Probl Perform Art* 2012, 27:219–223.
3. Lee A, Tominaga K, Furuya S, Miyazaki F, Altenmüller E: **Coherence of coactivation and acceleration in task-specific primary bowing tremor.** *J Neural Transm Vienna Austria 1996* 2014. epub ahead of print. doi:10.1007/s00702-014-1177-3.
4. Rothwell JC, Traub MM, Marsden CD: **Primary writing tremor.** *J Neurol Neurosurg Psychiatry* 1979, 42:1106–1114.
5. Bain PG, Findley LJ, Britton TC, Rothwell JC, Gresty MA, Thompson PD, Marsden CD: **Primary writing tremor.** *Brain J Neurol* 1995, 118(Pt 6):1461–1472.
6. Kachi T, Rothwell JC, Cowan JM, Marsden CD: **Writing tremor: its relationship to benign essential tremor.** *J Neurol Neurosurg Psychiatry* 1985, 48:545–550.
7. Rosenbaum F, Jankovic J: **Focal task-specific tremor and dystonia: categorization of occupational movement disorders.** *Neurology* 1988, 38:522–527.
8. Elble RJ, Moody C, Higgins C: **Primary writing tremor. A form of focal dystonia?** *Mov Disord Off J Mov Disord Soc* 1990, 5:118–126.
9. Minguez-Castellanos A, Carnero-Pardo C, Gómez-Camello A, Ortega-Moreno A, García-Gómez T, Arjona V, Martin-Linares JM: **Primary writing tremor treated by chronic thalamic stimulation.** *Mov Disord Off J Mov Disord Soc* 1999, 14:1030–1033.
10. Berg D, Preibisch C, Hofmann E, Naumann M: **Cerebral activation pattern in primary writing tremor.** *J Neurol Neurosurg Psychiatry* 2000, 69:780–786.
11. Racette BA, Dowling J, Randle J, Mink JW: **Thalamic stimulation for primary writing tremor.** *J Neurol* 2001, 248:380–382.
12. Modugno N, Nakamura Y, Bestmann S, Curra A, Berardelli A, Rothwell J: **Neurophysiological investigations in patients with primary writing tremor.** *Mov Disord Off J Mov Disord Soc* 2002, 17:1336–1340.
13. Byrnes ML, Mastaglia FL, Walters SE, Archer S-AR, Thickbroom GW: **Primary writing tremor: motor cortex reorganisation and disinhibition.** *J Clin Neurosci Off J Neurosurg Soc Australas* 2005, 12:102–104.
14. Papapetropoulos S, Singer C: **Treatment of primary writing tremor with botulinum toxin type a injections: report of a case series.** *Clin Neuropharmacol* 2006, 29:364–367.
15. Singer C, Papapetropoulos S: **Adult-onset primary focal foot dystonia.** *Parkinsonism Relat Disord* 2006, 12:57–60.
16. Ljubisavljevic M, Kacar A, Milanovic S, Svetel M, Kostic VS: **Changes in cortical inhibition during task-specific contractions in primary writing tremor patients.** *Mov Disord* 2006, 21:855–859.
17. Blomstedt P, Fytagoridis A, Tisch S: **Deep brain stimulation of the posterior subthalamic area in the treatment of tremor.** *Acta Neurochir (Wien)* 2009, 151:31–36.
18. Hai C, Yu-ping W, Hua W, Ying S: **Advances in primary writing tremor.** *Parkinsonism Relat Disord* 2010, 16:561–565.
19. Ondo WG, Satija P: **Task-specific writing tremor: clinical phenotypes, progression, treatment outcomes, and proposed nomenclature.** *Int J Neurosci* 2012, 122:88–91.
20. Meunier S, Bleton JP, Mazevet D, Sangla S, Grabli D, Roze E, Vidailhet M: **TENS is harmful in primary writing tremor.** *Clin Neurophysiol* 2011, 122:171–175.
21. Lederman RJ: **Tremor in instrumentalists: influence of tremor type on performance.** *Med Probl Perform Art* 2007, 22:70–73.
22. Altenmüller E, Jabusch H-C: **Focal dystonia in musicians: phenomenology, pathophysiology, triggering factors, and treatment.** *Med Probl Perform Art* 2010, 25:3–9.
23. Bain PG: **Task-specific tremor.** *Handb Clin Neurol Ed PJ Vinken GW Bruyn* 2011, 100:711–718.
24. Whitney N, Kareus S, Cetas JS, Chung K, Brodsky M: **Bilateral deep brain stimulation targeting ventralis intermedius nucleus to treat a professional musician's task-specific tremor.** *Mov Disord Off J Mov Disord Soc* 2013, 28:1896–1897.
25. Deuschl G, Bain P, Brin M: **Consensus statement of the movement disorder society on tremor. Ad Hoc scientific committee.** *Mov Disord Off J Mov Disord Soc* 1998, 13 Suppl 3:2–23.
26. Schiebler S, Schmidt A, Zittel S, Bäumer T, Gerloff C, Klein C, Münchau A: **Arm tremor in cervical dystonia–is it a manifestation of dystonia or essential tremor?** *Mov Disord Off J Mov Disord Soc* 2011, 26:1789–1792.

7

A novel scale to assess psychosis in patients with parkinson's disease

William G. Ondo[1*], Sana Sarfaraz[1] and MinJae Lee[2,3]

Abstract

Background: Organic psychosis effects up to 70 % of patients with PD at some point yet no widely accepted scale for this entity exists.

Methods: We developed a 10 question PD specific psychosis severity scale that we feel has good content validity. It asks about the presence, severity, frequency, and consequences of the hallucinations (visual, auditory, olfactory) and delusions.

Results: Fifty different PD patients with psychosis and 25 PD patients without psychosis were included, and serial information was available in 21 of those encounters with psychosis. In psychosis subjects, results were normally distributed: mean 17.23 (SD = 6.30). In those without psychosis 14 % scored >0, mean 0.36 [range0-7]. The intra-rater, inter-class correlation coefficient was excellent (N = 21 pairs of observations seven days apart, ICC = 0.87). Inter-rater reliability (two different raters, N = 46 pairs) was outstanding for the entire group, ICC = 0.92). As expected visual hallucinations were most common (mean = 3.13). The presence of delusions was associated with greater total scores.

Conclusions: This scale, specifically designed for PD psychosis is easy to administer and has impressive metrics.

Keywords: Parkinson's disease, Psychosis, Hallucinations, Delusions, Scale, Metrics

Background

Psychosis in Parkinson's disease (PD) affects up to 70 % of patients, and causes tremendous morbidity [1]. The phenotype is much different than psychosis associated with schizophrenia or delirium. Although many different hallucinations, illusions, and delusions are reported in PD, the majority of episodes are visual hallucinations (usually "benign" content of silent people or animals), and persecutory/infidelity delusions, which are usually more problematic [1].

Despite the prevalence and importance of PD psychosis, no widely accepted scale exists. A Movement Disorder Task Force evaluated scales used to assess psychosis in PD, and concluded that a novel PD specific scale is needed [2]. Several small scales designed specifically for PD were felt to be insufficiently inclusive or poorly validated [3, 4], whereas better known and validated psychosis scales were not designed for PD psychosis and were felt to have poor content validity [5–7].

The lack of a disease specific severity scale has probably hampered efforts to test treatments for PD psychosis. To this day only clozapine and pimavanserin have compelling published efficacy data [8, 9]. To better quantify PD psychosis and aid in future therapeutic trials, we designed a PD specific psychosis scale and undertook psychometric evaluations.

Methods

The main goals for this scale development were content validity (based on the most common psychosis symptoms in the literature and experience, as there is no gold standard scale to compare), ease of use (10–15 minutes), inter-rater validation to include both physicians and non-physicians, and intra-rater validity measured over time. It is not a specifically designed quality of life scale, although questions 6–10 investigate how the psychosis would likely effect quality of life (insight, affective consequences and actions, and impact on family), nor is it designed as a screening tool. The questions evolved over 10 years and included patient and family input. Earlier non-validated

* Correspondence: William.Ondo@uth.tmc.edu
[1]Department of Neurology, Methodist Neurological Institute, 6560 Fannin, Ste 802, Houston, TX 77030, USA
Full list of author information is available at the end of the article

versions of the scale have been used in previous clinical trials [10, 11].

The study received a waiver from full consent from the University of Texas Health Science Center Institutional Review Board. All PD patients were recruited from a movement disorder center. We included PD patients with psychosis, based on a rating of ≥1 on UPDRS question #2, as determined by interview with the investigator, and a comparator group of PD patients without psychosis, score = 0. There were no formal exclusion criteria other than complete inability to participate. We intentionally allowed subjects with clinical dementia but in all cases motor symptoms preceded cognitive symptoms by more than a year [12]. Dementia was diagnosed if patients had a chart documented diagnosis of dementia and/or were taking acetylcholinesterase inhibitors for dementia. All consecutively seen psychosis patients seen in our tertiary referral center were included, but the control group was a convenience sample from the same clinic seen over the same period.

The first five questions identify the type of hallucination (visual, auditory, olfactory, sense of presence) or delusion [Fig. 1: Scale]. The second five questions further quantify the intensity, frequency, insight and impact of the worst psychotic feature on the life of the patient and family. The source of the information (patient/family/both) is documented. Since insight varies among patients, some latitude in question semantics is allowed and we did not include a specific question on how the psychosis affects only the patient's quality of life. [Additional file 1: Instructions] The final answer (0–4 for each question) is the opinion of the interviewer. It is not self-administered.

The patients were interviewed by an experienced physician and an inexperienced coordinator who had just started working with PD patient, at least 15 minutes apart (inter-rater assessments). Physician interview preceded the "inexperienced" interview in all cases. Intra-rater reliability (test-retest) was also tested at a second point in time 7+/−3 days after the first administration, in patients who did not require therapeutic intervention (change in medications) prior to then. This was done by a single interviewer (WO).

The range of score for each specific question is 0–4 and the total score simply adds all 10 questions. Weighted kappa statistics were calculated for inter and intra-rater reliability on the scale ranged 0–4 for each question, and intra-class correlation coefficients were calculated for inter- and intra-rater reliability on total score and individual questions. We used the mixed effect model to account for correlation within subjects. Poisson and linear model were conducted for patients with/without psychosis and with psychosis respectively because the total score for those with psychosis is normally distributed but not for those with non-psychosis [Fig. 2]. Descriptive statistics are also

presented. Analyses were performed using SAS 9.3 (SAS Institute Inc, Cary, NC) at a statistical significance level of 0.05.

Results

On average the questionnaire required a 10 min interview and family input was obtained in 84.8 % of all interviews. Inter-rater testing was completed on 46 different subjects with psychosis and 25 PD patients without psychosis. One subject was excluded because psychosis status was not definitively marked, leaving 49, and three psychosis subjects had intra-rater serial data, but not inter-rater data. The mean age for all 75 subjects (51 male) was 70.0 ± 10.8 years and duration of PD motor features was 9.4 ± 5.1 years. Dementia was diagnosed in 26 of the 75 total subjects (34.7 %). The PD without psychosis and PD with psychosis groups had similar age (68.8 ± 9.1 vs 70.6 ± 11.6 years), duration of PD 8.5 ± 5.0 vs 9.9 ± 5.1 years), percent that were male (68 % vs. 70 %), and percent that were demented (36.0 % vs. 34.0).

For those with psychosis, the results were normally distributed with a mean score of 17.23 ± 6.30, [range: 3–32]. Only 7 of 50 questionnaires from subjects without psychosis scored greater than 0, and only 1 scored >3 [Fig. 2]. The inter-rater reliability was excellent for the entire group (71 pair including psychotic and non-psychotic subjects, ICC = 0.92). For just those with psychosis (46 pairs) the ICC was 0.87. The intra-rater, inter-class correlation coefficient (time 1 vs. time 2 with same administrator) was excellent, N = 21 pairs of observations, ICC = 0.88. As expected, visual hallucinations were most common (mean = 3.13), followed by sensing a presence (mean = 2.06), auditory (mean = 1.16), and olfactory (mean = 0.29) [Table 1]. A delusion (question #5) was scored as >0 in 36/100 PD psychosis questionnaires. The total score in these cases with any delusion was much higher than those with pure hallucinations without delusions (mean = 22.51 vs. 14.49, $p < 0.001$, powered by higher responses in questions #6–10 (mean of 12.53 vs 7.73, $p < 0.001$).

Discussion

We report very good intra-rater reliability and excellent inter-rater reliability on a 10 question scale designed specifically for PD associated psychosis. Several content features warrant comment. We did not include a separate question on illusions because subjects often have difficulty differentiating these from true hallucinations so it could be "double scored". We instruct that illusions be included with hallucinations (almost always visual). We did not include tactile hallucinations. These have been reported [13, 14], but in our experience are essentially impossible to differentiate from "actual" sensations, which are very common in parkinsonism, and do not

1. How frequently do you <u>see</u> things that other people do not see (hallucinations) ?
    0. Never
    1. Rarely
    2. Occasionally (about once per week)
    3. Frequently (more than three times per week, 50% of days)
    4. Almost always (every day)

2. How frequently do you <u>smell</u> things that other people do not smell, and that possibly are not there (hallucinations) ?
    0. Never
    1. Rarely
    2. Occasionally (about once per week)
    3. Frequently (more than three times per week, 50% of days)
    4. Almost always (every day)

3. How frequently do you <u>hear</u> things that other people do not hear, and that possibly are not there (hallucinations) ?
    0. Never
    1. Rarely (less than once per week)
    2. Occasionally (at least once per week)
    3. Frequently (more than three times per week, 50% of days)
    4. Almost always (more than once per day)

4. How frequently do you <u>sense a presence</u> that other people do not sense, for example someone is behind you but you don't actually see them (hallucinations) ?
    0. Never
    1. Rarely
    2. Occasionally (about once per week)
    3. Frequently (more than three times per week, 50% of days)
    4. Almost always (more than once per day)

5. Do you ever feel cheated or persecuted by people, examples include a spouse that is unfaithful or that some people are trying to harm you for no reason?
    0. No
    1. Occasionally I feel this but I know it is not true
    2. Often I feel this but I know it is not true
    3. Occasionally I feel this and am sure it is true
    4. Often I feel this and am sure it is true

6. When you do, for example, see, hear smell, sense a presence, or feel cheated, for how long will it typically last during that episode? (score the worst of Questions 1-5)
    0. I do not see, hear of sense any presence
    1. just a second
    2. seconds (2-59 seconds)
    3. minutes (1-59 minutes)
    4. hours (>59 minutes)

7. Can you tell that these things (hallucinations/delusions) [ask about whichever is most prominent] are not real ?
    0. I am not having any now
    1. I have them, but can always tell they are not real
    2. after talking to other people who say they are not real, I am convinced they are definitely <u>not</u> real
    3. after talking to other people who say they are not real, I am not sure if they are real
    4. after talking to other people who say they are not real, I still definitely feel that they <u>are</u> real

8. When you have the hallucinations, do the hallucinations ever threaten you in any way ? This means their actions against you, not just the fact that they are there.
    0. I don't have any hallucinations now
    1. Never
    2. Sometimes
    3. Usually
    4. Always

9. Do you try to communicate or interact with the hallucinations ?
    0. I don't have any hallucinations now
    1. Never
    2. Sometimes
    3. Usually
    4. Always

10. How upset or concerned is your family about the hallucinations. If your family does not know about them, how upset do you think they would be about the hallucinations ?
    0. Not concerned at all
    1. Mildly concerned
    2. Moderately concerned
    3. Markedly concerned
    4. Extremely concerned

Fig. 1 Actual Scale

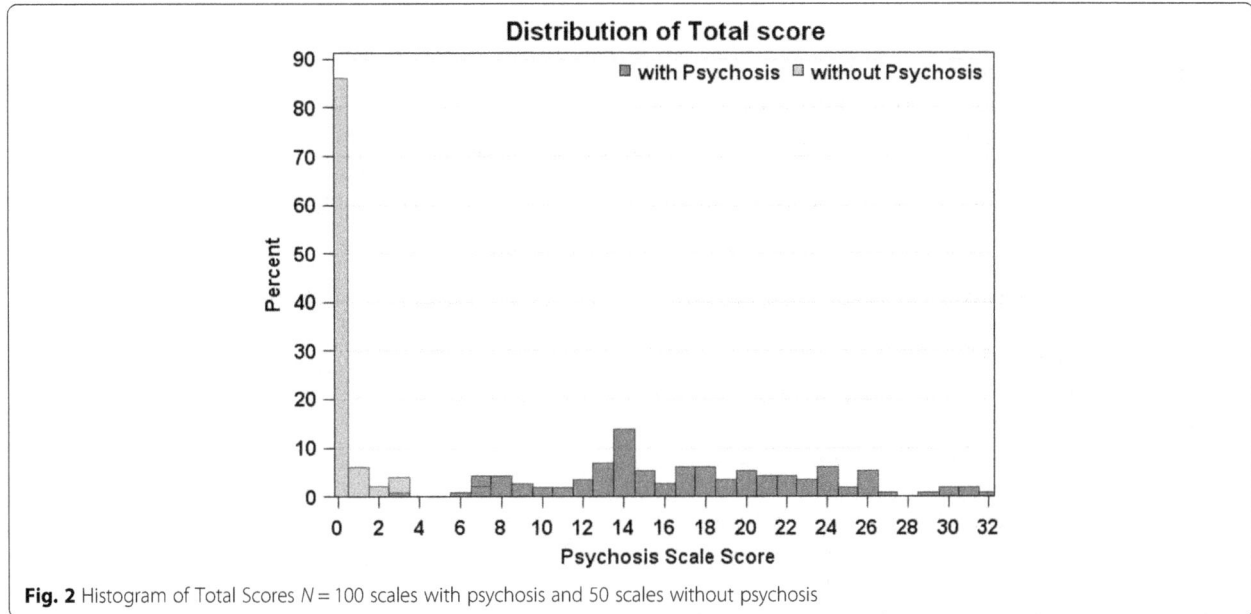

Fig. 2 Histogram of Total Scores N = 100 scales with psychosis and 50 scales without psychosis

respond similarly to interventions to reduce psychosis (dopamine dose reduction, addition of anti-psychotic medications), suggesting they are intrinsically different and perhaps not best thought of as "hallucinations". It is also our opinion that they do not contribute much to morbidity. "Passage" (very brief) hallucinations/illusions are differentiated from more prolonged visual hallucinations in the duration score. Delusions are usually the most problematic psychosis. We have only a single question on amount of delusions, compared to four regarding different hallucinations, but hypothesized that the

final five questions regarding how the psychosis affects the patient would score higher on subjects with delusions, and compensate for the single delusion question. Even if question #5 (delusions) is excluded from the total score summation, patients who scored >0 on #5 had significantly higher scores ($p < 0.001$). The last question regarding impact on family was included to account for the poor insight many patients possess, the fact that families are often more disturbed by psychosis than the patient, and because some of the major consequences of psychosis, such as nursing home placement, are often

Table 1 Summary of Data

	Mean Score in Psychosis Subjects, mean (SD)	Number of questionnaires in Control Subjects with a score of >0 (out of 50 assessments)	Inter-Rater Reliability (95 % CI)[a]		Intra-Rater Reliability (95 % CI)[b]
			All (N = 71)	Psychosis patients (N = 46)	Psychosis (N = 17)
1. Frequency Visual	3.13 (0.98)	1	0.85 (0.79, 0.91)	0.62 (0.47, 0.77)	0.51 (0.23, 0.80)
2. Frequency Olfactory	0.29 (0.65)	2	0.85 (0.70, 1.00)	0.84 (0.66,1.00)	0.66 (0.47, 0.86)
3. Frequency Auditory	1.16 (1.50)	0	0.76 (0.66, 0.85)	0.72 (0.60, 0.83)	0.68 (0.51, 0.85)
4. Frequency Presence	2.06 (1.41)	4	0.79 (0.71, 0.87)	0.70 (0.58, 0.82)	0.72 (0.54, 0.90)
5. Delusion Assessment	0.97 (1.41)	2	0.64 (0.47, 0.81)	0.59 (0.40, 0.45)	0.65 (0.33, 0.97)
6. Duration of Psychosis	2.66 (0.90)	4	0.82 (0.73, 0.90)	0.59 (0.42, 0.77)	0.46 (0.15, 0.77)
7. Insight	2.03 (0.97)	2	0.75 (0.65, 0.86)	0.58 (0.41, 0.76)	0.65 (0.48, 0.82)
8. Threatening	1.34 (0.60)	0	0.82 (0.73, 0.91)	0.62 (0.43, 0.80)	0.77 (0.47, 1.00)
9. Interaction	1.71 (0.82)	0	0.81 (0.73, 0.90)	0.62 (0.45, 0.80)	0.37 (0.07, 0.66)
10. Family Concern	1.90 (1.42)	0	0.86 (0.78, 0.94)	0.80 (0.68, 0.92)	0.86 (0.73, 0.99)
TOTAL	17.23 (6.30)	7	0.92 (0.89, 0.94)	0.87 (0.80, 0.92)	0.86 (0.80, 0.91)

Weighted kappa statistics for each of 10 specific questions and intra-class correlation coefficients (ICC) for total score were shown as Inter- [a]and Intra-rater [b]reliability determined by the caregivers. Since patients themselves have markedly variable insight into their own hallucinations, asking impact of their own psychosis would be difficult to quantify. We also did not exclude patients with varying degrees of cognitive impairment, who may further require family input. We did not formally assess cognition at time of assessment so can't statistically compare "demented" vs "not-demented" subject results.

Our scale has several potential weaknesses. Data on test-retest reliability was skewed towards subjects with less severe psychosis, as more severe subjects required immediate interventions, and therefore could not be reassessed for this purpose. We did not compare our results to any validated general psychosis study (content validity) because their content was not designed for the PD psychosis phenotype so any subsequent interpretation of "content" validity would have limited utility. Content validity was excellent based on UPDRS psychosis question (mean 17.23 for score >0 vs. 0.36 for 0) We did not formally assess sensitivity to change with intervention, although several subjects started on clozapine showed marked reduction in scores (data not shown).

The final 10 question set was created over a decade and included patient and family input, however they were not formally culled from a larger set and did not undergo cognitive pre-testing. We included subjects with dementia, as this is common in hallucinating patients, so family input was absolutely necessary in this group, as demented subjects could not understand or respond to some of the questions by themselves. No subject had psychosis in the absence of dopaminergic medications, but we did not attempt to exclude the clinical diagnosis of dementia with Lewy bodies, except by onset of motor vs. cognitive symptoms. Importantly, the questionnaire is not meant to be self-administered and some interpretation of response is needed by the interviewer (discussed more fully in the Additional file 1: Instructions), nor is it meant to be a screening tool to diagnose psychosis. Future research could formally assess sensitivity to treatment response, correlations with other scales assessing quality of life, other scales for psychosis, formal comparison of demented vs. non-demented patients, comparison of patient vs family scores, and neurophysiology correlates.

Conclusion
We feel this scale offers very good content valisity, inter- and intra-rater reliability and ease of use.

Competing interest
There was no specific funding for this project. There are no conflicts of interest related to this article.
William Ondo:

speaker- Lundbeck, TEVA, Merz, UCBPharma, Avanir, IMPAX
advisory board – Lundbeck, Auspex, UCBPharma, Abbvie, ACADIA
Sana Sarfaraz, BA none
MinJae Lee, PhD none

Authors' contribution
WO, All aspects. SS, data acquisition and critical review. ML statistical analysis and critical review. All authors read and approved the final manuscript.

Author details
[1]Department of Neurology, Methodist Neurological Institute, 6560 Fannin, Ste 802, Houston, TX 77030, USA. [2]Biostatistics/Epidemiology/Research Design (BERD) Core, Center for Clinical and Translational Sciences, The University of Texas Health Science Center at Houston and Division of Clinical and Translational Sciences, Houston, TX 77030, USA. [3]Department of Internal Medicine, The University of Texas Medical School at Houston Center for Clinical and Translational Sciences, University of Texas Health Science Center at Houston, Houston, TX 77030, USA.

References
1. Friedman JH. Parkinson's disease psychosis 2010: a review article. Parkinsonism Relat Disord. 2010;16(9):553–60. doi:10.1016/j.parkreldis.2010.05.004.
2. Goetz CG. Scales to evaluate psychosis in Parkinson's disease. Parkinsonism Relat Disord. 2009;15 Suppl 3:S38–41. doi:10.1016/S1353-8020(09)70777-1.
3. Friedberg G, Zoldan J, Weizman A, Melamed E. Parkinson Psychosis Rating Scale: a practical instrument for grading psychosis in Parkinson's disease. Clin Neuropharmacol. 1998;21(5):280–4.
4. Brandstaedter D, Spieker S, Ulm G, Siebert U, Eichhorn TE, Krieg JC, et al. Development and evaluation of the Parkinson Psychosis Questionnaire A screening-instrument for the early diagnosis of drug-induced psychosis in Parkinson's disease. J Neurol. 2005;252(9):1060–6. doi:10.1007/s00415-005-0816-x.
5. Cummings JL, Mega M, Gray K, Rosenberg-Thompson S, Carusi DA, Gornbein J. The Neuropsychiatric Inventory: comprehensive assessment of psychopathology in dementia. Neurology. 1994;44(12):2308–14.
6. Kay SR, Opler LA, Lindenmayer JP. The Positive and Negative Syndrome Scale (PANSS): rationale and standardisation. Br J Psychiatry Suppl. 1989;7:59–67.
7. Overall JE, Gorham DR. The brief psychiatric rating scale. Psychol Rep. 1962;10:799–812.
8. Anonymous. Low-dose clozapine for the treatment of drug-induced psychosis in Parkinson's disease. The Parkinson Study Group. Eng J Med. 1999;340(10):757–63.
9. Cummings J, Isaacson S, Mills R, Williams H, Chi-Burris K, Corbett A, et al. Pimavanserin for patients with Parkinson's disease psychosis: a randomised, placebo-controlled phase 3 trial. Lancet. 2014;383(9916):533–40. doi:10.1016/S0140-6736(13)62106-6.
10. Ondo WG, Levy JK, Vuong KD, Hunter C, Jankovic J. Olanzapine treatment for dopaminergic-induced hallucinations. Mov Disord. 2002;17(5):1031–5. doi:10.1002/mds.10217.
11. Ondo WG, Tintner R, Voung KD, Lai D, Ringholz G. Double-blind, placebo-controlled, unforced titration parallel trial of quetiapine for dopaminergic-induced hallucinations in Parkinson's disease. Mov Disord. 2005;20(8):958–63.
12. McKeith I, Mintzer J, Aarsland D, Burn D, Chiu H, Cohen-Mansfield J, et al. Dementia with Lewy bodies. Lancet Neurol. 2004;3(1):19–28.
13. Chou KL, Messing S, Oakes D, Feldman PD, Breier A, Friedman JH. Drug-induced psychosis in Parkinson disease: phenomenology and correlations among psychosis rating instruments. Clin Neuropharmacol. 2005;28(5):215–9.
14. Gallagher DA, Parkkinen L, O'Sullivan SS, Spratt A, Shah A, Davey CC, et al. Testing an aetiological model of visual hallucinations in Parkinson's disease. Brain. 2011;134(Pt 11):3299–309. doi:10.1093/brain/awr225.

8

Lexical diversity in Parkinson's disease

Charles Ellis[*], Yolanda F Holt and Thomas West

Abstract

Background: Parkinson's disease (PD) is a neurodegenerative syndrome of the basal ganglia (BG) believed to disrupt cortical-subcortical pathways critical to motor, cognitive and expressive language function. Recent studies have shown subtle deficits in expressive language performance among individuals with PD even in the earliest stage of the disease. The objective of this study was to use measures of lexical diversity to examine expressive language performance during discourse production in a sample of individuals with PD.

Methods: Twelve individuals with idiopathic Parkinson's disease (PD) were compared to twelve matched, neurologically intact controls on measures of lexical diversity. Three minute discourse samples describing a typical day were collected and analyzed for lexical diversity with the CHILDES program using measures of type token ratio (TTR) and voc-D (D).

Results: Comparisons of three minute discourse samples indicated non-significant differences between individuals with PD and controls in word productivity (387 vs 356; p = .48). Similarly, there were also non-significant differences on measures of lexical diversity between the two groups (TTR = .45 vs.44; p = .50 and D 74 vs 68; p = .23).

Conclusions: These results suggest that lexical diversity during discourse production among individuals with PD is similar to non-neurological controls. These findings indicate that lexical diversity is an aspect of expressive language performance that is not impacted by the disease process in the earliest stages.

Keywords: Parkinson's disease, Basal ganglia, Discourse, Language

Background

Parkinson's disease (PD) is a neurodegenerative syndrome most often associated with reductions in motor performance. In the United States, 50,000-60,000 new cases are diagnosed annually [1]. The disease process associated with PD centers on the basal ganglia, however the disease progressions courses through multiple systems affecting the brainstem and eventually affecting the cerebral cortex [2]. In addition to motor deficits, many individuals with PD experience changes in cognitive and language skills. Declines in motor performance are readily detectable in PD and correlate with reported neuropathological stages of PD [2]. In contrast, although expressive language deficits have been identified in PD, they are not reported as frequently as more commonly observed motor speech deficits.

The basis of hypothesized expressive language production deficits in PD emerges from models of basal ganglia (BG) function which indicate critical connections between the BG and other areas of the brain. More specifically, the BG are connected to the cerebral cortex via a collection of cortical-BG-thalamic-cortical circuits that vary in function [3,4]. These connections offer support for an anatomical basis for expected deficits in expressive language which is primarily governed by the cerebral cortex [5,6]. Using these models of BG function in PD, studies of language production in PD have identified expressive language performance deficits. For example two reviews of expressive language in PD noted morphosyntactic, lexical semantic and language production breakdowns as linguistic complexity increased [7,8].

Language and other cognitive deficits are not as easily identifiable until later in the PD disease process. However, they too, appear to develop gradually and concurrently with the neuropathological stages of the disease beginning with the cortical-BG-thalamic-cortical circuits connecting subcortical structures to motor areas [2-4,9,10]. The disease process is then believed to disrupt cortical-BG-thalamic-cortical circuits subsequently diminishing non-motor connections to the cerebral cortex, particularly the frontal lobes which are vital to cognitive performance.

* Correspondence: ellisc14@ecu.edu
Department of Communication Sciences and Disorders, East Carolina University, 3310H Health Sciences Building, MS 668, Greenville, NC 27834, USA

It has been hypothesized that in addition to early motor symptoms, subtle cognitive declines that are not severe enough to justify a diagnosis of dementia can be present (i.e. at the onset of initial motor symptoms) [9,10]. It is tenable then that impairments in expressive language performance may be a specific example of declines in cognitive performance in PD that are more difficult to detect. The relative influence of PD on expressive language performance in PD has yet to be adequately examined. To test the hypothesis of early cognitive declines in PD, novel diagnostic measures sensitive to subtle changes in cognitive performance on skills such as expressive language in PD are required.

Discourse analyses have been suggested as a method to characterize expressive language performance deficits in a range of neurological diseases [11,12]. According to Fergadiotis & Wright, discourse analyses allow researchers to observe complex cognitive/linguistic behaviors during a common form of communication therefore offering a functional analysis of language skills [13]. Discourse is a complex goal directed activity requiring intent, planning and task persistence (i.e. executive function). Discourse production represents the highest level of expressive language use or language procedures designed to serially assemble complex utterances determined by context and a specific goal [14,15]. Discourse is a dynamic cognitive process comprised of microlinguistic (language features that occurs within sentences) and macrolinguistic (language features that that crosses sentence borders) levels of organization [16]. Consequently, any compromise of this dynamic process may result in impaired discourse production that is independent of coexisting motor speech difficulty [15].

Discourse production has been previously examined in PD [17,18]. However, conclusions drawn were based on studies that included participants with more advance disease stages or did not consider specific language deficits in favor of concomitant cognitive and speech impairments. To address these issues the objective of this study was to examine a specific language outcome, lexical diversity (LD), in a sample of individuals with PD to determine if LD is influenced by PD early in the disease process. The rationale for examining lexical diversity emerges from studies that suggest disruptions in how language is used occurs in PD. For example, Holtgraves and colleagues found that individuals with PD exhibited more "under-informativeness" than non-PD controls during interviews. Under-informativeness or too little information provided was hypothesized as the result of decreased executive control, mental status and speech comprehension. Similarly, because Rogers and colleagues observed executive deficits in PD patients, we believe the temporal aspect of discourse may result in differences when compared to those without PD [19]. Consequently, we hypothesized

that lexical diversity, a microlinguistic feature that occurs during discourse production might offer additional insights into the contributions of PD to disruptions in expressive language performance.

LD is defined as "a range of vocabulary deployed in a text by a speaker that reflects his/her capacity to access and retrieve target words from a relatively intact knowledge base i.e., lexicon for the construction of higher linguistic units (p.1415) [13]. It is believed that LD depends on word frequency and the interaction of phonologic, semantic and syntactic language subsystems [13]. Measures of LD are well documented in the child language literature. The most basic measure of LD is the number of different words (NDW) in a sample calculated as a division of the number of different words by the total number of words in the sample. NDW is significantly influenced by sample length and individuals who generate more verbal output exhibit higher levels of LD [20].

The most commonly used measure of LD is the type-token ratio (TTR). TTR is the ratio of the total number of different words to the total number of words in the sample. TTRs that are closer to zero are an indication of limited vocabulary diversity whereas values closer to one reflect greater LD or more diverse vocabulary use. Similar to NDW, TTR is also sensitive to sample length in that as the sample increases the probability of producing new words decreases and the TTR decreases [20]. Consequently, comparisons between speakers who produce samples varying in length are confounded by the length of the samples that are produced.

A third measure that has emerged and developed to address issues related to sample length experienced with the use of NDW and TTR is voc-D. voc-D (D) is a an estimate of LD derived from a combination of an algebraic transformation model and curve fitting. D allows a more accurate comparison of LD in discourse samples because it does not rely on sample length [21]. D can be calculated in discourse samples using the voc-D program in Computerized Language Analysis (CLAN). D has been previously used as a measure of lexical diversity in individuals with neurogenic communication disorders such as aphasia [13,20,22].

The purpose of this study was to use discourse in individuals with PD and non-neurological controls to examine the influence of PD on LD. Discourse production requires an integration of multiple cognitive skills including: linguistic organization, linguistic planning and working memory, which is sensitive to neurological disease [15]. We hypothesized that an analysis of discourse would provide samples of sufficient length to evaluate LD in PD where dementia was not a contributing factor. We sought to test the hypothesis that individuals with PD would have less LD when compared to matched non-neurologically impaired controls. We examined subjects classified in Hoehn & Yahr (H&Y) stages II and III which are individuals with bilateral involvement yet are absent of significant motor impairment and are physically independent [23]. Individuals at these stages tend to have limited reductions in overall communication ability due to motor declines relative to more advance disease stages. Thus, we wanted to ensure that speech production issues would not mask overall expressive language performance and subsequently measures of lexical diversity. Therefore, it was expected that the measures of LD in individuals with PD would not be related to any reductions in motor speech performance.

Method
Description of the subjects
Participants consisted of 12 community dwelling individuals diagnosed with idiopathic PD (hereafter referred to as experimental subjects) by a movement disorders neurologist using the strict criteria of the UK Brain Bank [24] and 12 individuals who were age, education, ethnicity and gender matched and neurologically intact (hereafter referred to as control subjects). All participants were recruited from the North Florida/South Georgia Veterans Health System. The study was approved by the University of Florida IRB and VA Research and Development Committee and all participants gave written informed consent. All participants were male, right handed, and had no history of prior stroke, dementia, brain tumor, or head trauma. All had at least a seventh grade education, functional hearing for normal conversation, functional vision for reading tasks, spoke English as their primary language, and demonstrated expressive language skills within intact range for normal conversation. Functional hearing and expressive language was determined by the first author (CE) a certified and licensed speech-language pathologist. All subjects (experimental and control) exhibited scores of 26 or better on the Mini Mental Status Exam (MMSE) [25].

Each experimental subject presented with a minimum of 3 of 4 cardinal features of PD (resting tremor, rigidity, bradykinesea, postural instability) and had no history of deep brain stimulation or brain lesion therapy. The parkinsonism of each experimental subject was rated with the Hoehn & Yahr (H&Y) Staging Scale for PD and classified by predominate feature (tremor vs. rigidity) [23].

Standardized assessments
The Boston Naming Test (BNT) [26] and Wechsler Memory Scale – Logical Memory I (WMS-LMI) [27] were administered to examine potential group differences relative to language form (BNT) and the influence of short term memory on language form and use (WMS-LMI).

Discourse data collection
Discourse samples were collected from experimental subjects by the first author in their homes prior to their first daily dose of anti-parkinsonian medication (levadopa, dopamine agonists, amantadine, and/or selegiline). The duration of time since their last dose was at least 12 hours. Collecting samples prior to their first daily dose of anti-parkinsonian medication ensured they were in their "off" medication state to maximize dopamine depletion, a major putative cause of cognitive dysfunction in PD. Five of the 12 experimental subjects were newly diagnosed with PD and had no history of PD medication use at the time of the study. Control subjects were also examined primarily in their homes.

All subjects were instructed to discuss a typical day for a minimum of three minutes. In the event that subjects stopped before 3-minutes, a standardized verbal cue ("Tell me more about that") was provided to continue the narrative until the 3-minute minimum was achieved. A Sony VN-480 PC digital voice recorder was used to record each subject's samples. The investigator provided the subjects instructions for each sample followed by a restatement of the topic. Audio-taping began at the point when the topic was restated.

Motor speech performance ratings
After completion of data collection, the motor speech performance of all subjects was rated. An independent judge (certified and licensed speech language pathologist) blind to the neurological status of the subjects rated each audio sample. Each sample was rated on a 5-point scale of speech intelligibility [28]. Ratings ranged from 1 (no detectable disorder) to 5 (no functional speech).

Motor speech ratings reliability
Transcription and segmentation
The first three minutes of all language samples were transcribed verbatim by a professional transcription service. Each sample was divided into communication units (CU), defined as the shortest allowable independent clause and related dependent clauses [29]. Individual CU's were defined primarily by syntax, however prosodic and semantic features were used at times when the unit could not be determined entirely by syntax. All unintelligible words were excluded from the analysis. In instances where the location of coordinating conjunctions such as "and", "but" and "or" was unclear, their prosodic feature determined their final location at the beginning or ending of the communication unit. One-word responses were not considered in the communication unit calculation.

CU reliability
Three trained raters participated in the project to establish reliability for identification of CU's. Raters were blinded to the neurological status of subjects that generated the

samples used for the analyses. One trained rater analyzed 100% of the samples that were used for the analysis. Two additional trained raters independently analyzed 15% of the total sample. Intra-class correlation coefficients (ICC) were calculated by using a two-way mixed model with repeated measures to evaluate scoring agreement among the raters for CU's. The ICC score for words was .99.

Computerized analysis of discourse language variables
Sample preparation and calculation of LD
The first author entered the transcribed samples into the CHILDES CLAN program using the CHAT format specified in the Tools for Analyzing Talk – Electronic Edition [30]. The Mac-based CLAN program was used on a Macbook Pro computer. In brief summary, samples were entered with emphasis on content words (i.e. nouns, verbs, adjectives and adverbs). Repetitions, repairs and fillers were not entered and thereby excluded from analysis. To estimate lexical diversity the CLAN "voc-D" function was used which generates total number words and two measures of LD; D and TTR.

LD reliability
The third author entered 15% of randomly selected samples into the CLAN program using the same CHAT format. Measures of lexical diversity were calculated independently for comparisons. Simple correlations of TTR and D were calculated as a measure of reliability. Correlations of .91 for TTR and .96 for D were achieved for each measure indicating a high agreement.

Statistical analysis
For group comparisons, independent samples t-tests were conducted for continuous variables and Chi-square for categorical variable with the criterion for significance set at p < .05 for all variables.

Results
Demographic comparisons
Table 1 lists demographic, cognitive and language comparisons for subjects in the study. Two-tailed t-test (p < .05), revealed non-significant differences between the two groups for age, education, short term memory (WMS-LMI), and language form (BNT) and general cognitive ability (MMSE).

Motor speech performance ratings
Group comparisons revealed a significant difference between the PD group (M = 2.2, SD .72) and control group (M = 1.3, SD .62) on intelligibility ratings, ($X^2 = 10.7$; p = .003). Scores ranged from 1–3 for each group [1 (no detectable disorder), 2 (obvious speech disorder with intelligible speech), and 3 (reduction in speech intelligibility)].

Table 1 Demographic, cognitive, and language comparisons for PD and control subjects

Variable	PD subjects		Controls		
	M	SD	M	SD	p
Age	71.8	13.2	72.6	13.5	.89
Education	12.0	1.3	12.8	2.8	.36
Parkinson years	3.6	4.6			
H & Y stage	2.4	.5			
BNT	52.8	6.7	51.8	8.4	.75
MMSE	28.6	1.4	28.8	1.7	.80
WMS-LMI	27.5	11.5	30.6	14.4	.57

Values are means ± S.D. p values are derived from comparisons of PD subjects to normal controls. Parkinson Years = the number of years since PD subjects were initially diagnosed with PD. H & Y = Hoehn and Yahr; BNT = Boston Naming Test, all items administered; MMSE = Mini Mental Status Exam; WMS-LMI = Wechsler Memory Scale – Logical Memory I subtest.

Computerized analysis of lexical diversity
Table 2 list measures of word productivity and lexical diversity. Two-tailed t-test (p < .05), revealed non-significant differences between the two groups on the number of words produced (PD = 387 vs controls = 357; p = .48). No significant differences were made on measures of TTR (PD TTR = .45 vs controls TTR = .44; p = .50) and D (PD D = 74 vs controls D = 68; p = .23).

Discussion and conclusions
The results of this study did not support the hypothesis that individuals with PD would exhibit less LD during discourse production when compared to matched non-neurological controls. Comparisons to non-neurologically impaired control subjects did not yield statistically significant differences. Although reductions in lexical diversity have been observed in other neurological populations who experience language deficits, we found that individuals with PD exhibited very similar lexical diversity whether measured with TTR or D. These findings are important because they add to current lines of research which indicate expressive language issues in PD a disorders primarily related to motor deficits. Although this analysis did not yield groups differences and support recent studies that suggest disruptions in language skills exist early in PD, it

Table 2 Group performances on measures of lexical diversity

Variable	PD subjects		Controls		
	M	SD	M	SD	p
Words	356.8	77.5	387.0	120.9	.48
TTR	.45	.04	.44	.05	.50
D	73.8	12.6	67.5	12.3	.23

Values are means ± S.D. p values are derived from comparisons of PD subjects to normal controls.

does support the current literature that suggests specific deficits are related "language use" issues rather than "language structure" issues (word and sentence productivity, syntax, grammaticality, etc.). For example, in previous work, we found that although individuals with PD did not differ from controls on measures of language structure in discourse (narrative productivity, communication units, and number of cohesive ties produced), they did differ on measures of cohesive adequacy [31]. These data are also supported by studies of language pragmatics or the use of verbal and non-verbal social communication among individuals with PD [19].

These preliminary findings may suggest that LD is a measure that may not be sensitive to changes in PD. It is possible that LD measures lack the sensitivity to differentiate changes in expressive language in patients early on in PD. The lack of observed differences may alternately suggest fronto-basal ganglia disruptions that influence linguistic processing for expressive language do not occur in the earliest H&Y stages of PD. We expected that the temporal aspects of discourse production would elicit group differences. This hypothesis is based on findings by Rogers and colleagues that report executive deficits in patients functioning at H & Y stages I & II [32]. Therefore, our results suggest that even though cognitive skills may be affected in PD populations, H & Y stages I-III may not be associated with the level of neuropathologic disease required to negatively influence expressive language performance.

It is also possible that other features of discourse production (i.e. cohesion and coherence) may be more sensitive to PD and probably should be considered in future studies. Similarly, the literature related to language performance in PD suggests that measures of language structure (word and sentence productivity, syntax, grammaticality, etc.) have failed to consistently differentiate PD from normal language performance. Therefore, some propose that measures of language use (language pragmatics) may be more sensitive to language related in PD [33,34].

The non-significant findings in light of recent hypotheses of earlier cognitive deficits in PD highlight two specific issues. First, although the neuropathological progression of PD has been described extensively, the exact impact of disease progression on cognitive skills such as language remains unclear. Braak and colleagues propose that individuals with PD may progress through a phase similar to mild cognitive impairment (MCI) prior to overt dementia [9]. However, it is important to note that the disease progression described by Braak and colleagues does not correlate specifically with clinical disease staging using the H&Y scale. Therefore, the cognitive changes that occur in patients with PD/MCI and the changes that occur during the transition from MCI to overt dementia are unclear. Consequently, difficulty exists in attempts to distinguish

the level of cognitive ability across the continuum of the two cognitive disorders. Second, the impact of cognitive deterioration in PD on expressive language and other cognitive skills is unknown.

A minor secondary finding of this study was although there were differences in motor speech performance, word productivity (number of words produced) did not differ between the two groups. On average, the participants with PD produced a greater number of words over the course of three minutes. We considered that the greater but non-significant difference in words produced may have been a function of the greater number of cues required among individuals with PD (45 vs 18) to elicit the three minute samples. However, because the focus of this study was measures of LD and LD is primarily a reflection of the range of words produced rather than the total, the increased need for verbal cuing likely did not influence the results reported here.

Future studies should be designed to evaluate individuals at all disease stages as well as equivalent representation of tremor and rigid predominant features would provide additional information about influence of PD disease progression on expressive language. It would additionally be better to divide patients for clinical studies by disease duration rather than stage as a majority of all patients are in stage II and III. We also acknowledge that alternate explanations such as reduced attention, depression, medication state, and apathy should be measured and correlated with changes in discourse production. However, the results of this study offer a number of future research possibilities that will increase our understanding of the influence of PD on expressive language production. Comparisons of PD and other basal ganglia diseases would help differentiate language disruptions that may occur. A detailed examination of all possible ways expressive language can be impaired following disease will be required to clarify the influences of PD on expressive language.

Competing interests
The authors declare that they have no competing interests.

Authors' contributions
CE conceived the study, participated in the design of the study, participated in the lexical diversity analysis and performed the statistical analysis. YFH participated in the draft of the manuscript and interpretation of the findings. TW participated in the lexical diversity analysis and draft of the manuscript. All authors read and approved the final manuscript.

Acknowledgements
This work was funded by a Pre-Doctoral Fellowship from the VA Office of Academic Affairs awarded to the first author (CE) while a predoctoral fellow in the Brain Rehabilitation Research Center, VAMC, Gainesville, FL.

References

1. National Parkinson Foundation. 2014. http://www.parkinson.org/parkinson-s-disease.aspx. Accessed on September 3, 2014

2. Braak H, Del Tredici K, Rub U, de Vos RA, Jansen Steur EN, Braak E. Staging of brain pathology related to sporadic Parkinson's disease. Neurobiol Aging. 2003;24(2):197–211.

3. Middleton FA, Strick PL. Basal ganglia and cerebellar loops: motor and cognitive circuits. Brain Res Brain Res Rev. 2000;31(2–3):236–50.

4. Middleton FA, Strick PL. Basal ganglia output and cognition: evidence from anatomical, behavioral, and clinical studies. Brain Cogn. 2000;42(2):183–200.

5. Alexander MP. Disorders of language after frontal lobe injury: evidence for the neural mechanisms of assembling language. In: Stuss DT, Knight, editors. Principles of frontal lobe function. Oxford: Oxford University Press; 2002. p. 159–67.

6. Salmon DP, Heindel WC, Hamilton JM. Cognitive abilities mediated by frontal-subcortical circuits. In: Litcher DG, Cummings JL, editors. Frontal-subcortical circuits in psychiatric and neurological disorders. New York: Guilford Press; 2001. p. 114–50.

7. Murray L. Language and Parkinson's disease. Annu Rev Appl Linguist. 2008;28:113–27.

8. Altmann LJ, Troche MS. High-level language production in parkinson's disease: a review, Parkinson's Disease. 2011.

9. Braak H, Rub U, Jansen Steur EN, Del Tredici K, de Vos RA. Cognitive status correlates with neuropathologic stage in Parkinson disease. Neurology. 2005;64(8):1404–10.

10. Braak H, Rub U, Del Tredici K. Cognitive decline correlates with neuropathological stage in Parkinson's disease. J Neurol Sci. 2006;248(1–2):255–8.

11. Glosser G, Deser T. Patterns of discourse production among neurological patients with fluent language disorders. Brain Lang. 1991;40(1):67–88.

12. Wilson BM, Proctor A. Oral and written discourse in adolescents with closed head injury. Brain Cogn. 2000;43(1–3):425–9.

13. Fergadiotis G, Wright HH. Lexical diversity for adults with and without aphasia across discourse elicitation tasks. Aphasiology. 2011;25(11):1414–30.

14. Alexander MP. Impairments of procedures for implementing complex language are due to disruption of frontal attention processes. J Int Neuropsychol Soc. 2006;12:236–47.

15. Ash S, Moore P, Antani S, McCawley G, Work M, Grossman M. Trying to tell a tale: discourse impairments in progressive aphasia and frontotemporal dementia. Neurology. 2006;66(9):1405–13.

16. Marini A, Carlomagno S, Caltagirone C, Nocentini U. The role played by the right hemisphere in the organization of complex textual structures. Brain Lang. 2005;93:46–54.

17. Illes J, Metter EJ, Hanson WR, Iritani S. Language production in Parkinson's disease: acoustic and linguistic considerations. Brain Lang. 1988;33(1):146–60.

18. Murray LL. Spoken language production in Huntington's and Parkinson's diseases. J Speech Lang Hear Res. 2000;43(6):1350–66.

19. Holtgraves T, Fogle K, Marsh L. Pragmatic language production deficits in parkinson's disease. Adv Park Dis. 2013;2:31–6.

20. Wright HH, Silverman SW, Newhoff M. Measures of lexical diversity in aphasia. Aphasiology. 2003;17(5):443–52.

21. McKee G, Malvern D, Richards B. Measuring vocabulary using dedicated software. Literacy Linguist Comput. 2000;15(3):323–3338.

22. Fergadiotis G, Wrigh HH, West T. Measuring lexical diversity in narrative discourse of people with aphasia. Am J Speech Lang Pathol. 2013;22:S397–408.

23. Hoehn MH, Yahr MD. Parkinsonism: onset, progression and mortality. Neurology. 1967;17:427–42.

24. Bower JH, Maraganore DM, McDonnell SK, Rocca WA. Influence of strict, intermediate, and broad diagnostic criteria on the age- and sex-specific incidence of Parkinson's disease. Mov Disord. 2000;15(5):819–25.

25. Folstein MF, Folstein SE, McHugh PR. "Mini-mental state". A practical method for grading the cognitive state of patients for the clinician. J Psychiatr Res. 1975;12(3):189–98.

26. Kaplan E, Goodglass H, Wientraub S. Boston naming test scoring booklet. Philadelphia: Lea & Febiger; 1983.

27. Wechsler D. Wechsler Memory Scale III. New York: Psychological Corporation; 1997.

28. Yorkston KM, Beukelman DR, Strand EA, Bell KR. Management of Motor Speech Disorders in Children and Adults. 2nd ed. Austin: Pro-Ed; 1999.

29. Hunt KW. Grammatical structures written at three grade levels. (Research Report No. 3). Urbana, IL: National Council of Teachers of English; 1965.

30. MacWhinney B. The CHILDES project: Tools for analyzing talk, Vol 1: Transcription format and programs. 3rd ed. Mahwah, NJ: Erlbaum; 2000.

31. Ellis C, Okun MS, Gonzalez-Rothi LJ, Crosson B, Rogalski Y, Rosenbek JC. Expressive language use after PD: deficits in use but not form. Mov Disord. 2006;21(S13):97–8.

32. Rogers RD, Sahakian BJ, Hodges JR, Polkey CE, Kennard C, Robbins TW. Dissociating executive mechanisms of task control following frontal lobe damage and Parkinson's disease. Brain. 1998;121(Pt 5):815–42.

33. Hall D, Ouyang B, Lonnquist E, Newcombe J. Pragmatic communication is impaired in Parkinson disease. Int J Neurol. 2011;121(5):254–6.

34. McNamara P, Durso R. Pragmatic communication skills in patients with Parkinson's disease. Brain Lang. 2003;84(3):414–23.

9

Divergent oral cavity motor strategies between healthy elite and dystonic horn players

Peter W. Iltis[1,3*], Jens Frahm[2*], Dirk Voit[2], Arun Joseph[2], Erwin Schoonderwaldt[3] and Eckart Altenmüller[3]

Abstract

Background: This paper describes the use of real-time magnetic resonance imaging in visualizing and quantifying oral cavity motor strategies employed by 6 healthy, elite horn players and 5 horn players with embouchure dystonia.

Methods: Serial images with an acquisition time of 33.3 ms were obtained from each performer during execution of an 11-note harmonic series encompassing 2.5 octaves on a magnetic resonance imaging-compatible horn. A customized MATLAB toolkit was employed for the extraction of line profiles from magnetic resonance imaging films allowing comparative analyses between elite and dystonic horn players.

Results: The data demonstrate differing motor strategies, particularly in moving from the 6th through 9th harmonics. The elite horn player strategy features elevation and anterior displacement of the tongue during ascending sequences, whereas dystonic players showed significantly less movement. The elite horn players thus narrowed the air channel on higher notes, presumably affording faster airflow for vibration of the lips at higher frequencies.

Conclusions: We postulate that failure to employ this strategy by dystonic horn players may require greater tension in the embouchure muscles to compensate for slower air speed. Though this may simply be an expression of or adaptation for dystonia, the possibility that it may be a contributing factor in the development of embouchure dystonia is suggested.

Keywords: Brass instrument players, Tongue movements, Oral cavity, Real-time (RT) magnetic resonance imaging (MRI), Tongue displacement

Background

Focal task-specific dystonia is a movement disorder characterized by the loss of fine motor control which only occurs when executing very specific movement patterns. When it is expressed in the execution of movement patterns required to play a musical instrument, it is often termed musicians' dystonia [1, 2]. With a reported incidence of about 1 % among professional musicians [3], the etiology of this disorder is complex. It often involves the muscles that have been extensively trained in the finest level of motor control. Repetitive movements requiring high temporal and spatial precision as well as synchronous demands of the musculature seem to be triggering factors. Thus, the expression of dystonic movement in the fingers of guitarists and pianists is common among those affected [1]. Suspected triggers for the development of this disorder include not only the repetition of fine motor activity, but also intrinsic (e.g. genetic predisposition, perfectionism and anxiety) and extrinsic (e.g. complexity of workload-specific movements) factors [4].

Embouchure dystonia is a subcategory of musician's dystonia affecting the muscles of the lower face, jaw, and tongue which control air flow into the mouthpiece of a wind instrument [5–11]. This painless disorder typically has its onset in the fourth decade, is often restricted to specific technical aspects of playing, may be limited to particular note frequency ranges, and has a variety of phenotypes including lip lock (inability to start notes), tremor, lip pulling (tendency of lips to be drawn out of

* Correspondence: peter.iltis@gordon.edu; jfrahm@gwdg.de
[1]Department of Kinesiology, Gordon College, Wenham, MA, USA
[2]Biomedizinische NMR Forschungs GmbH am Max-Planck-Institut für biophysikalische Chemie, Göttingen, Germany
Full list of author information is available at the end of the article

their normal configuration), jaw lock, and tongue-specific variants [6]. A recent cross-sectional study by Steinmetz et al. [11] suggests that the relative frequency of embouchure-related disorders in a sample of 585 professional brass players was 59 %, resulting in sick leave in 16 % of this population. The prevalence ratios were twice as great in females and in those brass players implementing voluntary mechanical changes in embouchure such as altering mouthpiece placement or lip conformation, or voluntary alterations in breathing technique involving posture and mechanics. The authors suggest that the resulting embouchure disorders (though not embouchure dystonia, per se) may be harbingers of more serious things to come.

Studies of embouchure problems in brass players have been conducted in several ways. Early work focused on descriptive case studies or cross-sectional studies [5, 8, 9, 12], identifying and characterizing various embouchure problems, including embouchure dystonia. Later work specifically targeted embouchure dystonia in an attempt to identify underlying physiologic mechanisms. For example, Hirata et al. [13] compared somatosensory homuncular representations in embouchure dystonia patients and controls and found aberrancies in the dystonic performers suggesting that abnormal somatosensory mapping had occurred. These data were confirmed by subsequent work conducted by Haslinger et al. [14] in which sensorimotor hyperactivity was detected in embouchure dystonia patients. The authors suggest that deficient subcortical and intracortical inhibition accompanied by aberrant sensorimotor integration and reorganization are possible mechanisms. Still other work has attempted to characterize the expression of embouchure dystonia using surface EMG [15] or measurements of tone instability [16].

Despite the suspected involvement of the tongue in embouchure dystonia, there are no published studies that have attempted to describe or quantify activity within the oral cavity in these subjects. The difficulty of imaging dynamic activity inside the mouth during playing is obvious. Conventional radiological techniques, such as computerized axial tomography or magnetic resonance imaging can provide high detail of static positions, but are incapable of assessing dynamic motor activity, and moreover are impractical in assessing movements within the oral cavity during musical performance. Sonography has been utilized to monitor dynamic activity during wind instrument performance [17, 18]. While this method allows some quantitative measures to be obtained (e.g. tongue motion amplitudes), the anatomical resolution provided is somewhat limited, falling short of that provided by MRI.

Recently developed real-time MRI and analysis techniques provide a powerful tool for describing and quantifying dynamic movement patterns of the oral cavity during brass performance. Whether examining discrete snapshots of oral cavity phenomena during movement, slow dynamic movements, or very fast articulatory movements discernable only with 10 msec acquisition rates, the ability to perform accurate quantitative analyses is now possible [19, 20]. It is suggested that such methods may be of use in studying embouchure dystonia. If it is assumed that elite brass performers utilize successful and sustainable motor strategies in executing various performance tasks, then studying this population may provide reference standards against which brass players with dystonia may be compared. Further, if dystonic brass players utilize alternate strategies, it may be possible to draw inferences that contribute to the understanding of embouchure dystonia.

The purpose of the current investigation is to examine these hypotheses by using real-time MRI to characterize, quantify, and compare motor strategies between a sample of elite horn players and a sample of horn players suffering from embouchure dystonia in executing a simple performance task.

Methods
Subjects, performance device and testing protocol

Six healthy elite horn players and five horn players diagnosed with embouchure dystonia served as subjects for this study. The elite performers are horn players of international reputation, four currently performing with major U.S. or European symphony orchestras, and two with an active international solo career. The embouchure dystonia players are former professional horn players whose voluntary participation was solicited from a pool of patients who had previously been diagnosed by a movement disorders specialist (author EA) at the Institute of Music Physiology and Musician's Medicine in Hannover, Germany. The subject characteristics of both groups are documented in Table 1. All testing was performed at the Max-Planck-Institute for Biophysical Chemistry, and prior to participation, all subjects gave written informed consent as approved by the ethics committee of that institution.

All subjects performed on a MRI-compatible horn pitched in the key of Eb (Richard Seraphinoff, builder). This horn consists of graded diameter segments of plastic tubing with a plastic mouthpiece at one end, and a non-ferromagnetic brass horn bell at the other end. The horn has no valves, but its acoustical properties allow the performance of an entire harmonic series spanning three octaves. This is an exercise that is commonly practiced by horn players on typical horns, and was famliar to the subjects. The bell was positioned near the feet of the subjects and fixed to the examination table, and the

Table 1 Subject characteristics of elite and dystonic horn players

Gender	Age	Disorder duration (months)	Playing history (years)	Daily practice hours prior to ED	Daily practice hours with ED	Dystonia score
M	60	144	52	3	2	5
M	53	48	43	4.5	1.5	4
M	62	26	53	4.5	3.5	3
M	44	48	35	4.5	1	5
M	45	72	34	4	2	4
M	50	N.A.	48	N.A.	N.A.	N.A.
M	31	N.A.	19	N.A.	N.A.	N.A.
M	63	N.A.	50	N.A.	N.A.	N.A.
F	50	N.A.	35	N.A.	N.A.	N.A.
M	48	N.A.	34	N.A.	N.A.	N.A.
M	57	N.A.	45	N.A.	N.A.	N.A.

Dystonia score key - 5: unable to play the brass instrument due to cramping and dystonic movements, 4: still able to produce sound in certain registers, visible cramping, lip-pull, lip stop, tongue-lock, 3: still able to produce sound in all registers, however sound quality reduced in all registers, subtle visible signs of dystonia such as lip pull and leaks, 2: able to produce sound in all register, however, reduction of sound quality in certain registers, subjective discomfort and cramping, not necessarily visible, 1: professional sound quality, no visible sign of dystonia. (N.A. indicates not applicable)

tubing leading to the mouthpiece was extended caudally into the magnet itself so that the subject could play while in the supine position during imaging. Despite the noise generated by the MRI scanner, the subjects were able to hear their playing during all tests, and communication with the investigators was possible due to 2-way intercom system between the control room and the MRI scanner. This also provided a way for recorded examples of each exercise to be played for the subjects prior to their performance.

Two exercises comprised this study: 1) performing a slurred, ascending 11-note harmonic sequence beginning on concert Eb2 and terminating on concert C5 (77.78, 116.54, 155.56, 196, 233.08, 277.18, 311.11, 349.23, 392, 440, and 523.25 Hz, respectively), and 2) performing the same sequence again, but with each note initiated with the tongue. Because the MRI horn has no valves, all note changes were achieved by altering lip tension, air speed, and oral cavity configuration, well-documented strategies typical of horn players [21–23]. The music score for the slurred trials only (horn) is illustrated in Fig. 1. Copies of the exercises were available to the subjects for practice at least three weeks prior to testing. In addition, familiarization with the MRI horn and the exercises was

accomplished by allowing 5–10 min of practice outside the scanner. Once in the scanner, practice of individual exercises was also allowed. In both cases, the performers indicated when they felt comfortable and were ready. Each exercise was performed two times, and the trial with the fewest missed notes was chosen for analysis.

Real-time MRI

All experiments were performed on a 3 T MRI system (Magnetom Prisma, Siemens Healthcare, Erlangen, Germany) using the standard 64-channel head coil. RT-MRI was based on highly undersampled radial FLASH acquisitions with temporally regularized nonlinear inverse (NLINV) reconstruction as previously described [24]. All measurements were performed with an in-plane resolution of 1.5 mm, slice thickness of 10 mm, FOV = 192×192 mm^2 and base resolution 128×128 mm^2. Acquisitions at 30 fps employed the following parameters: TR = 1.96 ms, TE = 1.25 ms, flip angle = 5°, 17 radial spokes per image and $n = 5$ different sets of complementary radial spokes for consecutive acquisitions. Post-processing involved the application of a temporal median filter extending over $n = 5$ frames to reduce residual streaking artifacts and ensure optimum image quality for

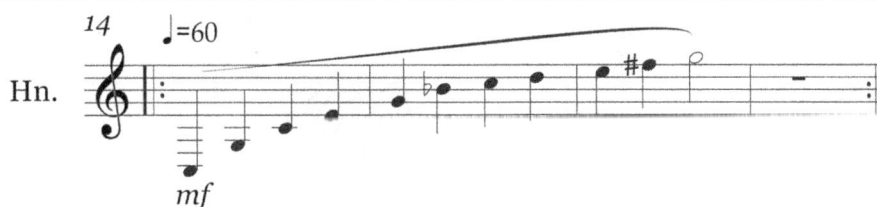

Fig. 1 Ascending, slurred harmonic sequence exercise. A single selection from a set of exercises developed for the MRI-horn. Tongued exercise not shown

quantitative analyses. The resulting temporal accuracy of the RT-MRI method has recently been evaluated for small objects moving with velocities of up to 30 cm/s, and movements in the current investigation were well-within the range established for temporal accuracy in previous studies [25].

Online reconstruction and display of real-time images with minimal delay was achieved by a parallelized version of the NLINV algorithm [26] and a bypass computer (sysGen/TYAN Octuple-GPU, 2× Intel Westmere E5620 processor, 48GB RAM, Sysgen, Bremen, Germany) which was fully integrated into the reconstruction pipeline of the commercial MRI system and equipped with two processors (CPUs, SandyBridge E5-2650, Intel, Santa Clara, CA) and 8 graphical processing units (GPUs, GeForce GTX, TITAN, NVIDIA, Santa Clara, CA).

In this study, RT-MRI acquisitions of horn playing tasks were recorded for a period of 30 s corresponding to 900 images. Acoustic recordings relied on a MR-compatible optical microphone (Dual Channel-FOMRI, Optoacoustics, Or Yehuda, Israel) attached to the bell of the French horn, which was placed at about the end of the patient table outside the bore of the magnet. Sound recording was triggered by the radial FLASH sequence and thus synchronized to image acquisition. Further details are provided elsewhere [27].

Prior to conducting data analysis, the audio track for each selected trial was examined using standard audio processing software (Audacity: http://audacity.sourceforge.net/) to determine the moment for each note change.

These timings were matched to the exact frame number in the RT-MRI films which then provided an index for determining the number of frames comprising the duration of each note. In this way, it was possible to perform subsequent quantitative measurements during the performance of each note using the custom MATLAB toolbox (RT-MRI toolbox) described later in this paper.

Data analysis and statistical procedures

The procedures used for obtaining quantitative information from RT-MRI films have been detailed elsewhere [20], so only a brief description will be provided here highlighting unique procedures employed for this study. We utilize a custom RT-MRI toolbox developed for MATLAB (MATLAB R2014a, including the Image Processing and Signal Processing Toolbox) that allows for dynamic data analysis. This toolbox creates a grid over the image of the oral cavity identifying 7 line profiles, each with their own spatial orientation, allowing changes in pixel luminescence across time during each performance task to be studied (see Fig. 2). Within MATLAB, this grid is created by identifying two anatomical landmarks (lower edge of the upper incisor and the anterior edge of the third intervertebral disc) to define a baseline, followed by the automatic creation of an array of 7 segments oriented at 0, 30, 60, 90, 120, 150, and 180° relative to that baseline. Each line was thereby associated with a different region of the oral cavity, thus allowing the study of movements involving different parts of the tongue and throat. Because consistent patterns were seen

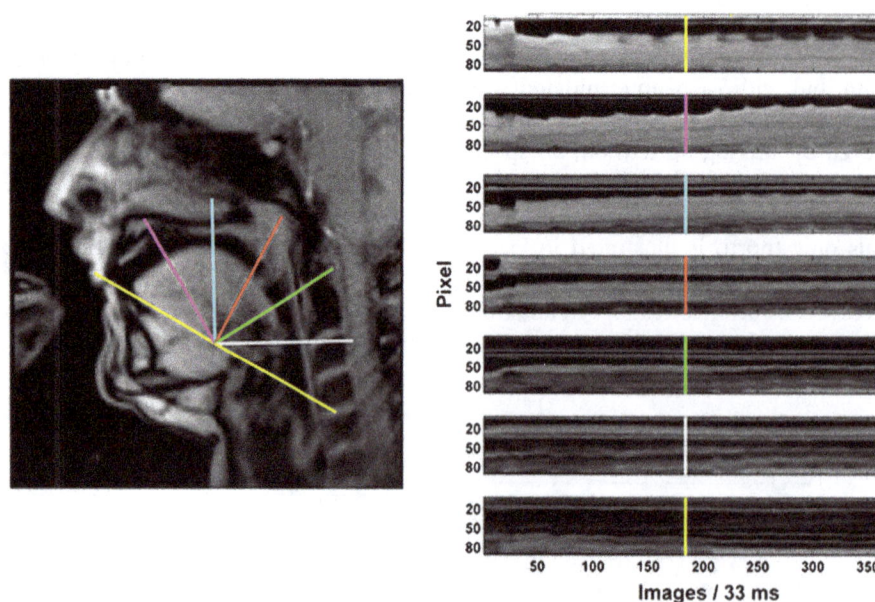

Fig. 2 Sagittal view (*left panel*) of an elite horn player at the moment of initiating the 6th note in the harmonic sequence. Seven grid lines are positioned for analysis, and the resulting line profiles (*right panel*) illustrate changes in pixel luminescence along each line during the entire 11-note sequence. Text refers to line profile 2, and the highlighted *vertical marker line* indicates the beginning of the 6th note in the harmonic sequence

within the elite subjects in line profile 2 representing the anterior 1/3 of the tongue (second from top, right panel), this line was chosen for all subsequent quantitative analyses comparing the elite to the dystonic performers.

As an example, Fig. 2 and Additional file 1 illustrate an elite performer playing the slurred, ascending 11-note sequence. In line profile 2, vertical undulations appear at the beginning of each note change (for example, frames 97, 124, 154, 184 for the 4th–7th harmonics) and the subsequent baseline between consecutive notes (i.e. the period while each note is sustained) tends to rise with time, particularly during the last half of the exercise. The RT-MRI toolbox allows calculation of the edge position of the anterior-dorsal tongue surface [20], and the precise position of the tongue over time. Thus, for the duration of each note played, the average position of the tongue along the selected line profile was calculated for each subject in each group. Statistical comparisons were made by pooling data within groups, i.e. by calculating the average tongue position on each note within the elite and dystonic performer groups.

The experiment is a repeated measures design having one within-subjects factor (harmonic played, 11 levels) and one between-subjects factor (elite group vs. dystonia group). All statistical tests were executed at the 0.05 significance level. In cases where the assumption of data sphericity was violated, Greenhouse-Geisser adjustments to the degrees of freedom were made to increase the robustness of the analysis.

Results

Visual comparisons of RT-MRI films prior to exercise performance revealed no differences between groups in the resting position of the tongue, teeth, jaw and oral cavity. However, this was not the case during task performance. Figure 3 depicts a sagittal view of one of the dystonic horn players performing the slurred 11-note ascending sequence. Comparing line profile 2 of this performer with that of an elite subject in Fig. 2, there is clear discrepancy in terms of tongue mechanics. While both performers show vertical undulations at the change of each note suggesting tongue elevation, the progressive note-wise elevation of the baseline between inflections identified in Fig. 2 is less evident or absent in the dystonic performer, particularly from the 5th to the 11th harmonics. This observation was typical regardless of whether the notes were slurred or tongued.

For the definition of oral cavitation, a brief referral to line 2 in Fig. 2 (an elite player/slurred sequence) is helpful. In this and all line profile plots, the Y axis has its zero origin position at the top-left, and the vertical length of that axis represents the length of the line in pixels. In this figure, it is about 80 pixels long. The edge created between the oral cavity and the dorsal tongue surface is approximately at the 25 pixel mark in frame 1, drops slightly at the initiation of the first note (Eb2, image 31) rises very slightly over the next 5 notes (6th note, Db4, image 184), and then rises at a greater rate

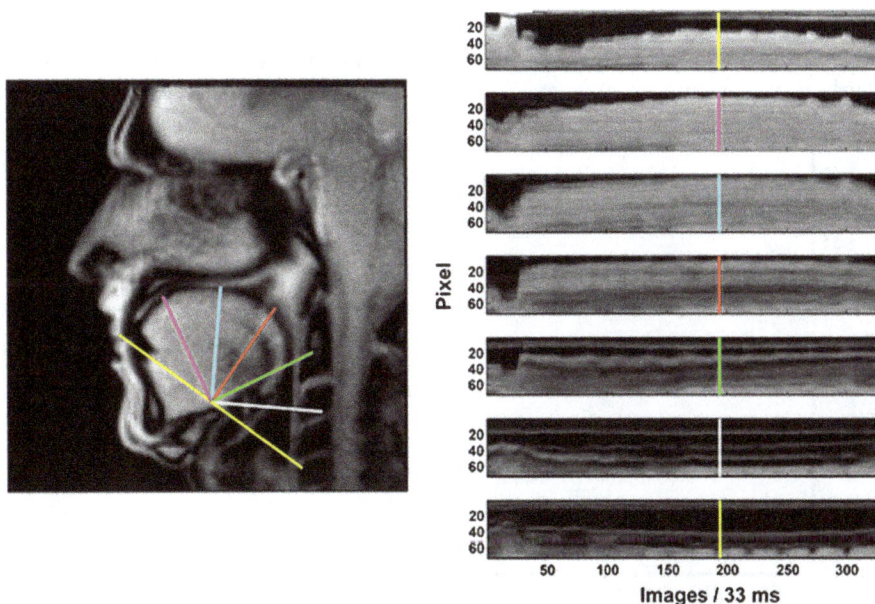

Fig. 3 Sagittal view (*left panel*) of a dystonic horn player at the moment of initiating the 6th note in the harmonic sequence. Seven grid lines are positioned for analysis, and the resulting line profiles (*right panel*) illustrate changes in pixel luminescence along each line during the entire 11-note sequence. Text refers to line profile 2, and the highlighted *vertical marker line* indicates the beginning of the 6th note in the harmonic sequence

from the 6th through the 9th note (G4, image 268), showing little additional change through the rest of the exercise. Movements toward the origin indicate a decrease in oral cavitation (the tongue moves upward and forward along line 2), while movements away indicate the opposite.

Figure 4 summarizes these movements for the slurred trials across all subjects by group. In this figure, the height along the Y axis indicates the amount of oral cavitation present during each note. The analysis results in three major findings: 1) in general, the elite players create a larger oral cavity in the lower notes than the dystonic players, 2) both groups tend to reduce the oral cavity moving from low to high notes, and 3) the degree to which the oral cavity is reduced is more pronounced and precipitous in the elite players. Repeated measures ANOVA revealed that the group by harmonic interaction was highly significant ($p < 0.001$ after Greenhouse-Geisser adjustment of the degrees of freedom, observed power = 0.917).

The same tendency was true during the tongued trials, as shown in Fig. 5, though in this case, the repeated measures ANOVA failed to show a significant group by harmonic interaction effect after applying the corresponding Greenhouse-Geisser adjustment of the data ($p = 0.112$, observed power 0.485). Nonetheless, a significant group main effect was demonstrated, with the elite performers having a larger oral cavity than the dystonic players (estimated marginal means of 30.3 and 20.9 pixels for elite and dystonic performers, respectively, $p = 0.039$, observed power, 0.579).

Discussion

The findings of this investigation suggest that elite horn players utilized a fairly consistent motor strategy across subjects with respect to the anterior-dorsal aspect of the tongue when performing a slurred, ascending 11-note harmonic series. On the lowest notes, the tongue was positioned low within the oral cavity creating a large cavitation until the 5th harmonic was reached. Subsequently higher notes involved a progressive upward and forward movement of the dorsal surface of the tongue that decreased the size of the oral cavity.

These adjustments are similar to those used when phonating the English vowel sounds: (as in "law"), u (as in "mud"), e (as in "ten"), i (as in "is"), ē (as in "he"). Purposeful use of these vowel/tongue adjustments is advocated by several horn teachers [21, 22, 28]. Among these, the American teacher and artist, Eli Epstein, advocates a systematic association of various notes in the range of the horn to specific vowel/tongue positions, postulating that narrowing the airway results in acceleration of the air column and higher vibration frequencies of the lips. He further suggests that this may reduce excess tension in the muscles supporting the embouchure. Though the degree to which the elite performers adhere to such an approach is not as systematic throughout the range as Epstein recommends, it is apparent that the general pattern is present, particularly in the upper range of the instrument. There, oral cavitation measured along line profile 2 is nearly one-half of that utilized on the lower notes.

In contrast, the dystonic players, though less consistent across subjects, generally display smaller oral cavities on the lower notes, and a less precipitous reduction in cavitation as they move to the higher notes, decreasing oral cavitation by approximately one-third. Though in most cases these performers could execute the appropriate note frequency, their sound was thinner and less stable. Such tonal features are noted by Lee et al. who

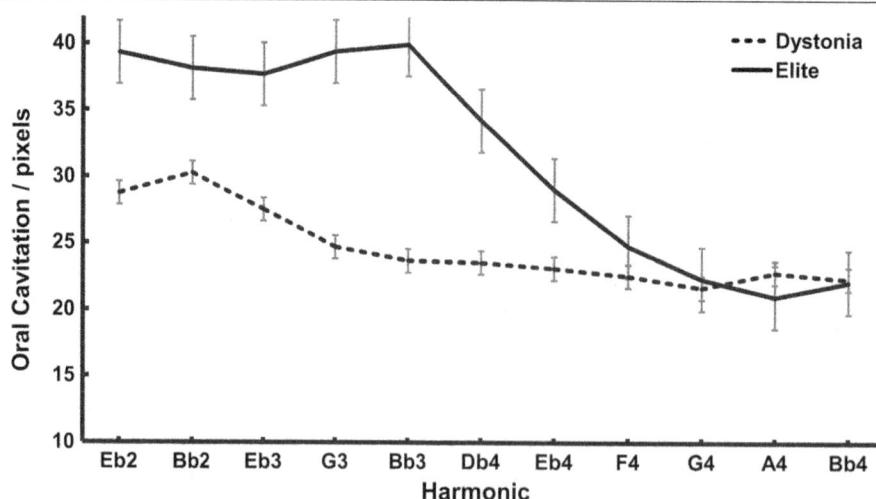

Fig. 4 Oral cavitation changes across a slurred 11- note harmonic series. Significant group by harmonic interaction ($p < 0.001$, Greenhouse-Geisser adjusted df)

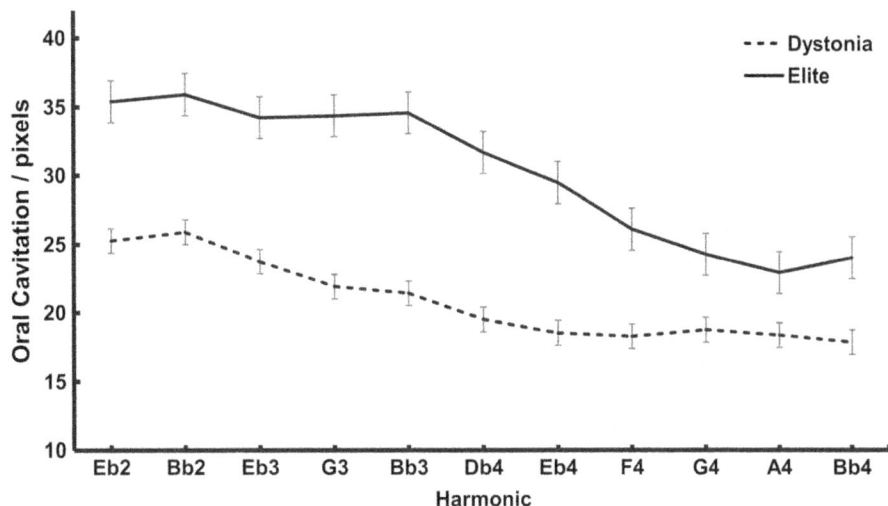

Fig. 5 Oral cavitation changes across a tongued 11- note harmonic series. Group main effect is statistically significant ($p = 0.039$, observed power 0.579). No significant group by harmonic interaction

recently compared tone stability of dystonic players to non-dystonic players [16]. Similar findings have been reported by Iltis and Givens who recorded both audio signals and surface EMG in a dystonic horn player [15]. In that study, both EMG and audio measures showed stochastic patterns in the dystonic horn player indicating marked instability compared to a normal horn player.

The scientific literature to date is limited with regard to describing activity within the mouth during brass performance comparable to the present study. One of the first papers utilizing MRI by Schumacher et al. [29] studied trumpet players, and found that there are concomitant increases in posterior oral cavity area with increasing pitch and loudness. It is noteworthy that these increases were not present in the anterior oral cavity of the performers as these remained small throughout the studied note range. Subsequently, Iltis et al. [20] compared changes in total, anterior, and posterior oral cavity size in performing an ascending 5-note harmonic sequence between a trumpet, horn, trombone, and tuba player. These data suggest that there are between-instrument differences in tongue movements. Specifically, for a trombone and tuba player, the trend was for a decrease in total area as a function of both anterior and posterior oral cavity reduction in moving from low to higher notes. In contrast, the trumpet player showed an increase in total oral cavity area, primarily due to increases in the posterior cavity size. Anterior oral areas were unchanged. In contrast, the horn player (an advanced amateur), showed no change in total, anterior, or posterior oral cavitation during the exercise.

When compared to data in the current study, it is clear that our elite horn players deviate from the horn player described above. This may be explained, at least

in part, by the difference in level of expertise. However in addition, the performance devices were considerably different, the former study utilizing a mouthpiece and a plastic resistance attachment (The B.E.R.P., Fairfax, CA) and the current study using an MRI-compatible horn. The MRI-compatible horn mimics an actual instrument and possesses similar acoustical properties. These properties reinforce particular resonant frequencies and provide unique sensory feedback to the player, while pitches performed on the B.E.R.P. are dependent solely on lip tension and air flow, and provide different afferent information. This requires the performer to match pitches without the aid of any the corresponding tactile and acoustical reinforcement properties present in an actual horn.

As mentioned above, the dystonic players do not employ the same tongue movements as the elite performers. They fail to elevate the tongue to the degree shown by the elite players during the ascending exercise, and yet still play the same notes, though with much less stability and tone quality. We propose that in failing to employ the elite strategy, greater tension in the muscles of the embouchure is required in order to increase the vibration frequency of the lips required to play notes of higher frequency. Increased facial muscular tension and co-contraction of non-task-specific muscles is a hallmark of embouchure dystonia [5–8]. This raises the question of whether the increased muscular tension in embouchure dystonia is a compensatory maneuver employed by these players to accommodate a less efficient airway configuration. If it may be assumed that the careers of world-class elite performers are successful and sustainable in part because of employing efficient motor strategies, then it may also be possible that dystonic players habitually use less efficient strategies to compensate for poor technique. Further, the repeated practice of such poor technique may contribute to maladaptive plastic changes in sensory-motor processing [1, 3, 30]. While this idea has some appeal, it must be noted that it is also possible that these less efficient motor strategies are consequences of embouchure dystonia rather than triggers for it. Finally, it must be acknowledged that the expression of symptoms in embouchure dystonia may be seen in structures other than the tongue. Future studies should utilize RT-MRI to study pharyngeal and laryngeal movements in a wider variety of brass and wind instruments, and there is a clear need for obtaining data on larger numbers of subjects.

Conclusions

We have shown that real-time MRI films can be useful in describing and quantifying movement of the tongue within the oral cavity during performance on an MRI-compatible horn in both elite and dystonic players. Further we have illustrated significant differences in movement strategies between these sample groups that may provide insight into possible triggers for or consequences of embouchure dystonia. Future studies should examine a variety of performance tasks challenging more diverse playing skills in an effort to develop a more complete understanding of this phenomenon. Additionally, studies examining similar comparison groups among different brass instrumentalists (i.e. trumpet, trombone, and tuba) will be useful in extending our understanding.

Competing interests

J. Frahm holds a patent about the real-time MRI acquisition and reconstruction technique used here. E. Altenmüller serves on the editorial board of BMC Movement Disorders. There are no other potential competing interests in any of the other authors.

Authors' contributions

PWI: Principle investigator, corresponding author taking full responsibility for the integrity of the data and the accuracy of the data analysis. Research project: conception, organization, execution of testing sessions, all data processing. Statistical Analysis: design, execution. Manuscript: writing of first draft and all subsequent revisions, submission. JF: Research project: execution (all MRI aspects). Statistical Analysis: review and critique. Manuscript: review and critique, writing of MRI methods. DV: Research project: execution (MRI operator), formatting MRI films. Manuscript: review. AJ: Research project: execution (MRI operator), formatting MRI films. Manuscript: final preparation of figures, Review. ES: Research project: development of RT-MRI MATLAB toolbox. Manuscript: review. EA: Research project: provision of dystonic subjects, project conception. Manuscript: review and critique. All authors read and approved the final manuscript.

Authors' information

Peter W. Iltis: Faculty member, full professor, Gordon College, Wenham, MA
Jens Frahm: Director of Biomedical NMR Research, The Max Planck Institute for Biophysical Chemistry, Gottingen, Germany
Dirk Voit: Scientist, Biomedical NMR Research, The Max Planck Institute for Biophysical Chemistry, Gottingen, Germany
Arun Joseph: Scientist, Biomedical NMR Research, The Max Planck Institute for Biophysical Chemistry, Gottingen, Germany
Erwin Schoonderwaldt: Post-doctoral researcher, The Institute of Music Physiology and Musician's Medicine, Hannover, Germany
Eckart Altenmüller: Full professor, the University of Music, Drama and Media, Hannover, Germany.

Acknowledgments

We wish to acknowledge Stefan Dohr, Andrej Just, and Fergus McWilliam of the Berlin Philharmonic Orchestra as well as Marie-Luise Neunecker, Jeff Nelsen, Eli Epstein, and Amanda Kleinbart for their enthusiastic support.

Author details

[1]Department of Kinesiology, Gordon College, Wenham, MA, USA. [2]Biomedizinische NMR Forschungs GmbH am Max-Planck-Institut für biophysikalische Chemie, Göttingen, Germany. [3]Hochshule für Musik, Theater und Medien, Hannover, Germany.

References

1. Altenmüller E, Baur V, Hofmann A, Lim VK, Jabusch HC. Musician's cramp as manifestation of maladaptive brain plasticity: arguments from instrumental differences. Ann N Y Acad Sci. 2012;1252:259–65. doi:10.1111/j.1749-6632.2012.06456.x.
2. Iltis PW. Dystonia. In: Auday BC, editor. Salem Health Magill's Medical Guide, vol II. 7th ed. Ispwich Massachusetts: Salem Press; 2014. p. 692–4.
3. Altenmüller E, Jabusch HC. Focal dystonia in musicians: phenomenology, pathophysiology, triggering factors, and treatment. Med Probl Perform Art. 2010;25(1):3–9.
4. Altenmüller E, Jabusch HC. Focal dystonia in musicians: phenomenology, pathophysiology and triggering factors. Eur J Neurol. 2010;17 Suppl 1:31–6. doi:10.1111/j.1468-1331.2010.03048.x.
5. Frucht SJ, Fahn S, Ford B. French horn embouchure dystonia. Mov Disord. 1999;14(1):171–3.
6. Frucht SJ. Embouchure dystonia–portrait of a task-specific cranial dystonia. Mov Disord. 2009;24(12):1752–62. doi:10.1002/mds.22550.
7. Frucht SJ, Estrin G. "Losing one's chops": clues to the mystery of embouchure dystonia. Neurology. 2010;74(22):1758–9. doi:10.1212/WNL.0b013e3181e0f85d.
8. Frucht SJ, Fahn S, Greene PE, O'Brien C, Gelb M, Truong DD, et al. The natural history of embouchure dystonia. Mov Disord. 2001;16(5):899–906.
9. Lederman RJ. Embouchure problems in brass instrumentalists. Med Prob Perfom Art. 2001;16:53–7.
10. Satoh M, Narita M, Tomimoto H. Three cases of focal embouchure dystonia: classifications and successful therapy using a dental splint. Eur Neurol. 2011;66(2):85–90. doi:10.1159/000329578.
11. Steinmetz A, Stang A, Kornhuber M, Rollinghoff M, Delank KS, Altenmüller E. From embouchure problems to embouchure dystonia? A survey of self-reported embouchure disorders in 585 professional orchestra brass players. Int Arch Occup Environ Health. 2014;87(7):783–92. doi:10.1007/s00420-013-0923-4.
12. Brevig P. Losing one's lip and other problems of the embouchure. Med Prob Perfom Art. 1991;6:105–7.
13. Hirata Y, Schulz M, Altenmüller E, Elbert T, Pantev C. Sensory mapping of lip representation in brass musicians with embouchure dystonia. Neuroreport. 2004;15(5):815–8.
14. Haslinger B, Altenmüller E, Castrop F, Zimmer C, Dresel C. Sensorimotor overactivity as a pathophysiologic trait of embouchure dystonia. Neurology. 2010;74(22):1790–7. doi:10.1212/WNL.0b013e3181e0f784.
15. Iltis PW, Givens MW. EMG characterization of embouchure muscle activity: reliability and application to embouchure dystonia. Med Probl Perform Art. 2005;20(1):25–34.

16. Lee A, Furuya S, Morise M, Iltis P, Altenmüller E. Quantification of instability of tone production in embouchure dystonia. Parkinsonism Relat Disord. 2014;20(11):1161–4. doi:10.1016/j.parkreldis.2014.08.007.

17. Angerstein W, Isselstein A, Lindner C. Ultraschalluntersuchungen der zunge beim spielend von blasinstrumenten. Musikphysiologie und Musikermedizin. 2009;16:7–8.

18. Zielke A, Muth T, Massing T. Zungenbewegungen und gesichts-hals-motorik beim spielen von blasinstrumenten. Musikphysiologie und Musikermedizin. 2012;3(19):189–95.

19. Iltis P, Frahm J, Val JD, Joseph A, Schoonderwaldt E, Altenmüller E. High-speed real-time magnetic resonance imaging of fast tongue movements in elite horn players. Quant Imag Med Surg. 2015. doi:10.3978/j.issn.2223-4292.2015.03.02.

20. Iltis P, Frahm J, Voit D, Joseph A, Schoonderwaldt E, Altenmüller E. Real-time MRI comparisons of brass players: a methodological pilot study. Hum Mov Sci. 2015; in press

21. Epstein E. Horn playing from the inside out : a method for all brass musicians. Eli Epstein Productions. 2013.

22. Farkas P. The art of brass playing; a treatise on the formation and use of the brass player's embouchure. Bloomington, Ind: Brass Publications; 1962.

23. Rider W. Real world horn playing. 2nd ed. San Jose, Calif: W. Rider Publications; 2006.

24. Uecker M, Zhang S, Frahm J. Nonlinear inverse reconstruction for real-time MRI of the human heart using undersampled radial FLASH. Magn Reson Med. 2010;63(6):1456–62.

25. Frahm J, Schaetz S, Untenberger M, Zhang S, Voit D, Merboldt KD, et al. On the temporal fidelity of nonlinear inverse reconstructions for real-time MRI - The motion challenge. The Open Med Imaging J. 2014;8:1–7.

26. Schaetz S, Uecker M. A multi-GPU programming library for real-time applications. Algorithms and Architectures for Parallel Processing. 2012;7439:114–28.

27. Niebergall A, Zhang S, Kunay E, Keydana G, Job M, Uecker M, et al. Real-time MRI of speaking at a resolution of 33 ms: undersampled radial FLASH with nonlinear inverse reconstruction. Magn Reson Med. 2013;69(2):477–85.

28. Gardner R. Mastering the horn's low register. Richmond, Virginia: International Opus; 2002.

29. Schumacher M, Schmoor C, Plog A, Schwarzwald R, Taschner C, Echternach M, et al. Motor functions in trumpet playing-a real-time MRI analysis. Neuroradiology. 2013;55(9):1171–81.

30. Altenmüller E. Focal dystonia: advances in brain imaging and understanding of fine motor control in musicians. Hand Clin. 2003;19(3):523–38. xi.

10

Detecting position dependent tremor with the Empirical mode decomposition

André Lee[*] and Eckart Altenmüller

Abstract

Background: Primary bowing tremor (PBT) occurs in violinists in the right bowing-arm and is a highly nonlinear and non-stationary signal. However, Fourier-transform based methods (FFT) make the a priori assumption of linearity and stationarity. We present an interesting case of a violinist with PBT and apply a novel method for nonlinear and non-stationary signals for tremor analysis: the empirical mode decomposition (EMD). We compare the results of FFT and EMD analyses.

Methods: Tremor was measured and quantified in a 50-year-old professional violinist with an accelerometer. Data were analyzed using the EMD, the Hilbert transform, the Hilbert spectrum and the marginal Hilbert spectrum. Findings are compared to the FFT-spectrum and FFT-spectrogram.

Results: We could show that the EMD yields intrinsic mode functions, which represent the tremor and IMFs, which are associated with voluntary movement. The instantaneous frequency and amplitude are obtained. In contrast the low time frequency resolution and the artifacts of voluntary movements are seen in the FFT results.

Conclusions: PBT may present itself as a highly non-stationary and nonlinear phenomenon, which can be accurately analyzed with the EMD, since it gives the instantaneous amplitude and frequency and can identify voluntary from involuntary (tremor) movement.

Keywords: Essential tremor, Dystonia, Dystonic tremor, EMD, Hilbert spectrum, Musician

Background

Tremor is defined as an involuntary rhythmical oscillation of a body part [1]. Particularly pathological tremors are time-varying [2] and highly nonlinear and non-stationary in nature [1,3,4]. Task-specific tremors (TST) are pathological tremors that occur predominantly during certain tasks [1]. Primary bowing tremor (PBT) [5] occurs unilaterally in the right arm of bowed string-instrument players while playing the instrument. This is a highly disabling condition and may threaten the musician's professional career. We describe a violinist in whom PBT occurred when he played a fast movement from the tip of the bow to the frog (the part of the bow held by the violinist), brought the movement to a sudden stop and tried to maintain the hand in a stable position (Additional file 1: Video). In that position tremor

appeared and decreased in amplitude over the next 10–20 seconds, giving a highly non-stationary and non-linear signal.

The disadvantage of applying the Fourier transform (FFT) to these kinds of signals is the *a-priori* assumption of a linear and periodic or stationary signal i.e. a sine or cosine of constant amplitude and frequency spanning the whole signal. The FFT gives reliable results therefore only in case of linear and stationary signals [6]. However, periodicity cannot be assumed for tremors, since frequency not only changes with the waves in a dispersive system (interwave modulation) but likewise within one oscillation cycle or wave (intrawave modulation) [7]. Therefore the wave-profile cannot be considered a sine or cosine function. Furthermore FFT has a limited time-frequency resolution. Thus potentially meaningful local (in a temporal sense) oscillations may not be detected. Finally the FFT does not distinguish between noise (e.g. voluntary movement in this study) and the actual

* Correspondence: andre.lee@hmtm-hannover.de
Institute of Music Physiology and Musicians' Medicine, Hannover University of Music, Drama and Media, Emmichplatz 1, 30175 Hannover, Germany

signal (e.g. tremor, as in this study), making the result less reliable. In recent studies a new method that takes into account the nonlinearity and non-stationarity of signals has been introduced [8] and has been applied in tremor research [2,9,10]. This approach combines two tools: Empirical mode decomposition (EMD) and the Hilbert transform.

EMD decomposes signals into basic components, called intrinsic mode functions (IMFs, Figure 1). In contrast to the FFT, the EMD is an adaptive, data-driven, *a-posteriori* approach, which does not need a-priori assumptions with regard to the signal [7,8]. The IMF can be regarded as a more general counterpart of the simple harmonic functions obtained by the FFT that may have a variable amplitude and frequency [7]. It has been shown that IMFs can be used to identify distinct frequency bands associated with physical or physiological phenomena, for example particular types of tremor, [9,11,12] however it has been noted that mainly tremor data from gyroscopes was analyzed [9,11,12], but not from accelerometers. Furthermore, the EMD may separate noise from the actual data [8].

The Hilbert transform yields the Hilbert spectrum, i.e. the instantaneous amplitude and frequency. It is thus a measure of the contribution of each frequency over time, from which the marginal Hilbert spectrum (MHS), a measure of the total amplitude contribution for each frequency value [7,8], can be derived. The advantage of this method over the FFT is that it is a windowing independent time-frequency representation with a high time-frequency resolution.

The aim of this paper was thus threefold: 1. to present an interesting case of a task-specific tremor in a violinist; 2. to investigate, whether the EMD and Hilbert transform can identify the tremor signal from the highly non-stationary and nonlinear signal obtained from the accelerometer and to separate artifacts from voluntary movements inherent to the task from the involuntary tremor (see Methods) 3. to demonstrate the advantages of the EMD over the FFT.

Methods

The study was approved by the ethics committee of the Hanover medical school and written informed consent was obtained by the participant. Tremor was measured in a 50-year-old professional violinist who had played in a prestigious orchestra for more than 20 year. He was asked to play a fast up-bow-movement, which triggered tremor at the end of that movement when trying to hold the hand in a stable position. He then took back the bow from the frog of the bow to the tip to prepare another fast up-bow movement. The fast up-bow movement and retaking the bow are referred to as voluntary movement. This was repeated for five times. Measurement occurred with a 3D accelerometer (biovision, Wehrheim, Germany, 8×8×11 mm; 4 gram; DC–500 Hz; max 50 g),

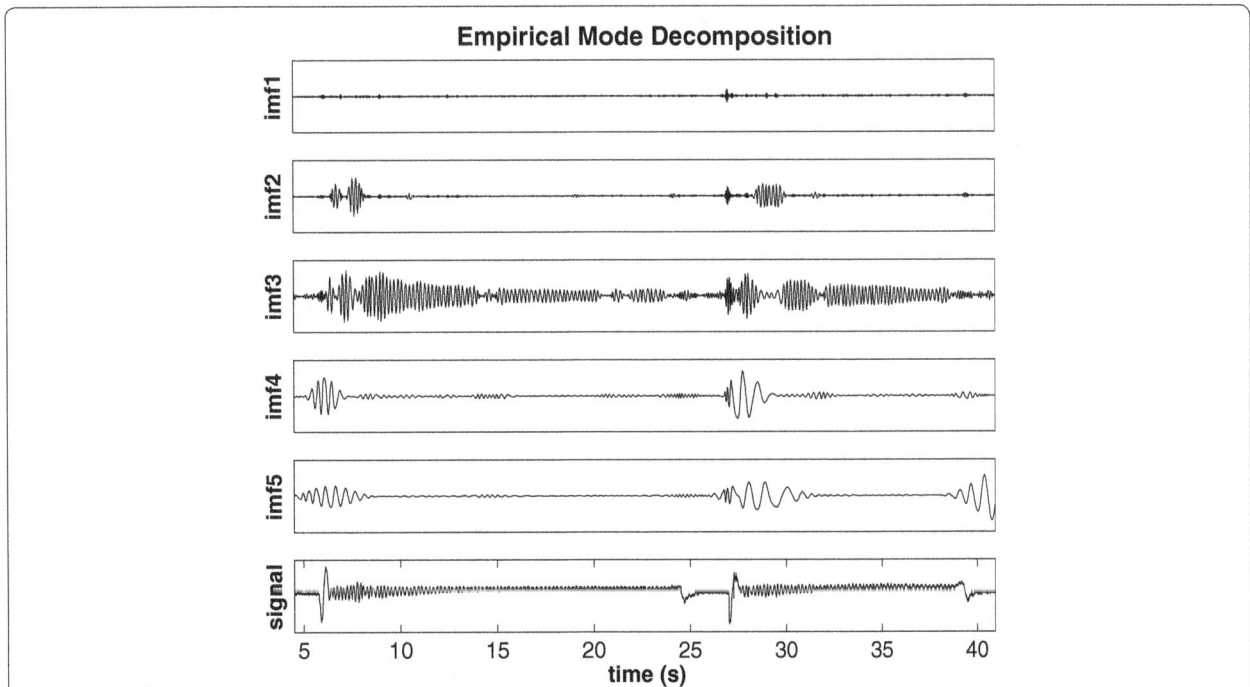

Figure 1 Empirical mode decomposition of the original signal with the intrinsic mode functions (imf) 1–5 and the original signal at the bottom. The x-axis displays the time in seconds. Details are described in the text.

which was attached to the metacarpo-phalangeal (MCP) joint of the index finger of the right hand. Data were band-pass filtered using a 4th degree butterworth-filter (cutoff 1–50 Hz), applied back and forth to compensate for phase shift. With the accelerometer signal onset and end of the fast up-bow movement as well as retaking the bow could be identified.

Empirical mode decomposition

The EMD consists of a sifting process of the original signal [X(t)], in which the intrinsic mode functions (IMF) are obtained. The EMD algorithm as described by Huang et al. is as follows [7,8].

An envelope is created by connecting the local maxima and minima of X(t) with a cubic spine interpolation. The mean value is calculated by taking the average of the upper and lower limit of the envelope (m_1) and subtract it from X(t):

$$X(t) - m_1(t) = h_1(t) \tag{1}$$

In order to be considered an IMF two conditions must be fulfilled: 1) the number of extrema and the number of zero crossings must be either equal or differ at most by one, and 2) at any time the mean value of the envelope defined by the local maxima and the envelope defined by the local minima is zero [7,8]. If $h_1(t)$ does not fulfill the criteria for an IMF, this procedure is repeated n-times until $h_{(1n)}(t)$ fulfills the criteria and is thus defined as the first IMF [$c_1(t)$]:

$$c_1(t) = h_{1n}(t) \tag{2}$$

Next, $c_1(t)$ is subtracted from X(t):

$$X(t) - c_1(t) = r_1(t) \tag{3}$$

$r_1(t)$ is called the residue which is substituted for X(t) in formula (1) and the first steps are repeated m-times until a residual r_m is reached that is a monotonic function of which no more IMFs can be extracted [7,8]. Thus, the original signal can be obtained by

$$X(t) = \sum_{i=1}^{m} c_i(t) + r_m \tag{4}$$

The frequency ranges of the IMF are ordered in such a way that IMF1 contains the highest and IMF_m the lowest frequencies. Being a data-driven approach, the frequency ranges depend on the original signal.

Hilbert transform, Hilbert spectrum and marginal Hilbert spectrum

The Hilbert transform is applied to the IMFs to obtain the instantaneous frequency and amplitude (Hilbert-spectrum) i.e. the amplitude and frequency at each moment in the movement. The MHS h(ω) is obtained by

$$h(\omega) = \int_0^T H(\omega, t) dt \tag{5}$$

where H(ω,t) is the Hilbert spectrum derived by

$$H(\omega, t) = \sum_{j=1}^{n} a_j(t) \exp\left[i \int \omega_j(t) dt\right] \tag{6}$$

$a_j(t)$ is the instantaneous amplitude, $\omega_j(t)$ the instantaneous frequency.

A detailed description can be found in Huang et al. [8] and Huang [7].

We expected to find an IMF, that would display the onset of tremor after stopping the up-bow movement with a decreasing amplitude without the artifact of the fast up-bow movement itself.

EMD was performed in Matlab using the EMD package by Rilling et al. [http://perso.ens-lyon.fr/patrick.flandrin/emd.html], applying the default stopping criterion [13].

FFT for comparison

To compare the results of the EMD and Hilbert transform with the FFT we performed an FFT with a window of 5096 data points and an overlap of 1024 data points.

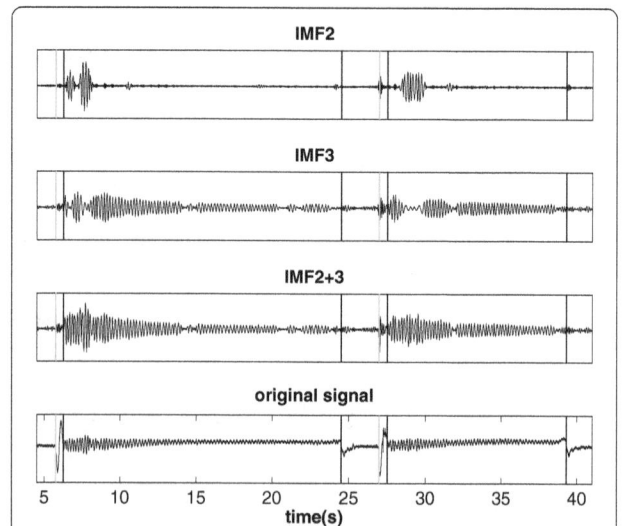

Figure 2 Depicted are IMF2, IMF3, the combination of IMF2 plus IMF3 = IMF2 + 3 and the original signal. The x-axis shows the time in seconds. The vertical green line shows the onset and the vertical red line the end of the fast up-bow movement as identified from the acceleration signal in the original signal. The vertical black line shows the moment, when the bow is retaken from the frog of the bow to the tip for the second fast up-bow movement. One fast up-bow movement took about 0.5 seconds, whereas retaking the bow took about 2 s.

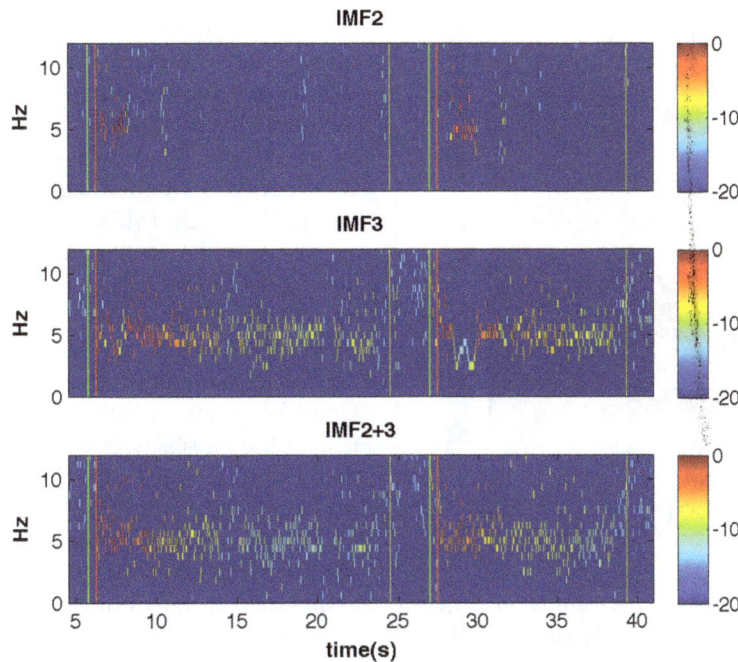

Figure 3 Hilbert spectrum of IMF2, IMF3 and IMF2 + 3. The x-axis shows the time in seconds. The vertical green and red line are as in Figure 2, for visibility reasons the vertical black line of Figure 2 is shown in yellow here. The instantaneous frequency can be seen around 5 Hz. The amplitude of the tremor is color-coded; the colorbar units are dB. The onset of tremor after stopping the bow (vertical red line) and the decrease of amplitude until the bow is taken back to the tip (vertical yellow line) can be clearly seen and is best represented in IMF2 + 3. Higher frequency of low amplitude can be seen when the bow is taken back (between the vertical yellow and green line).

Results

Tremor detection

Empirical mode decomposition

Figure 1 displays the EMD with 5 IMFs and the original signal for the first two fast up-bow movements. In the original signal the artifact voluntary movements (i.e. at the onset of the fast up-bow movement and when taking back the bow) are visible, showing the non-stationarity of the signal. IMF3 best represents the tremor signal, however, part of signal becomes apparent in IMF2, known as mode-mixing. No tremor is detected in IMF1. Low-frequency tremor can be seen in IMFs 4 and 5. To investigate the mode mixing we chose the combination of IMF2 and IMF3 (IMF2 + 3) for further evaluation (see below).

Figure 2 displays IMF2 and IMF3, the combination of both, IMF2 + 3, as well as the original signal. IMF2 + 3 give a more accurate representation of the tremor signal. In the IMFs and the original signal the moments where voluntary movements occur are indicated by vertical lines (see legend).

Hilbert spectrum and marginal Hilbert spectrum

Figure 3 shows the Hilbert spectrum i.e. the time-frequency representation of IMF2, IMF3 and IMF2 + 3. The instantaneous frequency and amplitude are shown, as described in the methods part. Figure 4 depicts the MHS of IMFs 1 to 5 as well as IMF2 + 3. The peak amplitude of both, IMF3 and IMF2 + 3 is 4.7 Hz. Lower frequencies are detected in IMF4 and IMF5.

Comparison with FFT

Figure 5 depicts the FFT-spectrogram of the original signal. The low time-frequency resolution becomes apparent.

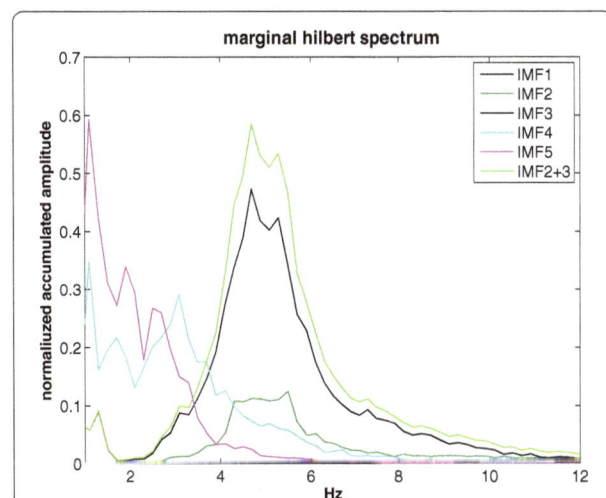

Figure 4 Marginal Hilbert spectrum of IMF1 – IMF5 and IMF2 + 3. IMF1 is not visible due to the large scale. The main contribution of IMF3 to tremor-detection becomes visible and the mode mixing of IMF2 + 3 does not alter the peak frequency.

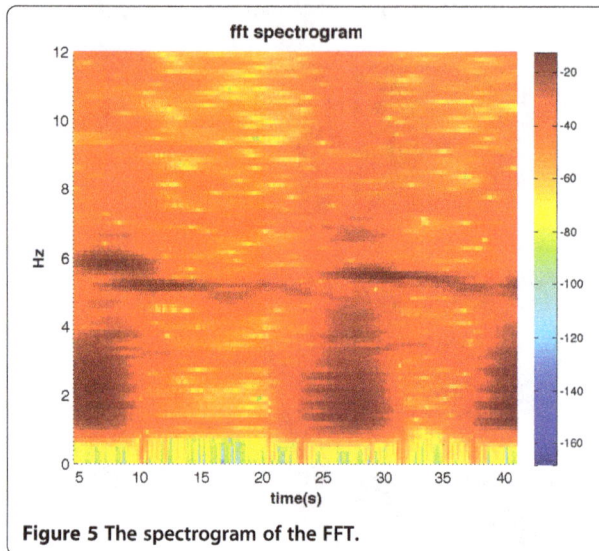

Figure 5 The spectrogram of the FFT.

Figure 6 depicts the FFT power spectrum of the original signal with a peak amplitude at 5.2 Hz and the MHS of IMF2 + 3 for comparison.

Discussion

We describe a patient with an unusual form of task specific bowing tremor that appeared only when a sudden up-bow movement was brought to a sudden stop at the frog of the bow and held there as steadily as possible. The peak frequency was at 4.7 Hz (Figure 4) and thus was in the range of PBT described before [14,15]. Since we had a highly non-stationary signal with artifacts from voluntary movements (i.e. the fast up-bow movement as

well as the movement for returning the bow to the tip) as seen in Figures 1 and 2, we applied a novel method for analyzing the signal, the EMD and Hilbert transform that do not require stationarity and linearity as a prerequisite. We could show that the EMD and the Hilbert transform are able to correctly identify the tremor signal. As expected the tremor signal was mainly contained in one IMF, namely IMF3. One interesting aspect of our analysis was the finding of a mode mixing, which has been described by Huang [7]. It describes the finding of part of the tremor signal being distributed between two (or more) IMFs, in our case between IMF2 and IMF3. According to formula (4), the original signal can be obtained by adding all IMF and the final residual r_m, which implies the possibility of adding two (or more) IMF. We therefore added IMF2 + IMF3. The Hilbert spectrum of this combined IMF2 + 3 (Figure 3, bottom) corroborates this finding, since the tremor amplitude of very precisely represents the course of the tremor observed during clinical examination at the instrument (Additional file 1: Video): It is highest after the up-bow movement and diminishes over time. Virtually no tremor is present when retaking the bow.

Importantly, our expectation that the EMD can reduce artifacts, e.g. from voluntary movement as has been shown before [9], was confirmed. As shown in Figure 2, the low frequency artifacts of the up-bow movement and of retaking the bow are removed in the IMFs. The up-bow movement lasted for 0.5 s, giving a low frequency artifact of 2 Hz. Even lower frequencies were to be expected from retaking the bow. Peaks at around 2 Hz and below are visible in IMF4 and IMF5. We therefore interpret the low frequency signal of these

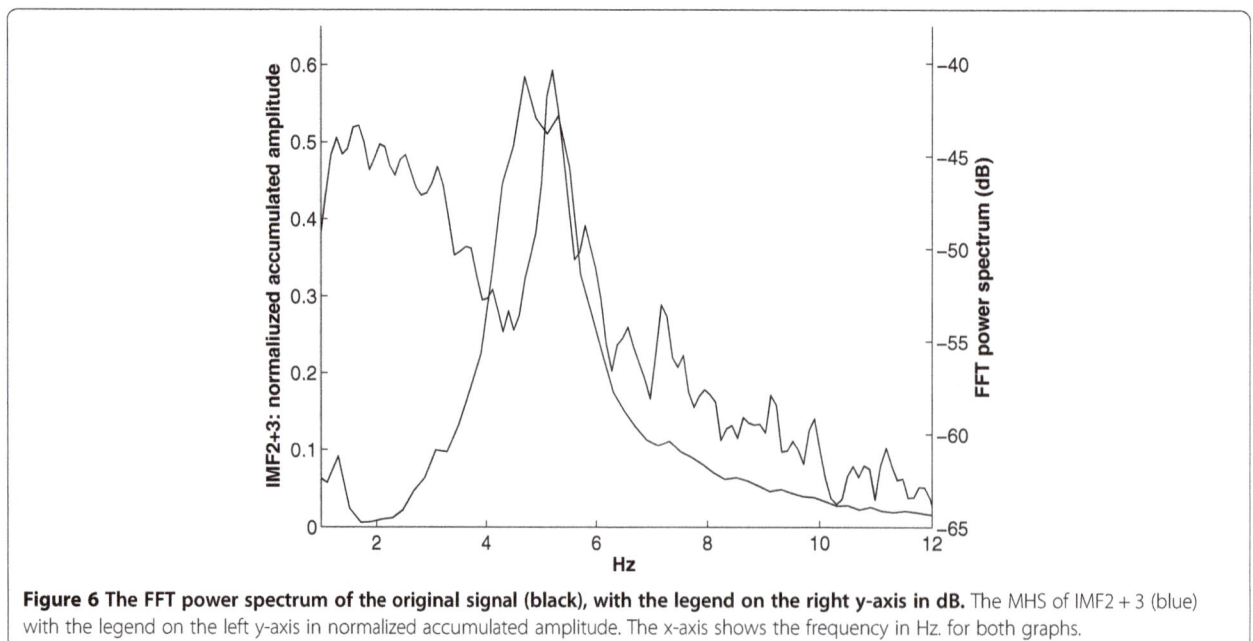

Figure 6 The FFT power spectrum of the original signal (black), with the legend on the right y-axis in dB. The MHS of IMF2 + 3 (blue) with the legend on the left y-axis in normalized accumulated amplitude. The x-axis shows the frequency in Hz. for both graphs.

IMFs (Figure 1) to be caused by the voluntary movements. This is important, because it suggests that discontinuities in tremor signals and voluntary movements have a small effect on the precision of the method.

Given the algorithm of the EMD, fast voluntary movements in music making with a high frequency (e.g. tremolo) would have been represented in IMF 1. Our paradigm did not include those kinds of movements and thus, as expected, almost no signal was detected here.

The comparison with results of an FFT analysis revealed similar peak frequencies for both methods. However, the limited time-frequency resolution of the FFT becomes apparent when comparing Figures 3 and 5. The instantaneous frequency and amplitude allows a more precise course of the tremor, whereas for FFT-based methods, a compromise between time and frequency resolution has to be made. In the FFT spectrogram (Figure 6) the low-frequency artifact of the voluntary movement is overestimated and taken into account in the FFT power spectrum (Figure 5). In the IMFs, however, the signal is separated into frequency ranges that cover both, tremor (IMF2 + 3) and lower frequency voluntary movement (IMF 4, IMF5, see Figure 4). We therefore conclude that IMF2 + 3 represents the frequency range and thus the intrawave frequency modulation of task-specific tremor than the frequency range covered by the FFT power spectrum (Figure 5). This is important, because it has been shown that the wave-profile deformation seen in the FFT-power spectrum that are usually interpreted as harmonic distortions, are more likely due to the intrawave frequency modulation [8].

Since the EMD has been applied so far only for tremor data derived from a gyroscope [2,9,10] we finally conclude that it is applicable for accelerometer data, as well.

Conclusion

We present an interesting and unusual case of a patient with a highly non-stationary and nonlinear PBT. We could show that the EMD can accurately detect and analyze the tremor, identify voluntary movement and is applicable for data obtained with an accelerometer. In comparison to the FFT, the EMD does not make a priori assumptions on the data, yields the instantaneous frequency and amplitude and is thus a more precise tool for analyzing tremor data.

Competing interests
The authors declare that they have no competing interests.

Authors' contributions
AL: Conception and design of the study, acquisition, analysis and interpretation of data. Drafting of the manuscript. Final approval. Agrees to be accountable for all aspects of the work in ensuring that questions related to the accuracy or integrity of any part of the work are appropriately investigated and resolved. EA: Conception and design of the study, interpretation of data. Revision of manuscript for important intellectual content. Final approval. Agrees to be accountable for all aspects of the work in ensuring that questions related to the accuracy or integrity of any part of the work are appropriately investigated and resolved.

Acknowledgements
Funding for AL and EA: Hannover University of Music, Drama and Media.

References
1. Deuschl G, Bain P, Brin M. Consensus statement of the Movement Disorder Society on Tremor. Ad Hoc Scientific Committee. Mov Disord. 1998;3 (13 Suppl):2–23.
2. De Lima ER, Andrade AO, Pons JL, Kyberd P, Nasuto SJ. Empirical mode decomposition: a novel technique for the study of tremor time series. Med Biol Eng Comput. 2006;44:569–82.
3. Gantert C, Honerkamp J, Timmer J. Analyzing the dynamics of hand tremor time series. Biol Cybern. 1992;66:479–84.
4. Timmer J, Haussler S, Lauk M, Lucking C-H. Pathological tremors: deterministic chaos or nonlinear stochastic oscillators? Chaos. 2000;10:278–88.
5. Lee A, Altenmüller E. Primary task-specific tremor: an entity of its Own? Med Probl Perform Art. 2012;27:224–6.
6. Oppenheim AV, Schafer RW. Discrete-Time Signal Processing. Prentice Hall: Englewood Cliffs, NJ; 1989.
7. Huang NE. Introduction to the Hilbert–Huang Transform and Its Related Mathematical Problems. In: Hilbert-Huang Transform and its Applications. Singapore; Hackensack, NJ; London: World Scientific; 2005. p. 1–26.
8. Huang NE, Shen Z, Long SR, Wu MC, Shih HH, Zheng Q, et al. The empirical mode decomposition and the Hilbert spectrum for nonlinear and non-stationary time series analysis. Proc R Soc A: Math Phys Eng Sci. 1998;454:903–95.
9. Rocon E, Pons JL, Andrade AO, Nasuto SJ. Application of EMD as a novel technique for the study of tremor time series. Conf Proc IEEE Eng Med Biol Soc. 2006, Suppl:6533–6536.
10. Gallego JA, Rocon E, Koutsou AD, Pons JL. Analysis of kinematic data in pathological tremor with the Hilbert-Huang transform. IEEE. 2011:80–83
11. Silchenko AN, Adamchic I, Pawelczyk N, Hauptmann C, Maarouf M, Sturm V, et al. Data-driven approach to the estimation of connectivity and time delays in the coupling of interacting neuronal subsystems. J Neurosci Methods. 2010;191:32–44.
12. Li K, Hogrel J-Y, Duchêne J, Hewson DJ. Analysis of fatigue and tremor during sustained maximal grip contractions using Hilbert-Huang Transformation. Med Eng Phys. 2011;34:832–40.
13. Hogan N. Adaptive control of mechanical impedance by coactivation of antagonist muscles. IEEE Trans Automatic Control. 1984;29:681–90.
14. Lee A, Chadde M, Altenmüller E, Schoonderwaldt E. Characteristics of task-specific tremor in string instrument players. Tremor Other Hyperkinet Mov (NY). 2014;4:198.
15. Lee A, Tominaga K, Furuya S, Miyazaki F, Altenmüller E. Coherence of coactivation and acceleration in task-specific primary bowing tremor. J Neural Transm. 2014;121:739–42.

11

The phenomenology and natural history of idiopathic lower cranial dystonia

Pichet Termsarasab[*], Donald R Tanenbaum and Steven J Frucht

Abstract

Background: Many patients with lower cranial dystonia (LCrD) are misdiagnosed, and recognition of this condition by general practitioners and dental health professionals is limited.

Methods: We define the phenomenology and natural history of idiopathic LCrD, presenting in 41 patients with the disorder, the largest series of these patients reported to date.

Results: Phenomenology of dystonia included lower cranial and pharyngeal involvement, jaw opening and jaw closing dystonia, and tongue dystonia. Of 25 newly described patients, 72% (18) were female, average age at onset was 56 years, and delay before correct diagnosis was 3.8 years (0-25 years, median 2 years). Eleven patients (44%) reported a precipitating event, the most common of which was recent dental work. Geste antagonistes were found in 18 patients (72%). Response to treatment was mixed, indicating an unmet therapeutic need.

Conclusions: Idiopathic LCrD is often missed and institution of effective therapy is often delayed. The clinical features and natural history of LCrD are similar to other forms of focal dystonia.

Keywords: Lower cranial dystonia, Oromandibular dystonia, Geste antagoniste

Background

Lower cranial dystonia (LCrD), focal dystonia of the muscles of the lower face, jaw, tongue and pharynx, may be seen in a variety of scenarios including tardive dystonia, DYT6 and DYT12, and in neurodegenerative disorders such as Wilson's disease and neurodegeneration with brain iron accumulation (NBIA). In contrast, isolated LCrD occurring without other abnormalities is distinctly rare. Many patients with LCrD are misdiagnosed, and recognition of this condition by general practitioners and dental health professionals is limited, delaying appropriate diagnosis and treatment. Two hundred and twenty eight patients with lower cranial dystonia have been reported in at least 8 prior case series/reports [1-8], however significant limitations in these reports include; 1) mixing of patients with tardive or other secondary forms of LCrD; 2) inclusion of patients with dystonia in other body regions such as the upper face or neck; and, 3) lack of detailed phenomenologic descriptions. We present 41 patients with idiopathic LCrD (25 newly reported), the largest report to date of

idiopathic LCrD, in order to increase awareness and facilitate diagnosis and treatment of this unusual condition.

Methods

Twenty-five patients with idiopathic LCrD were evaluated by the senior movement disorders neurologist (SJF) over a period of eight years. Many patients were referred by dentists or oral surgeons (DT). Patients with secondary dystonia or with exposure to dopamine receptor blocking agents were excluded. Clinical history, examination, and video review were performed (PT, SJF). Age at onset, duration of symptoms, precipitating factors, clinical phenomenology, the presence or absence of geste maneuvers, task-specificity, aggravating and relieving factors, and associated symptoms and treatment response are summarized in Table 1.

To make description of this entity more comprehensive, we have included the 16 patients with idiopathic LCrD from our previous publication in our series [4]. We excluded three patients from the previous publication who also had blepharospasm. The study was approved by the Mount Sinai Institutional Review Board. Video written-informed consent was obtained from all patients. We did not obtain separated informed consent as this is a retrospective chart review.

---

* Correspondence: Pichet.Termsarasab@mountsinai.org
Department of Neurology, Movement Disorders Division, Icahn School of Medicine at Mount Sinai, 5 East 98th St, first floor, New York, NY 10029, USA

Table 1 Summary of clinical features including phenomenology of 41 patients with idiopathic LCrD

Number	Gender	Age at onset	Duration	Areas affected	Primary movement	Task specificity	Precipitating event	Sensory trick	Associated symptoms	Treatment	Oral device; response
1	F	65	2	Jaw	Jaw opening	Speech, eating, chewing	Dental work	None	None	LD (no), BoNT (no, dysphagia), THP (no), CLZ (no), baclofen (unknown)	N
2	F	71	1	Jaw	L jaw deviation	Eating, chewing, speech	Mandibular fx after a fall	None	None	THP (yes, 2–4 mg/d)	N
3	F	59	2	Jaw	Jaw opening and protrusion	Speech -> eating, chewing	Maxillary bridge replacement	Plastic between teeth	Pain/clicking in TMJ	THP (no)	N
4	F	53	0	Jaw	Jaw opening	Speech -> eating	None	Plastic/tongue depressor between teeth > holding jaw	R ear clicking, lower jaw pain	THP (no), BoNT (no), Baclofen (no), TBZ (no, depression), CLZ (no, sedation), DZP (unknown)	N
5	F	46	2	Jaw	Jaw opening	Speech -> eating	None	Plastic between teeth, holding jaw	None	CLZ (no), THP (unknown), BoNT (yes, mild)	Y; initial response
6	M	61	1	Pharynx, larynx	Pharyngeal/laryngeal dystonia	Speech (worse with ke, ge sounds)	R sinus lift and dental implant	Plastic/tongue depressor between teeth	None	THP (yes, 6–15 mg/d)	N
7	F	73	1	Jaw	R jaw deviation	At rest	None	Plastic between teeth on the L	None	THP (no), CLZ (1 mg/d, unknown)	N
8	F	70	1	Jaw	Jaw opening	Speech	Cheering a football game	Tongue depressor between lip/teeth; holding jaw	None	CLZ (no), LD (no), THP (no), Baclofen (no), BoNT (no)	N
9	F	51	2	Jaw	L jaw deviation	Speech, eating	R crown replacement and repair	Tongue depressor between teeth on the L	Jaw pain	CLZ (unknown)	N
10	F	56	2	Jaw	R jaw deviation	Speech, chewing	None	Plastic between teeth on the right and in front, holding jaw	Mild pain	THP (yes, 6 mg/d)	N
11	F	58	1	Jaw	L jaw deviation	Speech, eating	3 wks after L subdural hematoma	Plastic between teeth	None	THP (unknown)	N
12	F	50	1	Jaw	L jaw deviation	Speech	None	Holding the L jaw, imagination about holding the jaw, tongue depressor/syringe between teeth	None	THP (unknown)	N
13	M	56	7	Jaw, tongue	Jaw opening and tongue mvmts	None	None	Straw in his mouth, lightly touching lips	Difficulty chewing	CLZ (no), BoNT (no), THP (unknown)	N

Table 1 Summary of clinical features including phenomenology of 41 patients with idiopathic LCrD (Continued)

No.	Sex	Age		Distribution	Phenomenology	Activating conditions	Precipitant	Sensory trick	Associated features	Treatment	Response
14	F	56	1	Jaw, tongue	Jaw opening, tongue protrusion, alternating tongue deviation	Speech → eating, chewing on the R side	3 mo after traumatic facial abrasion	None	Clicking in jaw	LVT (no), TBZ (no), THP (unknown)	Y; no response
15	F	44	11	Jaw, tongue	Jaw closing, tongue retraction	Speech, chewing	Ill-fitting new denture leading to painful jaw and facial swelling	None	None	CLZ (unknown), THP (no), Baclofen (unknown), BoNT (yes, mild)	N
16	M	41	3	Jaw	Jaw protrusion	At rest, speech, eating	Skull fx and extensive L orbital bone damage, R lower molar extraction 1 y later	Tongue depressor or a pen cap between teeth	None	CLZ (yes, mild, 3–4 mg/d), THP (unknown)	Y; no response
17	M	55	2	Tongue	Tongue protrusion with 90° clockwise rotation	At rest, absent during tasks	None	None	None	LD (no), CLZ (yes, mild, 3 mg/d), BoNT (no), THP (unknown)	N
18	F	78	4	Lower face	Multiple mvmts with coexisting ET	Arrhythmic facial movements (talking > at rest); rhythmic facial movements (at rest > talking)	Dental procedure to crown several lower molar teeth	Holding chin with hand	Voice straining (started after the dental procedure), facial movements started 2 years after.	TBZ (no), CLZ (no), THP (unknown)	N
19	F	67	7	Tongue	Tongue protrusion	At rest, chewing/eating	None	None	None	TBZ (unknown)	N
20	F	63	1	Jaw	Jaw opening, jaw protrusion	Speech (words with an "r" or "l", at rest		Holding a plastic syringe in the left corner of mouth	Difficulty swallowing liquids	LD (no), LZP (no), Baclofen (unknown)	N
21	M	45	1	Jaw	Jaw closing, jaw protrusion and L jaw deviation	At rest	None	Tongue depressor between teeth on the right side, touching L lower cheek	Clicking noise at the L jaw, jaw pain (L > R)	CLZ (no), Cyclobenzaprine (yes, mild), Jaw surgery (no), THP (unknown), BoNT (unknown)	Y; no response
22	M	45	2	Jaw, tongue	Jaw opening, tongue retraction	At rest, chewing	?cocaine abuse	None	None	Clonidine (yes, mild), CBZ (mild), CLZ (unknown), THP (unknown)	N
23	M	51	1	Jaw	L jaw deviation, mild jaw protrusion	At rest	None	Firm pressure on R cheek, holding object between teeth on the L side	None	LD (no), BoNT (unknown)	N

Table 1 Summary of clinical features including phenomenology of 41 patients with idiopathic LCrD *(Continued)*

#	Sex	Age		Distribution	Involuntary movement		Task specificity	Sensory trick	Associated features	Treatment	Response
24	F	51	15	Lip, tongue, perioral muscles	Invol. dystonic mvmt of face, lips and tongue; invol. sucking mvmt of mouth	None	Speech, eating	Tongue depressor between teeth, putting hand on face	Dysphagia, 8-lb wt loss, biting cheek->mouth ulcers	THP (no), CLZ (no, confusion, memory problem), BoNT (yes, mild)	N
25	M	25	25	Jaw, perioral muscles	Mouth closure with sl jaw opening and protrusion	None	Speech, praying, chewing	Tongue depressor between teeth (L > R), touching jaw/chin lightly	Pain at b/l lower jaw, burning sensation in buccal mucosa, biting buccal mucosa-> bleeding	CLZ (no, 1.5 mg/d), THP (no, 2 mg/d, dose inadequate)	N
26	M	50		Tongue	Tongue rolling		Speech	Toothpick in mouth; touch lips with finger		TBZ (no); THP (unknown)	Y; good response
27	M	38		Jaw	L jaw deviation		Speech, chewing	Pipette between left molars; touch left jaw		CLZ, THP (no)	Y; no response
28	F	60		Jaw	Jaw closure		Non-specific, worse with speech	Touch L cheek; plastic tube between teeth		BoNT (unknown)	N
29	F	43		Jaw	Jaw closure and L jaw deviation		Bassoon --> speech, chewing	Device over molar; plastic appliance between teeth		BoNT (yes)	Prior device; good response
30	M	41		Jaw	Jaw closure		French horn --> speech, drinking	Bite plate; straw between teeth on L		BoNT, CLZ, baclofen, THP (no to all)	Y; brief response
31	F	41		Jaw	Jaw protrusion and left jaw deviation		Speech	Straw between teeth, L > R		BoNT (unknown)	Y (bite blocks); help when bite
32	M	33		Lip	Lip pulling to the corners of the mouth		Speech	Straw between upper lip-teeth; hold upper lip with 2 fingers		THP (yes, 6–18 mg/d)	N
33	F	51		Platysma, face	Neck pull forward, grimacing		Non-specific	Straw between teeth on either side		CLZ (yes, 0.5 mg/d), BoNT (no)	N
34	M	64		Pharynx, larynx	Pulling		Paradoxical; worse at rest, speech better	Plastic between teeth		CLZ (unknown)	N
35	F	68		Jaw, tongue	Lateral movements of jaw, tongue rolling		Non-specific	Straw/spoon between teeth		THP (no); CLZ (yes, 1 mg/d)	Y; good response
36	F	66		Tongue	Tongue pushing against teeth (protrusion?)		Non-specific	Paper towel over lower front teeth; toothpick		Unknown	Unknown
37	M	48		Perioral muscles	Rotation of perioral muscles		Speech	Straw in his mouth		BoNT (yes)	Y; unknown

Table 1 Summary of clinical features including phenomenology of 41 patients with idiopathic LCrD *(Continued)*

38	M	44	Tongue	Tongue rolling	Flute – >speech	Plastic pipette in cheek	THP (yes, 4–6 mg/d)	N
41	M	30	Embouchure	Lowering, protrusion	Trombone	Touch chin or L side of face	None	N
42	M	66	Jaw, tongue	Jaw opening, tongue movements	Paradoxical; worse at rest, speech better	Straw between teeth	THP, CLZ, BoNT (no to all)	Not yet referred to M.G.
43	F	42	Jaw, lips	Jaw and lip opening	Speech, chewing	Touch R temple	CLZ, THP, BoNT, baclofen (no to all)	Y; brief response

Data on our new patients (number 1–25) is presented with previously published patients (number 26–43; shown in italics).

Legend: Patient number, gender, age at onset (years), duration of the disease (years), areas that are affected (arrow shows the pattern of spreading from one region to another), primary movement, task specificity, precipitating events, sensory trick, associated symptoms, treatment employed, and trial of oral devices and response are listed in columns. Patients 1 to 25 were new and patients 26 to 43 (shown in italics) were previously published [4]. Patients 39, 40 and 44 were excluded due to co-existing blepharospasm. There is no information on precipitating event in patients 26 to 43.

M, male; F, female; L, left; R, right; mvmt, movement; invol., involuntary; >, had greater effect than; fx, fracture; wk, week; mo, month; y, year; TMJ, temporomandibular joint; sl, slight; wt, weight; b/l, bilateral; LD, levodopa; BoNT, botulinum toxin injections; THP, trihexyphenidyl; CLZ, clonazepam; mg/d, milligram per day; DZP, diazepam; LVT, levetiracetam; TBZ, tetrabenazine; N, no; Y, yes. In treatment column, response is shown in the brackets (yes, no, unknown): "yes" (in patients 1 to 25), a good response; "yes, mild", mild response, effective dose indicated in the brackets. In the oral device column, response is shown as Y and N (yes and no).

Results

Of 25 patients identified in the current series, 18 (68%) were female, and the mean age at evaluation was 60 years (range 44–82). Mean age at onset of symptoms was 56 (range, 25–78), 59.5 years in women and 48.6 in men. Only one patient had a positive family history, a patient with a son with an identical phenotype of rightward jaw deviation. The most common primary phenotype was a mixed dystonia (12 patients, 48%). Of the mixed phenotypes, jaw opening was the most common primary movement (4 patients). The second most common primary phenotype was jaw deviation (6 patients, 24%), followed by jaw opening (4 patients, 16%). Of 6 patients with pure jaw deviation, the jaw was deviated to the left in 4 patients and to the right in 2 patients. There was one patient each with pure jaw protrusion, pure tongue protrusion and pharyngeal/laryngeal dystonia.

In almost all patients (24/25, 96%), dystonia was task-specific. The most common task triggering dystonia was speaking (16/25, 64%), followed by eating or chewing (15/25, 60%). Thirteen patients had dystonia related to both speaking and eating/chewing. Four of these 13 demonstrated a pattern of progression of task-specificity, with dystonia initially involving speech and then progressing over time to involve eating as well. Some patients who had dystonia with chewing had difficulty specifically with hard objects. A few patients with dystonia related to speaking described a trigger with particular sounds, such as "r" or "l" sounds in one patient, and "ke" or "ge" sounds in another. Dystonia also occurred at rest in 9 patients.

Eleven patients (44%) reported a precipitating event before onset of dystonia, the most common of which was dental work within the preceding several weeks (5 patients, 20%). Two precipitating events related to injury or manipulation of maxillofacial bones included a traumatic mandibular fracture after a fall and maxillary bridge replacement. The latter patient was required to hold her mouth open for 2 hours while the temporary bridge was fit. Other precipitating events included a history of a left subdural hematoma 3 weeks prior, and a skull fracture with extensive left orbital bone damage from a car accident.

Geste antagonistes were found in 18 patients (72%). The most common one observed on examination was holding an object such as a piece of plastic, a tongue depressor, syringe or straw between the teeth, in 17 out of 18 patients. Six patients demonstrated marked side specificity of the geste: improvement when placing the trick device between teeth on one side but not the other side. Complete data on side specificity in all patients could not be assessed due to lack of testing. There was no clear relationship between the phenomenology of dystonia (for example, the side that the jaw deviated to) and the side specificity of this geste antagoniste. Ten patients also had improvement in dystonia when lightly touching the jaw, chin or face with finger(s) or a hand. One of these ten patients had improvement even when he imagined holding his jaw. Three reported improvement with chewing gum, one of which had side specificity on the left.

Stress and fatigue were aggravating factors in some patients. The most common associated symptom was jaw pain (5 patients, 20%). A clicking noise in the jaw or ear was found in 4 patients (16%). Dysphagia was found in 2 patients: one had severe weight loss and the other had dysphagia only with liquids. Two patients reported mouth ulcers or bleeding from biting buccal mucosa.

Oral medication and botulinum toxin injections were employed in treatment. Oral medications included trihexyphenidyl (21 patients, 84%), clonazepam (15 patients, 60%), baclofen (5 patients, 20%) and levodopa (4 patients, 16%). Propranolol, carbamazepine and clonidine were each also used in one patient. The most common daily dose of trihexyphenidyl was 6 mg/day in 10 patients (range 1–19 mg). Of 21 patients treated with trihexyphenidyl, three had response with very good benefit at the dose of 2–15 mg/day, seven did not have benefit and the response was unknown in 11 patients. Of 15 patients treated with clonazepam, two had response that was only mild at the dose of 1.5-3 mg/day, nine had no response and the response was unknown in four patients. Baclofen was employed in 5 patients, none of whom had a good response, three had no response and the response was unknown in the other two patients. Of data available, the dose of baclofen employed was 10–30 mg/day.

Ten patients (40%) underwent botulinum toxin (BoNT) injections. The sites of the injections depended on the primary movement, mostly external or internal pterygoids. There was a response that was only mild in three patients, one of whom continued to have significant disability. Five patients had no response to BoNT injections and the response was unknown in two patients.

With regards to side effects, confusion, mild tendency to sadness and anxiety each were found in one patient each taking trihexyphenidyl at 3–6 mg/day. Side effects from clonazepam included anxiety, confusion/memory problem, and sedation, each found in one patient taking the dose of 1–1.5 mg/day. One patient who received BoNT injections was complicated by marked dysphagia. Depression and rash each were found in one patient taking tetrabenazine.

Table 2 illustrates the comparison of results combining our 25 new patients with 16 patients from the previously published series, when analyzing the new patients compared to all 41 patients. The results with regards to sex predilection, areas affected, primary movement, task-specificity, geste antagoniste, treatment employed and response to the treatment were similar. Of note, 3 patients from the previously published series had task specificity related to performance on a brass or woodwind musical instrument (embouchure dystonia).

Table 2 Comparison of results between new patients and combined data with the previous publication

	New patients	Combined data
Number of the patients	25	41
Sex	Female 18/25 (72%)	Female 24/41 (58.5%)
	Male 7/25 (28%)	Male 17/41 (41.5%)
Female/male (F/M ratio)	2.6:1	1.4:1
Average age at onset (years)	**56**	**53.3**
In female subgroup	59.5	48.6
In male subgroup	48.6	47.2
Areas affected		
Jaw only (including mixed primary movements of jaw)	15 (60%)	20 (48.8%)
Lip or perioral only	0 (0%)	2 (4.9%)
Tongue only	2 (8%)	5 (12.2%)
Pharynx/larynx	1 (4%)	2 (4.9%)
Mixed	7 (28%)	11 (26.8%)
Jaw and tongue	4 (16%)	6 (14.6%)
Primary movement		
Pure jaw deviation	6 (24%)	7 (17%)
to the left	4 (16%)	5 (12.2%)
Pure jaw opening	4 (16%)	4 (9.8%)
Mixed	12 (48%)	17 (41.5%)
Task specificity		
Speech	18 (72%)	27 (65.9%)
Eating/chewing	15 (60%)	18 (43.9%)
At rest	9 (36%)	11 (26.8%)
Musical instrument	0 (0%)	4 (9.8%)
Geste antagoniste	**18 (72%)**	**34 (82.9%)**
Object between teeth	17 (68%)	31 (75.6%)
with side specificity	6 (24%)	8 (19.5%)
Holding body part lightly	10 (40%)	15 (36.6%)
with side specificity	4 (16%)	8 (19.5%)
Treatment		
THP	**21 (84%)**	**29 (70.7%)**
good response	3 (12%)	5 (12.2%)
CLZ	**15 (60%)**	**22 (53.7%)**
good response	2 (8%) - all mild	4 (9.8%)
Baclofen	**5 (20%)**	**7 (17%)**
good response	0 (0%)	0 (0%)
BoNT	**10 (40%)**	**18 (43.9%)**
good response	3 (12%) - all mild	5 (12.2%)
Dental device	**4 (16%)**	**11 (26.8%)**
good response	0 (0%)	2 (4.9%)

Legend: Data on our 25 patients and combined 41 is shown in the middle and right columns, respectively. Number of patients, sex, average age at onset, areas affected, primary movement, task specificity, geste antagoniste, and treatment employed are listed in the left column. With regards to areas affected, note that "jaw only" group also includes patients with mixed primary movement of the jaw such as mixed jaw opening and protrusion. With regards to geste antagoniste, data on side specificity, either left or right, is shown. Numbers of the patients on each treatment modality and the ones with a good response are shown. Data on "no-response" and "unknown" group is not shown here. All numerical data (except average age at onset) represent numbers of the patient with percentage (in the brackets) of total number of the patients in each group, 25 and 41, respectively, are shown.
THP, trihexyphenidyl; CLZ, clonazepam; BoNT, botulinum toxin injections.

The following case histories illustrate the clinical entity (see video in Additional file 1).

Patient 2: pure jaw deviation

A 72-year-old woman suffered a traumatic mandible fracture after a fall. Her jaw was wired shut for six weeks. On recovering from surgery, she immediately became aware of a change in the way her jaw felt. She noticed that her right molars were no longer contacting one another when she chewed; eating, chewing and speaking were difficult, and her jaw would move spontaneously to the left. She had no history of neuroleptic or anti-emetic exposure. She was not aware of any sensory tricks. Examination revealed mild jaw dystonia with leftward shift, mildly accentuated by speaking. There was no clear change with holding a plastic syringe between her teeth on either side. She was started on trihexyphenidyl 2 mg daily with titration to 2 mg twice a day. She had a very good sustained response even when decreasing the dose down to 2 mg/day.

Patient 17: pure lingual dystonia

A 57-year-old man developed involuntary movements of the tongue over a period of two years. He did not identify any sensory tricks, and there was no history of precipitating factors, neuroleptic or antiemetic exposure. Examination revealed mild protrusion and rotation of the tongue in a 90-degree clockwise fashion. Movements were not triggered by tasks, and indeed were absent when he spoke. We were not able to identify any sensory tricks such as placing a tongue depressor or a small plastic bite block between his teeth. He had been treated with botulinum toxin injections, without apparent benefit, and with clonazepam, with mild benefit at the dose of 3 mg/day. He was then started on trihexyphenidyl with a slow titration schedule up to 6 mg/day (in 3 divided doses) without either benefits or side effects. We increased the dose to 12 mg/day (in 3 divided doses). The response with this dose was unknown as further follow-up information was not available.

Patient 3: mixed dystonia

A 61-year-old woman underwent a maxillary bridge replacement four years prior to being seen. A temporary bridge was made and her mouth was open for two hours while this was fit. Since that time, she felt that her jaw alignment was incorrect, and she developed difficulty with her speech, jaw pain and clicking in her temporomandibular joints (TMJs). In the last year she noticed movements involving the tongue and jaw, initially limited to the task of speaking. Over time, movements spread to involve eating and chewing, sparing drinking. There was no history of neuroleptic or anti-emetic exposure. She saw a dentist and tried multiple oral devices without benefit. Examination revealed

a tendency of the jaw to open and push forward anteriorly at rest. When she spoke, movements were further activated causing mild dysarthria. Holding a piece of plastic between her teeth immediately improved her speaking. She was started on low dose trihexyphenidyl with slow titration to 2 mg three times daily without benefit. We then referred her for botulinum toxin injections.

Discussion

In this series, the largest of such patients reported, idiopathic LCrD was more common in women than men (2:1). This is similar to the pre-existing literature on LCrD and other forms of focal dystonia such as cervical dystonia (female/male; F/M ratio 1.2-1.92:1) [9-17], blepharospasm (F/M ratio 1.35-2:1) [9,18-20], spasmodic dysphonia (F/M ratio 1.35-15:1) [9,21-24], and oromandibular dystonia 3.28:1 [9], but opposite to what is seen in writer's cramp (F/M ratio of 1:2) [9]. Almost half of our patients had a mixed phenotype and the other half were simpler (pure). In the group with pure phenotype, the most common primary movement was jaw deviation, whereas jaw opening was the most common phenotype of mixed phenotype. Jaw protrusion, as well as tongue and pharyngeal dystonia was much less common.

Table 3 Practical guideline in evaluation of patients with LCrD

History

- Onset
- Description of the abnormal movement or sensation
- Precipitating factor (especially history of recent dental work or maxillofacial trauma) lower cranial
- Aggravating and relieving factors
- Associated symptoms such as pain, jaw clicking
- Sensory tricks
- History of previous treatment such as dental prosthesis
- History of secondary causes of dystonia especially dopamine receptor blocking agent exposure

Examination

- Identify the primary movement(s)
  o Jaw in each axis: opening/closing, lateral deviation (left/right), protrusion/retraction
  o Tongue: protrusion/retraction, torsion
- Determine task specificity (dystonia occurs with speaking, eating/chewing and/or at rest)
- Identify sensory tricks: light touch, placing objects such as plastic syringe or tongue depressor between teeth on each side and in the center
- Assess evidence of dystonia in other body parts especially in upper cranial region, voice and neck

Legend: Practical guideline in history taking and physical examination of patients with LCrD is described.

The anatomy and function of the jaw is unique. Embryologically the jaw muscles are derived from presomitic mesoderm of the first branchial arch [25], whereas limb muscles are derived from somites. The multiple functions of the jaw are complex as well. Chewing requires complex coordinated movements of various jaw muscles. Masticatory myosin is expressed in the jaw, and during evolution it is replaced with other types of myosin to tailor for eating habits or types of diet [26]. In humans jaw closing muscles contain rich muscle spindle innervation whereas jaw-opening muscles do not [27,28], possibly due to the strong proprioceptive input related to jaw closure for modifying bite strength. One possible reason for this is the evolutionary pressure that modifies the bite. For example, humans can modulate bite strength to match different consistencies of food, and many mammals and vertebrates must be able to exert tremendous force with the jaw to capture prey, but also modify their bite so as to gently carry their young. These unique features of the jaw muscles might explain the common and often robust sensory gestes observed in our patients.

Task specificity is a nearly universal feature of LCrD, and the most common triggering tasks were speaking, followed by eating or chewing. Often dystonia began with speaking, and then spread to eating or chewing. We did not observe other patterns of spread of dystonic tasks. Recent dental work or oral trauma may precipitate LCrD, as can manipulation of the facial bones, especially the maxilla and mandible. There may be a role of "osseoperception" [29,30]; afferent signal from periodontal mechanoreceptor is required in fine motor control of the mandible such as chewing or jaw closing. However, this concept can explain only some, but not all, patients such as in the ones who had tooth extraction as a precipitating event. In addition, it does not explain non-jaw related dystonia such as lingual dystonia after dental work.

3/4 of our patients possessed a geste antagoniste, and all of those had improvement of LCrD by holding an object between their teeth. Some improved when lightly holding the chin and jaw, and occasionally with imagination of the sensory trick. This feature is a key diagnostic aide, and the presence or absence of a sensory trick should be investigated in all such patients. The numbers are too small to support a clear relationship between the presence of a geste antagoniste and treatment response in our series. Of 9 patients with response to at least one treatment modality, six had at least one sensory trick, whereas 12 of 16 patients without treatment response did not have an identified sensory trick.

The most common treatment used in our patients was trihexyphenidyl, the response of which was more robust than the other modalities, but still disappointing. None of the patients had good response to baclofen or dental device in our series. Response to botulinum toxin injection

was less robust than in other series, for reasons that are not clear.

Conclusion

Idiopathic LCrD is often missed and institution of effective therapy is often delayed. The clinical features and natural history of LCrD are similar to other forms of focal dystonia.

We offer the following practical guidelines for clinicians who evaluate patients with LCrD. Table 3 illustrates clinical approach to patients with LCrD. The differential diagnoses of idiopathic LCrD includes other primary dystonia (such as primary segmental dystonia, Meige's syndrome), secondary dystonia (such as tardive dystonia from dopamine receptor blocking agents, infectious dystonia including anti-NMDA encephalitis), heredodegenerative dystonia (such as X-linked dystonia parkinsonism or Lubag's disease, neuroacanthocytosis, Lesch-Nyhan syndrome, SCA 8 [31], cerebrotendinous xanthomatosis) [32], and pseudodystonia. Pseudodystonia in the differential diagnoses of LCrD include Isaac's syndrome, tetanus, and musculoskeletal abnormalities such as Satoyoshi syndrome.

We hope that this paper will call attention to this entity, and aide dental professionals, general physicians and neurologists in securing the correct diagnosis.

Additional file

Additional file 1: Patient 2 demonstrates pure left jaw deviation, accentuated by speaking. Patient 3 demonstrates jaw-opening dystonia and mild jaw protrusion, more prominent when speaking. Dystonia improved when a plastic syringe is placed between her teeth. **Patient 23** has prominent left jaw deviation and mild jaw protrusion at rest. Dystonia improves when he places a plastic syringe between his teeth on the left, but not on the right, and holding firm pressure on the right cheek. **Patient 1** demonstrates jaw opening dystonia when chewing. **Patient 4** has jaw opening dystonia, worse when speaking and chewing. Whispering and singing are easier for her. Dystonia was mildly improved when holding a lower jaw. Dystonia and speech were markedly improved when placing a plastic syringe or a tongue depressor between her teeth. **Patient 5** shows severe jaw opening dystonia, triggered when she speaks. Dystonia is improved when holding bilateral jaw with her hands or an examiner's hands. **Patient 10** shows pure right jaw deviation, accentuated by speaking. Dystonia is improved when holding her lower jaw with a finger, and placing a plastic syringe between her teeth on the right and in front, but not on the left. **Patient 25** has mouth closure with slight jaw opening and protrusion when speaking, worse when praying. Dystonia is better when placing a tongue depressor between his teeth. Dystonia was also accentuated by chewing but to a lesser degree than speaking.

Abbreviations

BoNT: Botulinum toxin; F/M: Female/male; LCrD: Lower cranial dystonia; NBIA: Neurodegeneration with brain iron accumulation; NMDA: N-methyl-D-aspartate; SCA: Spinocerebellar ataxia; TMJ: Temporomandibular joint.

Competing interests

The authors declare that they have no competing interests.

Authors' contributions

PT contributed to data collection and analysis, as well as manuscript drafting and revision. DRT initially evaluated and referred some of the patients to SJF.

SJF contributed to study design and conceptualization, as well as manuscript drafting and revision. All authors read and approve the final manuscript.

References

1. Robertson-Hoffman DE, Mark MH, Sage JI: Isolated lingual/palatal dystonia. *Mov Disord* 1991, **6:**177–179.
2. Tan EK, Jankovic J: Tardive and idiopathic oromandibular dystonia: a clinical comparison. *J Neurol Neurosurg Psychiatry* 2000, **68:**186–190.
3. Singer C, Papapetropoulos S: A comparison of jaw-closing and jaw-opening idiopathic oromandibular dystonia. *Parkinsonism Relat Disord* 2006, **12:**115–118.
4. Lo SE, Gelb M, Frucht SJ: Geste antagonistes in idiopathic lower cranial dystonia. *Mov Disord* 2007, **22:**1012–1017.
5. Esper CD, Freeman A, Factor SA: Lingual protrusion dystonia: frequency, etiology and botulinum toxin therapy. *Parkinsonism Relat Disord* 2010, **16:**438–441.
6. Charous SJ, Comella CL, Fan W: Jaw-opening dystonia: quality of life after botulinum toxin injections. *Ear Nose Throat J* 2011, **90:**E9.
7. Costa AL, Campos LS, Franca MC Jr, D'Abreu A: Temporomandibular disorders in patients with craniocervical dystonia. *Arq Neuropsiquiatr* 2011, **69:**896–899.
8. Bakke M, Larsen BM, Dalager T, Moller E: Oromandibular dystonia–functional and clinical characteristics: a report on 21 cases. *Oral Surg Oral Med Oral Pathol Oral Radiol* 2013, **115:**e21–e26.
9. Soland VL, Bhatia KP, Marsden CD: Sex prevalence of focal dystonias. *J Neurol Neurosurg Psychiatry* 1996, **60:**204–205.
10. Friedman A, Fahn S: Spontaneous remissions in spasmodic torticollis. *Neurology* 1986, **36:**398–400.
11. Duane DD: Spasmodic torticollis: clinical and biologic features and their implications for focal dystonia. *Adv Neurol* 1988, **50:**473–492.
12. Jahanshahi M, Marion MH, Marsden CD: Natural history of adult-onset idiopathic torticollis. *Arch Neurol* 1990, **47:**548–552.
13. Jankovic J, Schwartz K: Botulinum toxin injections for cervical dystonia. *Neurology* 1990, **40:**277–280.
14. Chan J, Brin MF, Fahn S: Idiopathic cervical dystonia: clinical characteristics. *Mov Disord* 1991, **6:**119–126.
15. Jankovic J, Leder S, Warner D, Schwartz K: Cervical dystonia: clinical findings and associated movement disorders. *Neurology* 1991, **41:**1088–1091.
16. Deuschl G, Heinen F, Kleedorfer B, Wagner M, Lucking CH, Poewe W: Clinical and polymyographic investigation of spasmodic torticollis. *J Neurol* 1992, **239:**9–15.
17. Jamora RD, Tan AK, Tan LC: A 9-year review of dystonia from a movement disorders clinic in Singapore. *Eur J Neurol* 2006, **13:**77–81.
18. Cohen DA, Savino PJ, Stern MB, Hurtig HI: Botulinum injection therapy for blepharospasm: a review and report of 75 patients. *Clin Neuropharmacol* 1986, **9:**415–429.
19. Carruthers J, Stubbs HA: Botulinum toxin for benign essential blepharospasm, hemifacial spasm and age-related lower eyelid entropion. *Can J Neurol Sci* 1987, **14:**42–45.
20. Grandas F, Elston J, Quinn N, Marsden CD: Blepharospasm: a review of 264 patients. *J Neurol Neurosurg Psychiatry* 1988, **51:**767–772.
21. Jankovic J, Ford J: Blepharospasm and orofacial-cervical dystonia: clinical and pharmacological findings in 100 patients. *Ann Neurol* 1983, **13:**402–411.
22. Ludlow CL, Naunton RF, Sedory SE, Schulz GM, Hallett M: Effects of botulinum toxin injections on speech in adductor spasmodic dysphonia. *Neurology* 1988, **38:**1220–1225.
23. Rosenfield DB: Spasmodic dysphonia. *Adv Neurol* 1988, **50:**537–545.
24. Blitzer A, Brin MF, Fahn S, Lovelace RE: Clinical and laboratory characteristics of focal laryngeal dystonia: study of 110 cases. *Laryngoscope* 1988, **98:**636–640.
25. Noden DM: The embryonic origins of avian cephalic and cervical muscles and associated connective tissues. *Am J Anat* 1983, **168:**257–276.
26. Hoh JF: 'Superfast' or masticatory myosin and the evolution of jaw-closing muscles of vertebrates. *J Exp Biol* 2002, **205:**2203–2210.
27. Lennartsson B: Muscle spindles in the human anterior digastric muscle. *Acta Odontol Scand* 1979, **37:**329–333.
28. Kubota K, Masegi T: Muscle spindle supply to the human jaw muscle. *J Dent Res* 1977, **56:**901–909.
29. Trulsson M: Sensory and motor function of teeth and dental implants: a basis for osseoperception. *Clin Exp Pharmacol Physiol* 2005, **32:**119–122.
30. Klineberg I, Murray G: Osseoperception: sensory function and proprioception. *Adv Dent Res* 1999, **13:**120–129.
31. Ushe M, Perlmutter JS: Oromandibular and lingual dystonia associated with spinocerebellar ataxia type 8. *Mov Disord* 2012, **27:**1741–1742.
32. Alcalay R, Wu S, Patel S, Frucht S: Oromandibular dystonia as a complication of cerebrotendinous xanthomatosis. *Mov Disord* 2009, **24:**1397–1399.

12

Postural deformities in Parkinson's disease – Mutual relationships among neck flexion, fore-bent, knee-bent and lateral-bent angles and correlations with clinical predictors

Fumihito Yoshii[*], Yusuke Moriya, Tomohide Ohnuki, Masafuchi Ryo and Wakoh Takahashi

Abstract

Background: Various postural deformities appear during progression of Parkinson's disease (PD), but the underlying pathophysiology of these deformities is not well understood. The angle abnormalities seen in individual patients may not be due to distinct causes, but rather they may have occurred in an interrelated manner to maintain a balanced posture.

Methods: We measured the neck flexion (NF), fore-bent (FB), knee-bent (KB) and lateral-bent (LB) angles in 120 PD patients, and examined their mutual relationships, and correlations with clinical predictors such as sex, age, disease duration, Hoehn and Yahr (H&Y) stage, medication dose (levodopa equivalent dose, LED; total dose of dopamine agonists, DDA). The relationship between the side of the initial symptoms and the direction of LB angle was also investigated.

Results: Our main findings were: (1) Significant relationships between NF and KB, NF and LB, FB and KB, KB and LB were observed. (2) NF angle was larger in males than in females, but FB, KB and LB angles showed no significant difference between the sexes. (3) FB and KB angles became larger with advancing age. (4) NF and FB angles were associated with disease duration. (5) NF, FB, KB and LB angles all increased significantly with increase of H&Y stage. (6) FB angle was significantly associated with LED, but DDA did not show a significant relationship with any of the measured angles. (7) Direction of LB angle was not associated with the side of initial symptoms.

Conclusions: Postural abnormalities are interrelated, possibly to maintain a balanced posture.

Keywords: Parkinson's disease, Postural deformity, Hoehn and Yahr (H&Y) stage, Levodopa equivalent dose, Mutual correlations, Balance

Background

Postural deformities are frequent and disabling complications of Parkinson's disease (PD) and interfere with daily living activities, often leading to falls. These deformities include antecollis (dropped head), camptocormia (stooped or bent posture; marked bending of the thoraco-lumbar spine), and lateral flexion (Pisa syndrome) [1]. In addition, knee flexion is often observed.

Although various types of postural deformities have been reported in patients with PD, the underlying pathophysiology of these deformities is not well understood and a number of different causes have been proposed. However, the angle abnormalities seen in individual patients may not be due to distinct causes, but rather they may have occurred in an interrelated manner to maintain a balanced posture. For example, combinations of deformities, such as dropped head and lateral flexion, are often observed simultaneously. Here, we measured the neck flexion (NF), fore-bent (FB), knee-bent (KB)

* Correspondence: yoshii@is.icc.u-tokai.ac.jp
Department of Neurology, Tokai University Oiso Hospital, 21-1 Gakkyou, Oiso, Naka-gun, Kanagawa 259-0198, Japan

and lateral-bent (LB) angles in 120 PD patients, in order to establish their mutual relationships. We also examined the relationships of these angles to several clinical predictors, such as sex, age, disease duration, disease severity, and dose of medicine, in order to clarify possible contributory pathophysiological mechanisms.

Methods

Subjects

We enrolled 120 patients (age: 41–88 years old, average: 67 ± 10 years old) with PD who were able to maintain a standing position without assistance (66 males, age 41–87 years, average 66 ± 11 years; 54 females, age 43–88 years, average: 68 ± 8 years). A diagnosis of PD was made according to the United Kingdom Parkinson's Disease Society Brain Bank Clinical Diagnostic Criteria. Disease duration was 0–21 years (8.2 ± 5.1 years). Hoehn & Yahr's severity scale "on stage" (H&Y stage) was 2.7 ± 0.8. Information about the laterality of the initial symptom at onset was extracted from clinical records. Brain magnetic resonance imaging (MRI) was performed in all individuals to rule out multiple system atrophy (MSA) [2] or progressive supranuclear palsy (PSP) [3], which frequently show similar postural deformities. Comorbid orthopedic spinal lesions (compression fracture of the vertebrae, disc hernia, or spondylolisthesis of the vertebrae) were diagnosed on anteroposterior and lateral views of cervical, thoracic and lumbar spinal X-ray pictures and five patients with prominent spinal bone disorders were excluded prior to enrollment into the study. Patients who had undergone deep brain stimulation were also excluded, because DBS is used for amelioration of postural deformities in PD [4], and we

wished to focus on the intrinsic postural characteristics of PD.

The study was approved by Tokai University Review Board, and all eligible individuals were informed of the purpose and methods of the study. All of them provided written informed consent.

Measurement of NF, FB, KB and LB angles

In the present study, four body angles, i.e., neck flexion (NF), fore-bent (FB), knee-bent (KB) and lateral-bent (LB) angles, were defined with reference to the report of Oeda et al. [5]. NF, FB, KB and LB angles were measured on photographs of the lateral and back views of the patients in an upright position (in an "on" period if the patients had motor fluctuations). In lateral view photographs, the angle between two intersecting lines — the line connecting the external acoustic foramen and the acromion, and the line connecting the acromion and the greater trochanter—was defined as the NF angle. Similarly, FB angle was defined as the angle between the line connecting the acromion and the greater trochanter, and a vertical line. KB angle was defined as the angle between the line connecting the greater trochanter and knee, and the line connecting knee and lateral malleolus. In back view photographs, the angle between the line connecting the posterior process of the seventh cervical vertebra and that of the fifth lumbar vertebra, and a vertical line was defined as the LB angle (Fig. 1). NF and FB angles toward flexion and extension were expressed as positive and negative values, respectively, and LB angle was shown as an absolute value, because bending toward the left or right sides appears to occur by chance.

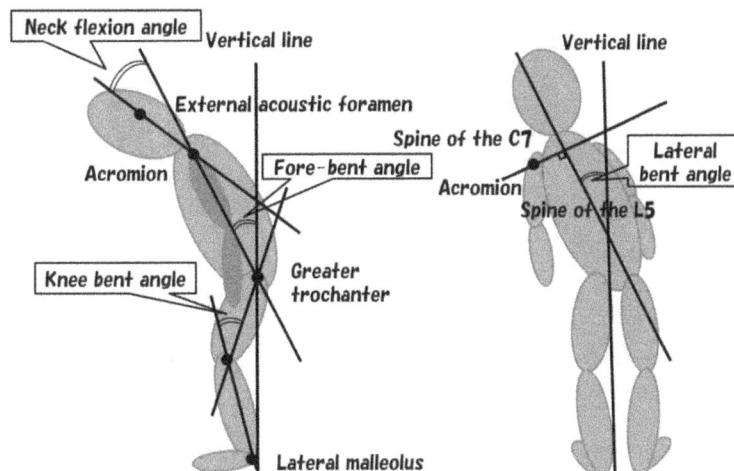

Fig. 1 Schematic representation of body angles. In lateral view photographs (left), NF (neck flexion) angle was defined as the angle between two intersecting lines: a line connecting the external acoustic foramen and the acromion, and another line connecting the acromion and the greater trochanter. Similarly, FB (fore-bent) angle was defined as the angle between a vertical line and the line connecting the acromion with the greater trochanter. KB (knee-bent) angle was defined as the angle between the line connecting the greater trochanter and knee, and the line connecting knee and lateral malleolus. In back view photographs (right), LB (lateral-bent) angle was defined as the angle between a vertical line and the line connecting the posterior process of the seventh cervical vertebra with that of the fifth lumbar vertebra

Data collection

Clinical data including sex, age, disease duration, H&Y stage, medication dose (levodopa equivalent dose, LED; total dose of dopamine agonists, DDA) and side of initial (prominent) parkinsonian symptoms (right or left) were collected as potential predictors of abnormal posture.

Daily doses of levodopa, dopamine agonists, selegiline entacapone and amantadine at study entry were also recorded. The LED was calculated according to the formula: LED (mg) = levodopa (mg) + pramipexole (mg) × 100 + ropinirole (mg) × 25 + pergolide (µg) × 0.1 + cabergoline (mg) × 67 + bromocriptine (mg) × 10. For patients treated with selegiline, their levodopa dose was multiplied by 1.30, and for those taking entacapone, by 1.25. The DDA was calculated according to the formula: pramipexole (mg) × 100 + ropinirole (mg) × 25 + pergolide (µg) × 0.1 + cabergoline (mg) × 67 + bromocriptine (mg) × 10.

Statistical analysis

Differences of NF, FB, KB and LB angles between male and female PD patients were compared using the Mann–Whitney U test. Correlations of the angles with age, disease duration, H&Y stage (on) and medication dose (LED, DDA) were examined using Spearman's rank correlation coefficients. The relationship between onset side and LB was examined with the Mann–Whitney U test. Mutual relationships of NF, FB, KB and LB angles were investigated using Spearman's rank correlation coefficients. We confirmed that the population was not

normally distributed by use of the Kolmogorov-Smimov test before running non-parametric tests. A value of $p < 0.05$ was considered statistically significant. Statistical analyses were performed using the SPSS-21 software package (IBM).

Results

Body angles in PD patients

NF, FB, KB and LB angles in male and female patients with PD are shown in Fig. 2. We found that age (male: 66 ± 11 years old, female: 68 ± 8 years old), disease duration (male: 7.8 ± 4.7 years, female: 8.6 ± 5.4 years), H&Y stage (male: 2.8 ± 0.8, female: 2.7 ± 0.7) and LED (male: 501 ± 253 mg, female: 436 ± 233 mg) were not significantly different between genders. NF angle for males (27.6 ± 11.8) was significantly greater than in females (22.9 ± 14.9) ($p = 0.01$). However, other angles were not significantly different between males and females (FB: 5.4 ± 11.6 and 2.2 ± 6.7, KB: 17.7 ± 7.7 and 19.6 ± 10.2, LB: 2.7 ± 3.9 and 3.5 ± 3.4, respectively).

Effects of age, disease duration, H&Y stage and LED

Correlations between NF, FB, KB, LB angles and clinical predictors (age, disease duration, H&Y stage and LED) are shown in Table 1.

FB ($r = 0.246$, $p < 0.01$) and KB ($r = 0.359$, $p < 0.001$) angles increased significantly with advancing age. Further, NF ($r = 0.197$, $p < 0.05$) and FB ($r = 0.196$, $p < 0.05$) angles were significantly associated with disease duration. All the

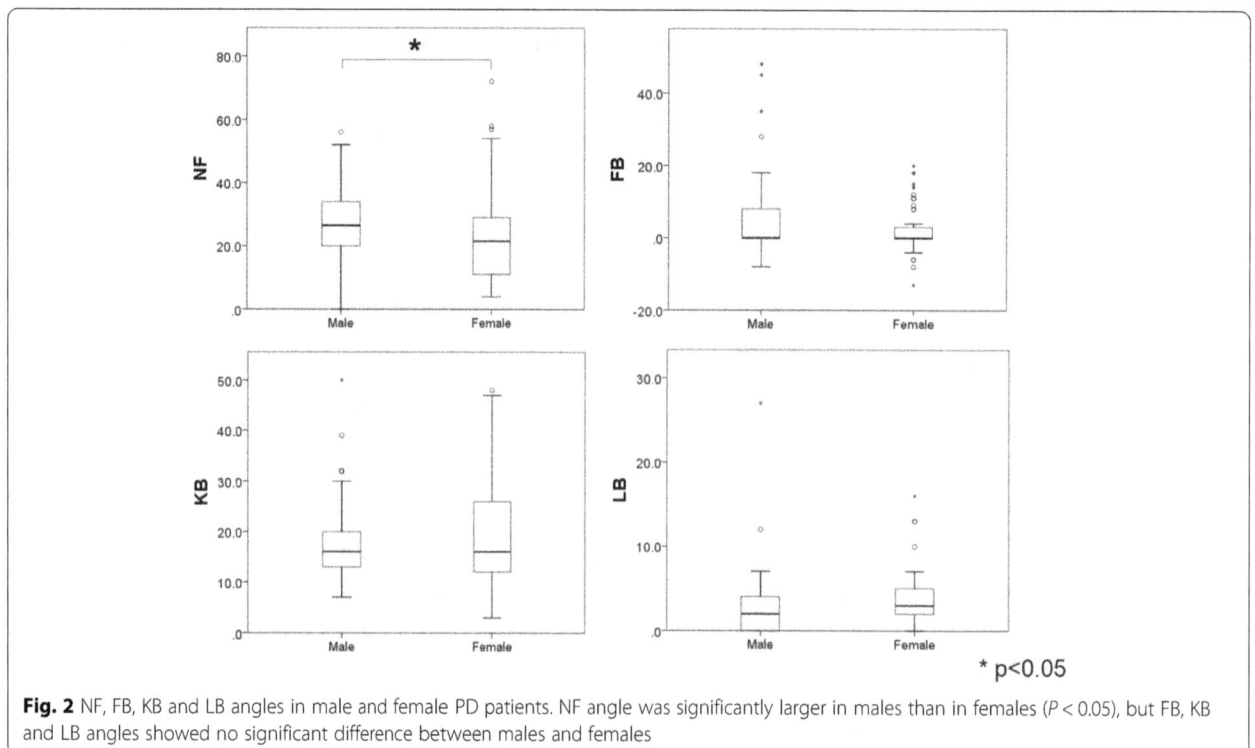

Fig. 2 NF, FB, KB and LB angles in male and female PD patients. NF angle was significantly larger in males than in females ($P < 0.05$), but FB, KB and LB angles showed no significant difference between males and females

Table 1 Correlation coefficients between NF, FB, KB, LB angles and clinical predictors

	Age	Disease Duration	H&Y stage	LED
NF	0.175	0.197 *	0.350 ***	0.135
FB	0.246 **	0.196 *	0.492 ***	0.243 **
KB	0.359 ***	0.098	0.381 ***	0.111
LB	0.162	0.103	0.213 *	0.173

FB and KB angles increased significantly with advancing age. NF and FB angles were significantly associated with disease duration. All the measured angles increased significantly with advancing H&Y stage. There was a significant association between LED and FB, but not the other angles
$^*P < 0.05$, $^{**}P < 0.01$, $^{***}P < 0.001$

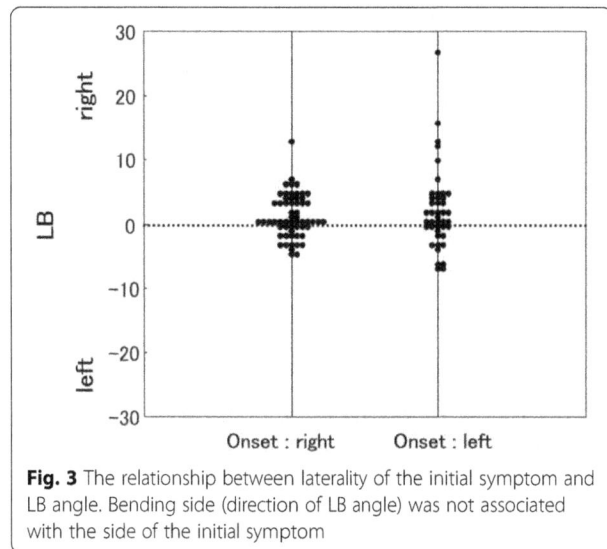

Fig. 3 The relationship between laterality of the initial symptom and LB angle. Bending side (direction of LB angle) was not associated with the side of the initial symptom

measured angles increased significantly with advancing H&Y stage: NF ($r = 0.350$, $p < 0.001$), FB ($r = 0.492$, $p < 0.001$), KB ($r = 0.381$, $p < 0.001$) and LB ($r = 0.213$, $p < 0.05$). Finally, there was a significant association between LED and FB ($r = 0.243$, $p < 0.01$), but not the other angles. DDA showed no significant relationship with any of the measured angles. Mean values of LED and DDA were 472 ± 248 mg/day and 123 ± 120 mg/day, respectively.

Multiple regression analysis was performed to assess the relationships among these four predictors as explanatory variables and each angle as a categorical response variable. H&Y stage was the most explanatory variable for NF (partial regression coefficient (B) = 6.578, $p < 0.001$), FB (B = 5.976, $p < 0.001$) and KB (B = 5.614, $p < 0.001$), while LED was the most explanatory variable for LB (B = 0.004, $p = 0.002$).

Laterality of initial symptom and LB angle
The relationship between laterality of the initial symptom and LB angle was examined. For 59 patients, the initial symptom was on the right side and for 43 patients, it was on the left (almost symmetrical 15, unknown 3). Bending side (direction of LB angle) was not associated with the side of the initial symptom (Fig. 3).

Mutual relationships among measured angles
Table 2 shows the relationships among the measured angles. NF and KB ($r = 0.275$, $p < 0.01$), NF and LB ($r = 0.250$, $p < 0.01$), FB and KB ($r = 0.335$, $p < 0.001$), KB and LB ($r = 0.225$, $p < 0.05$) were significantly positively correlated.

We also examined the relationships among the measured angles separately by age or gender, and the results are shown in Tables 3 and 4. When subjects were divided into a younger group (age less than 70 years old; $n = 57$) and an older group (age over 70 years old; $n = 63$), significant correlations were found only in the older group, between NF and LB ($r = 0.269$, $p < 0.05$) and between FB and KB ($r = 0.375$, $r < 0.01$). As to gender, different trends were found in men ($n = 66$) and women

($n = 54$), but significant correlations were seen between NF and LB and between FB and KB in both sexes.

Discussion
Postural deformities are frequent complications in PD: 5–6 % for dropped head (antecollis), 3–17.6 % for camptocormia and 8.5–60 % for lateral flexion (Pisa syndrome) [1]. However, frequency of knee flexion has not been reported. In general, epidemiological studies suggest that the prevalence of antecollis or camptocormia might be higher in Asian patients. As to the pathogenesis of these deformities, axial dystonia, muscle rigidity and myopathy have been suggested for camptocormia, and dopaminergic drugs may be associated with dropped head. However, the precise mechanisms have not been elucidated, although myopathy, skeletal and soft tissue changes have been proposed as peripheral processes. Furthermore, it is not clear whether each postural abnormality occurs independently, or whether the abnormalities occur in association at the same time.

We found that the NF angle was significantly larger in males than in females. Although Kashihara et al. found no gender effect on neck flexion (dropped head) [6], the NF angle of males has been reported to be greater than

Table 2 Mutual correlation coefficients among the measured angles (All)

	FB	KB	LB
NF	0.166	0.275 **	0.250 **
FB		0.335 ***	0.141
KB			0.225 *

NF and KB, NF and LB, FB and KB, KB and LB were significantly positively correlated. FB (camptocormia) showed a particularly strong correlation with KB (bending of the knee)
$^*P < 0.05$, $^{**}P < 0.01$, $^{***}P < 0.001$

Table 3 Mutual correlation coefficients among the measured angles (By age)

<70 years old (n = 57)	FB	KB	LB
NF	0.111	0.241	0.199
FB		0.234	0.070
KB			0.163
≧70 years old (n = 63)	FB	KB	LB
NF	0.166	0.245	0.269 *
FB		0.375 **	0.137
KB			0.190

Significant correlations were found only in the older group, between NF and LB, and between FB and KB

*P < 0.05, **P < 0.01

that of females even in normal healthy individuals [5]. In general, the development of PD symptoms in women may be delayed by higher physiological levels of striatal dopamine, possibly due to the activity of estrogens, as indicated by a SPECT imaging study using ^{123}I-FR-CIT tracer [7]. Milder motor deterioration or striatal degeneration suggests a more benign phenotype in women, and may be related to the gender difference of NF. We did not check MMSE (Mini-Mental State Examination) score, but another possibility is that men have more cognitive impairment [7], which also influences postural deformities [8]. On the other hand, no consistent trends concerning gender difference of camptocormia were found in previous studies [5, 6, 9, 10], as well as our study, suggesting that some other etiology, such as dystonia, rigidity or comorbid orthopedic spinal lesions, might be implicated in camptocormia.

Previous studies have identified many clinical parameters such as age [8, 10], disease duration [8], LED [10],

Table 4 Mutual correlation coefficients among the measured angles (By gender)

Male (n = 66)	FB	KB	LB
NF	0.271 *	0.228	0.305 *
FB		0.402 ***	0.222
KB			0.078
Female (n = 54)	FB	KB	LB
NF	−0.011	0.359 **	0.286 *
FB		0.295 *	0.095
KB			0.381 **

Significant correlations were found between NF and LB and between FB and KB in both sexes

*P < 0.05, **P < 0.01, ***P < 0.001

H&Y stage [8, 10], UPDRS (Unified Parkinson's Disease Rating Scale)-3 [5, 8, 10], MMSE scores [8], autonomic dysfunction [10], and history of vertebral surgery [5, 8] as risk factors for postural deformities. Most reports show a positive association between camptocormia and aging or disease severity. Tiple et al. [8] studied 275 consecutive PD patients and found that disease severity assessed by H&Y staging score or UPDRS part 3 score, levodopa dose and dementia (DSM-4) were associated with camptocormia. Kashihara et al. [6] reported that advancing age and disease severity may be the major risks for developing postural disorders. Seki et al. [10] showed that camptocormia had significant associations with aging, more severe motor symptoms, higher L-dopa daily dose and autonomic symptoms (severe constipation, urinary incontinence). In the study by Oeda [5], NF angle was associated only with H&Y stage ≥3. Our study revealed significant relationships of age with FB and KB angles, disease duration with NF and FB angles, H&Y stage with all of the measured angles, and LED with FB angle. Multiple regression analysis showed that H&Y staging was the most explanatory variable for NF, FB and KB angles, whereas LED was the most explanatory variable for LB angle.

Recent reports have drawn attention to a possible role of medication-induced changes in posture, particularly for dropped head. In particular, dopamine agonists can induce or aggravate abnormal posture [11, 12]. In our study, multiple regression analysis showed that LED had the greatest effect on LB angle, though DDA was not related to any of the measured angles. Although the dose of the drug is likely to parallel the severity of disease, we believe that there may be a need to consider the LED effect on LB. However, most cases of drug-induced postural changes have been reported from Japan, and this might suggest the involvement of a genetic difference in the expression of drug-metabolizing enzymes and/or transporters. In our study, we excluded patients who were considered to show postural changes potentially related to dopamine agonist treatment.

There has been debate about whether patients with lateral trunk flexion lean towards or away from the side with more prominent parkinsonian symptoms. Most investigators have found that patients tend to lean away from the most affected side. Although the number of subjects in the present study may be insufficient to allow a definitive conclusion, we found no association of LB angle with onset side (prominent parkinsonian symptom side), suggesting that lateral shift of the body in PD is not related to left-right difference of dopamine in the brain. The tilt to the side is thought not to be due to extrapyramidal symptoms such as axial rigidity or dystonia, but is believed to reflect impaired perception of the vertical position [13].

Although angle changes were associated with aging, increased disease severity, etc., it should be considered that they may occur in a compensatory manner in order to maintain postural stability. For example, when camptocormia becomes severe, the neck is flexed less because of compensatory hyperextension to obtain a normal visual field. In the present study, significant correlations were observed between NF and KB, NF and LB, FB and KB, and KB and LB. FB (camptocormia) showed a particularly strong correlation with KB (bending of the knee), suggesting that knee bending may serve to counteract a forward-inclined posture so as to prevent falling. We found that the correlations of the angles varied with age and gender. Significant correlations between NF and LB, and between FB and KB were seen only in the older group (Table 3). These results are consistent with the finding that significant aging-related changes of FB and KB angles occur in PD (Table 1). Interestingly, we found correlations between NF and LB and between FB and KB in both men and women, but other significant correlation found in women were not observed in men (Table 4). The reason for this is not clear, but may be related in part to the gender difference of aging-related motor deterioration [14].

Postural control is a complex system involving integration of sensory information (vestibular, visual and proprioceptive). Proprioception provides highly accurate information that helps to hold the body vertically in healthy people. Many studies have confirmed that proprioceptive function is abnormal in PD [15]. Proprioceptive defects affect axial motor or postural control in the sagittal and coronal planes, which makes turning movements difficult and may eventually lead to a fall or injury.

Abnormal postures often interfere with the daily life activities of PD patients and have many negative consequences. NF may cause difficulty in swallowing, excessive drooling or restricted vision. FB can cause of anorexia through pressure on the stomach or a sensation of tightening in the abdomen. Also, patients might complain of shortness of breath due to restricted lung capacity [16]. Seki et al. reported that FB may cause severe constipation and urinary frequency [10]. A recent study by Yamane et al. [17] showed that PD patients with FB and KB frequently have deep venous thrombosis of their lower extremities. With LB, patient can develop lumbar pain, dyspnea, unsteadiness leading to falls, or lower leg numbness due to radiculopathy.

Conclusion

Various postural abnormalities occur in patients with Parkinson's disease, and are influenced by gender, age, disease severity, anti-Parkinson drugs, and other factors. However, these postural abnormalities do not occur independently, but are interrelated. Thus, from the viewpoint of the underlying pathophysiology, early detection and management, e.g., by physiotherapy, of one mild deformity could help to prevent or at least delay exacerbation of postural abnormalities.

Abbreviations

PD: Parkinson's disease; H&Y stage: Hoehn & Yahr's stage; NF: Neck flexion; FB: Fore-bent; KB: Knee-bent; LB: Lateral-bent; LED: Levodopa equivalent dose; DDA: Total dose of dopamine agonists; MSA: Multiple system atrophy; PSP: Progressive supranuclear palsy; MMSE: Mini-Mental State Examination; UPDRS: Unified Parkinson's Disease Rating Scale.

Competing interests

The authors declare that they have no competing interest, and no funding was provided for this study.

Authors' contributions

FY designed and conducted the study, collected, analyzed and interpreted the data, and drafted the paper. YM, TO, MR and WT recruited the patients and interpreted the data. All authors read and approved the final manuscript.

Acknowledgements

We thank Saori Kohara and Isa Yoshinari at the Department of Neurology, Tokai University School of Medicine for their support in statistical analysis and technical assistance.

References

1. Doherty KM, van de Warrenburg BP, Peralta MC, Silveira-Moriyama L, Azulay JP, Gershanik OS, et al. Postural deformities in Parkinson's disease. Lancet Neurol. 2011;10:538–49.
2. Sławek J, Derejko M, Lass P, Dubaniewicz M. Camptocormia or Pisa syndrome in multiple system atrophy. Clin Neurol Neurosurg. 2006;108:699–704.
3. Solla P, Cannas A, Costantino E, Orofino G, Lavra L, Marrosu F. Pisa syndrome in a patient with progressive supranuclear palsy. J Clin Neurosci. 2012;19:922–3.
4. Umemura A, Oka Y, Ohkita K, Yamawaki T, Yamada K. Effect of subthalamic deep brain stimulation on postural abnormality in Parkinson disease. J Neurosurg. 2012;112:1283–8.
5. Oeda T, Umemura A, Tomita S, Hayashi R, Kohsaka M, Sawada H. Clinical factors associated with abnormal postures in Parkinson's disease. PLoS One. 2013. doi:10.1371/journal.pone.0073547.
6. Kashihara K, Imamura T. Clinical correlates of anterior and lateral flexion of the thoracolumbar spine and dropped head in patients with Parkinson's disease. Parkinsonism Relat Disord. 2012;18:290–3.
7. Miller IN, Cronin-Golomb A. Gender differences in Parkinson's disease: clinical characteristics and cognition. Mov Disord. 2010;25:2695–703.
8. Tiple D, Fabbrini G, Colosimo C, Ottaviani D, Camerota F, Defazio G, et al. Camptocormia in Parkinson disease: an epidemiological and clinical study. J Neurol Neurosurg Psychiatry. 2009;80:145–8.
9. Lepoutre AC, Devos D, Blanchard-Dauphin A, Pardessus V, Maurage CA, Ferriby D, et al. A specific clinical pattern of camptocormia in Parkinson's disease. J Neurol Neurosurg Psychiatry. 2006;77:1229–34.
10. Seki M, Takahashi K, Koto A, Mihara B, Morita Y, Isozumi K, et al. Keio Parkinson's Disease Database. Camptocormia in Japanese patients with Parkinson's disease: a multicenter study. Mov Disord. 2011;26:2567–71.
11. Suzuki M, Hirai T, Ito Y, Sakamoto T, Oka H, Kurita A, et al. Pramipexole-induced antecollis in Parkinson's disease. J Neurol Sci. 2008;264:195–7.
12. Uzawa A, Mori M, Kojima S, Mitsuma S, Sekiguchi Y, Kanesaka T, et al. Dopamine agonist-induced antecollis in Parkinson's disease. Mov Disord. 2009;24:2408–11. doi:10.1002/mds.22779.

13. Vaugoyeau M, Azulay JP. Role of sensory information in the control of postural orientation in Parkinson's disease. J Neurol Sci. 2010;289:66–8.

14. Haaxma CA, Bloem BR, Borm GF, Oyen WJ, Leenders KL, Eshuis S, et al. Gender differences in Parkinson's disease. J Neurol Neurosurg Psychiatry. 2007;78:819–24.

15. Carpenter MG, Bloem BR. Postural control in Parkinson patients: a proprioceptive problem? Exp Neurol. 2011;227:26–30.

16. Marinelli P, Colosimo C, Ferrazza AM, Di Stasio F, Fabbrini G, Palange P, et al. Effect of camptocormia on lung volumes in Parkinson's disease. Respir Physiol Neurobiol. 2013;187:164–6.

17. Yamane K, Kimura F, Unoda K, Hosokawa T, Hirose T, Tani H, et al. Postural abnormality as a risk marker for leg deep venous thrombosis in Parkinson's disease. PLoS One. 2013;8:e66984. doi:10.1371/journal.pone.0066984.

13

Repetitive finger movement performance differs among Parkinson's disease, Progressive Supranuclear Palsy, and spinocerebellar ataxia

Elizabeth L Stegemöller[1,2,3]*, Jennifer Uzochukwu[1], Mark D Tillman[2,4], Nikolaus R McFarland[3], SH Subramony[3], Michael S Okun[3] and Chris J Hass[2,3]

Abstract

Background: Differentiating movement disorders is critical for appropriate treatment, prognosis, and for clinical trials. In clinical trials this is especially important as effects can be diluted by inclusion of inappropriately diagnosed participants. In early disease duration phases, disorders often have overlapping clinical features, such as impairments in repetitive finger movement, making diagnosis challenging. The purpose of this pilot study was to examine and compare repetitive finger movement performance in participants diagnosed with idiopathic Parkinson's disease, Progressive Supranuclear Palsy, and spinocerebellar ataxias.

Methods: Participants completed an unconstrained index finger flexion/extension movement (i.e. finger tap) in time with an incremental acoustic tone. Measures of movement rate, movement amplitude, and coefficient of variation were compared among groups.

Results: Significant differences between groups were revealed for movement rate at faster tone rates. Participants with Parkinson's disease tended to tap faster than the tone rate while participants with Progressive Supranuclear Palsy and spinocerebellar ataxia tended to tap slower. No significant differences were revealed for movement amplitude, but participants with spinocerebellar ataxia demonstrated greater variance in amplitude than participants with Parkinson's disease.

Conclusion: Quantitative analysis of repetitive finger movement performance at faster rates may be helpful to differentiate Parkinson's Disease, Progressive Supranuclear Palsy and spinocerebellar ataxia.

Keywords: Finger tapping, Movement disorders, Movement rate, Movement amplitude, Coefficient of variation

Background

While Parkinson's disease (PD) is among one of the most common movement disorders, many other neurodegenerative syndromes display parkinsonian features and can present with similar deficits making accurate diagnosis challenging. Differentiation of other movement disorders from idiopathic PD is critical not only for appropriate treatment and prognosis, but also for clinical trials in which effects can be diluted by inclusion of inappropriately diagnosed subjects. As impaired control of

repetitive finger movements can significantly impact the performance of daily living activities, such as writing and buttoning clothing in these patients, the performance of repetitive finger movements is a clinical tool used to assess severity, progression, and treatment efficacy of various movement disorders. Thus, the purpose of this study was to examine and compare repetitive finger movement performance among three different movement disorders that present with similar deficits in repetitive finger movement performance: idiopathic PD, Progressive Supranuclear Palsy (PSP), and spinocerebellar ataxias (SCA).

While persons with PD, PSP, and SCA may present with similar clinical deficits in repetitive finger movement performance, the etiology of these movement disorders

* Correspondence: esteg@iastate.edu
[1]Department of Kinesiology, Iowa State University, 235 Forker, Ames, IA 50011, USA
[2]Department of Applied Physiology and Kinesiology, University of Florida, Gainesville, USA
Full list of author information is available at the end of the article

differs. In general, PD is attributed to the loss of neurons in the basal ganglia [1], while SCA is attributed to the loss of neurons in the cerebellum [2]. PSP is attributed to a loss of neurons in the basal ganglia, brain stem, and cerebellum [3]. However, many other brain areas are impacted by these diseases, and changes in movement performance cannot not be solely attributed to a loss of neurons in one region of the brain [2-4]. In any case, the differing etiology may contribute to differences in repetitive finger movement performance when quantitatively evaluated.

Previous research has revealed that persons with PD demonstrate impairments in repetitive finger movements at tone rates near to and above 2 Hertz (Hz) (i.e. 2 beats per second) compared to healthy control participants [5-8]. Impairments in repetitive finger movement performance at tone rates near to and above 2 Hz were not improved with dopaminergic medication [5]. However, differential effects of deep brain stimulation of the subthalamic nucleus (STN-DBS) on movement rate and movement amplitude were revealed [7]. Specifically, STN-DBS improved movement amplitude but not movement rate at tone rates near to and above 2 Hz. This would suggest that other non-dopaminergic mechanisms may mediate the impairments of repetitive finger movements that emerge at tone rates near to and above 2 Hz and may attribute to the clinical similarity of repetitive finger movements in persons with PD, PSP, and SCA.

Research is limited regarding repetitive finger movement performance in persons with PSP and SCA. One study has examined differences in repetitive finger movement performance between participants with PD and PSP [9]. Ling and colleagues [9] revealed that the performance of repetitive finger movements as big and fast as possible can distinguish between these two movement disorders. It is unclear if there are differences in repetitive finger movement performance over a range of movement rates between participants with PD and PSP. Many persons with SCA also present with or include parkinsonian features, which can be confused with PD [10]. Yet, research examining differences in repetitive finger movement performance between participants with PD and SCA is limited. Only one study has compared repetitive finger movement performance at rates above and below 2 Hz in persons with PD and spinocerebellar degeneration [11]. Kosaka and colleagues [11] revealed that performance differed between these two groups, suggesting that the cerebellum may play a role in the differential response. Research examining differences in repetitive finger movement performance in persons with PSP and SCA is limited.

Using the same paradigm in which the tone rate is systematically presented from low rates (i.e. 1 Hz) to high rates (i.e. 3 Hz), this study examined the differences in repetitive finger movement performance between participants with PD, PSP, and SCA across multiple tone rates.

Given that 1) persons with PD, PSP, and SCA demonstrate similar clinical deficits in repetitive finger movement performance and 2) impairments in repetitive finger movements that emerge at rates near to and above in persons with PD do not improve with dopaminergic medication suggesting the involvement of non-dopaminergic mechanisms, we hypothesized that participants with PSP and SCA would also demonstrate changes in repetitive finger movement performance at tone rates near to and above 2 Hz. However, we also hypothesize that given the differing pathophysiological mechanisms of each movement disorder, the changes in repetitive finger movement performance at tone rates near to and above 2 Hz would differ among participants with PD, PSP, and SCA.

Methods
Participants
Nineteen participants with PD (16 male/3 female; mean age = 72 ± 9 years; 18 right handed/1 left handed; disease duration = 6 ± 4 years), 10 participants with PSP (3 male/7 female; mean age = 70 ± 4 years; 10 right handed; disease duration = 5 ± 4 years), and 12 participants with SCA (5 male/7 female; mean age = 50 ± 17 years; 10 right handed/2 left handed; disease duration = 7 ± 7 years) were recruited from the University of Florida Center for Movement Disorders and Neurorestoration in Gainesville, Florida. The UPDRS motor scores for the PD and PSP group tested off medication were 29 ± 12 and 43 ± 11 respectively. For the SCA group, two patients were diagnosed with SCA1, two with SCA2, three with SCA3, one with SCA6, one with SCA8, one with sporadic ataxia (onset after 50 years of age), and one with ataxia not otherwise specified. Diagnosis was confirmed by a fellowship-trained movement disorders neurologist. All participants were tested on medication as previous research demonstrated that the impairments in movement performance using the same task as in this study were not significantly affected by optimal medication [5]. No dyskinesias were noted during data collection. Participants with PD were tested on the most affected side (13 right side/6 left side) and participants with SCA and PSP were tested on the dominant side. All participants gave their written informed consent prior to inclusion into the study, and the University of Florida Institutional Review Board approved the procedures.

Data collection
All participants completed three trials of an unconstrained finger flexion-extension movement (i.e. finger tap) in time with a series of acoustic tones presented at 1 Hz for 15 intervals and then increased by 0.25 Hz every 15 intervals until reaching 3 Hz [5-7] (Figure 1). The forearm (placed in a pronated position), wrist, thumb, and fingers 2–4 were supported by a brace. The index

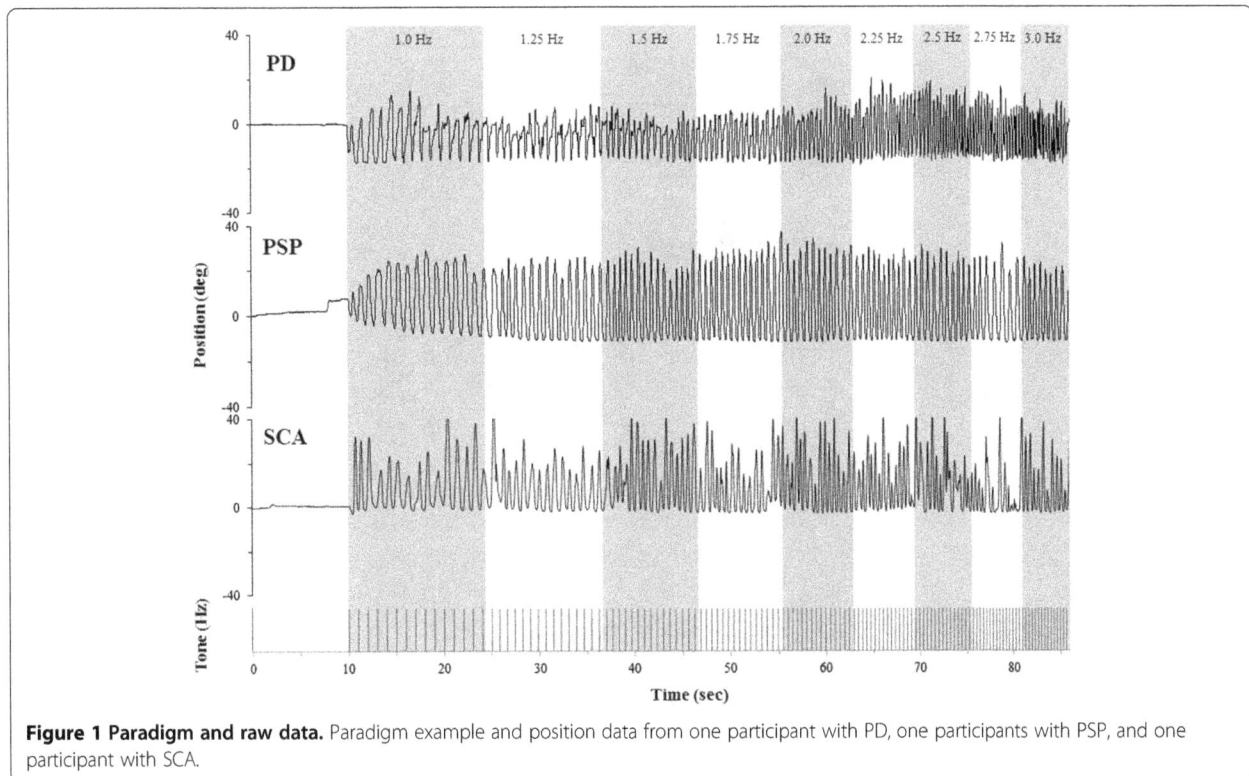

Figure 1 Paradigm and raw data. Paradigm example and position data from one participant with PD, one participants with PSP, and one participant with SCA.

finger remained unconstrained for full range of motion. A goniometer was used to collect position of the index finger. Movement rate, peak-to-peak amplitude, and corresponding coefficient of variation (CV) were obtained for each movement and averaged across each tone rate. Movement amplitude was normalized to the amplitude at 1 Hz to allow for comparison across tone rates since no constraints were placed upon range of motion. Movement rate difference (MRΔ) was calculated as the difference between the given tone rate and actual movement rate.

Statistical analyses

To examine repetitive finger movement performance in the PSP and SCA groups alone, a single factor repeated measures analysis of variation (ANOVA) model was completed to estimate differences in MRΔ and normalized peak-to-peak amplitude across tones rates for each group. To examine differences between MRΔ, normalized peak-to-peak amplitude and CV across all groups, a repeated measures ANOVA model was estimated. The between-group factor was PD vs. PSP vs. SCA, and the within-subjects factor was tone rate. Post hoc analysis was completed using Tukey's Honestly Significant Difference test. The level of significance was set at $\alpha < 0.05$.

Results

Figure 1 shows raw position data from one participant with PD, one participant with PSP, and one participant with SCA. Note that at approximately 2.25 Hz and above the participant with PD demonstrates an increase in movement rate with little decrement in movement amplitude. In contrast, the participant with PSP does not increment movement rate starting at approximately 2.0 Hz and maintains a relatively stable movement rate and movement amplitude until reaching 3.0 Hz. Finally, the participant with SCA demonstrated a much greater variation in movement performance across all tone rates, and at rates near to and above 2.0 Hz, this participant remains slower than the intended tone.

For comparison of the PSP and SCA groups alone, there was a significant effect of MRΔ for the PSP group ($F(8) = 7.48$, $p < 0.001$) and the SCA group ($F(8) = 13.809$, $p < 0.001$) (Figure 2A). For the PSP group, post hoc analysis revealed that MRΔ significantly differed between tone rates of 1.5 Hz and 3.0 Hz ($p = 0.03$), and 1.75 Hz and 3.0 Hz ($p = 0.05$) only. For the SCA group, post hoc analysis revealed that MRΔ significantly differed 1) from 1 Hz at tone rates of 2.75 Hz and above ($p < 0.01$), 2) from 1.25 Hz at tone rates of 2.75 Hz and above ($p < 0.01$), 3) from 1.5 Hz at tone rate of 2.75 Hz and above ($p < 0.03$), 4) between 1.75 Hz and 3.0 Hz ($p < 0.001$), 5) between 2.0 Hz and 3.0 Hz ($p = 0.004$), and between 2.25 Hz and 3.0 Hz ($p = 0.02$). There were no significant differences in normalized peak-to-peak amplitude for either the PSP ($F(8) = 0.02$, $p = 0.89$) or SCA ($F(8) = 0.17$, $p = 0.69$) group.

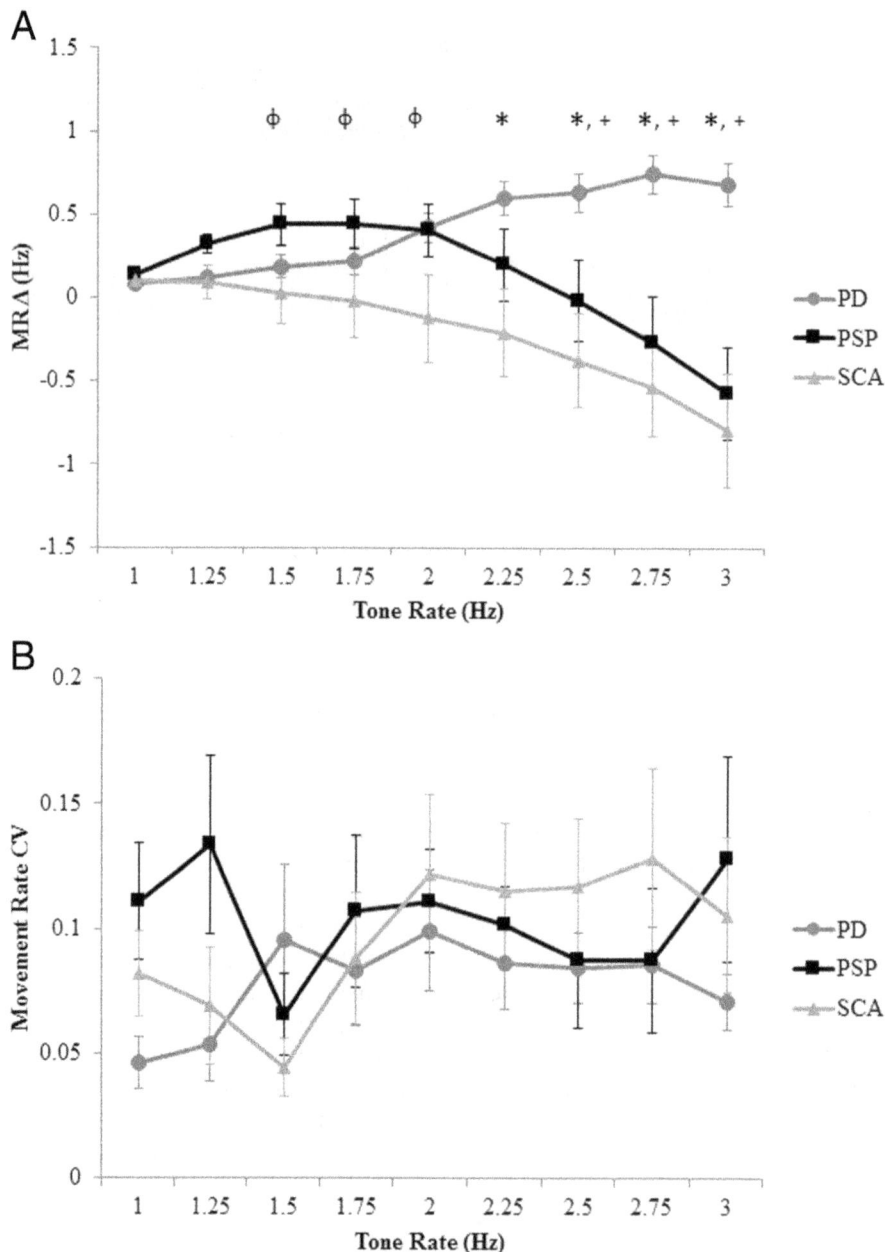

Figure 2 Movement rate difference and movement rate coefficient of variation. Mean and standard error for **(A)** movement rate difference (MRΔ) and **(B)** movement rate coefficient of variation across all tone rates for the PD, PSP, and SCA groups. Crossed ($^+$) designate significant differences between the PD and PSP groups. Asterisks (*) designate significant differences between the PD and SCA groups. Phi ($^\phi$) designates significant differences between the PSP and SCA groups.

When comparing performance across groups, it was observed that MRΔ between the three groups diverged at tone rates near to 2 Hz. Specifically, the PD group moved faster than the intended tone rate while both the PSP and SCA group moved slower than the intended tone rate (Figure 2A). Moreover, for both MRΔ and normalized peak-to-peak amplitude the standard error was larger in the PSP and SCA groups than the PD group.

Thus, a comparison of CV for both outcome measures was completed.

Statistical comparison revealed a significant rate effect ($F(8) = 7.12$, $p < 0.001$), a significant group effect ($F(2) = 8.21$, $p = 0.001$), and a significant interaction effect ($F(16) = 13.28$, $p < 0.001$) for MRΔ. Post hoc analysis revealed that MRΔ between the PD group significantly differed (moved faster) from the PSP group at tone rates of 2.5 Hz and above (p < 0.02) and significantly differed (moved faster) from the SCA group at tone rates of 2.0 Hz and above (p < 0.02). MRΔ between the PSP group significantly differed from the SCA group at tone rates of 1.5 Hz, 1.75 Hz, and 2.0 Hz (p < 0.05) (Figure 2A). For CV of MRΔ, there was no main effect of tone rate, group, or interaction effect (Figure 2B).

Figure 3 shows the normalized peak-to-peak amplitude and CV for all three groups. No main effect of tone rate or group, as well as no interaction effect, was revealed for normalized peak-to-peak amplitude (Figure 3A). However, there was a main effect of group for CV of normalized peak-to-peak amplitude. Amplitude variance in the SCA group significantly differed from the PD group (p = 0.04). There were no differences in amplitude variance between the SCA and PSP groups (p = 0.26) or the PSP and PD groups (p = 0.81). There was no main

effect of tone rate or interaction effect for normalized peak-to-peak amplitude CV (Figure 3B).

Discussion

This study is the first to examine differences in repetitive finger movement performance in persons with PD, PSP, and SCA. Results revealed significant differences in movement rate across groups and tone rates. The PD group tended to move faster than the tone, while the PSP and SCA groups moved slower than the intended tone at higher tone rates. While there were no differences among groups or across tone rates in movement amplitude, the SCA group demonstrated greater variance in movement amplitude compared to the PD group. Taking these characteristics together, the results of this study suggest that quantitatively evaluating the movement rate and amplitude variance of repetitive

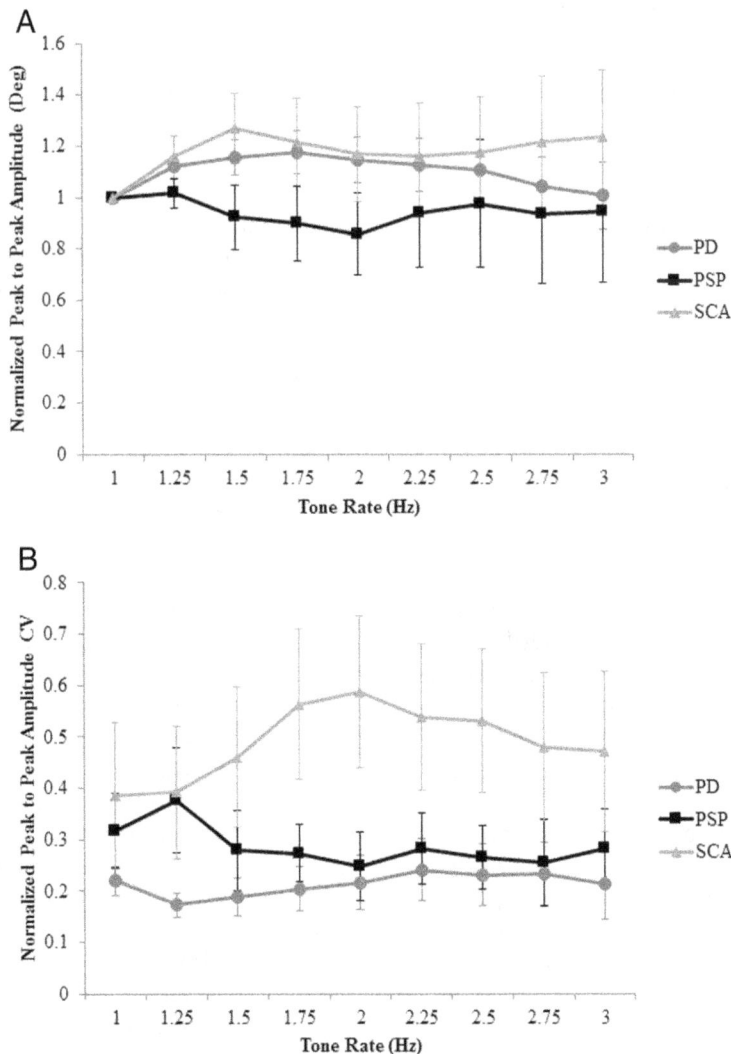

Figure 3 Amplitude and amplitude coefficient of variation. Mean and standard error for **(A)** normalized peak-to-peak amplitude and **(B)** normalized peak-to-peak amplitude coefficient of variation (CV) across all tone rates for the PD, PSP, and SCA groups.

finger movement performance at high rates may help distinguish among these three movement disorders. Future work should focus on testing patients early in disease and off medication.

There were no differences observed in movement amplitude across tone rates or across groups in this study. All participants were tested on medication which may account for the lack of detectable effect. However, when comparing peak-to-peak amplitude (not normalized to 1 Hz) across groups, peak-to-peak amplitude was largest across all tone rates in the SCA group (27.0 ± 0.6 degrees) and smallest in the PSP group (16.2 ± 0.8 degrees) compared to the PD group (21.3 ± 0.5 degrees). This is in keeping with previous research that has reported decreased movement amplitude for repetitive finger movements in persons with PSP compared to persons with PD [9]. No study has compared movement amplitude of repetitive finger movements between PD and SCA. However, the increased variance in movement amplitude for the SCA group compared to the PD group is consistent with previous findings comparing gait in PD and cerebellar ataxia [12], and may reflect ataxia/poor coordination. The main differences in repetitive finger movement performances between the PD, PSP, and SCA groups were related to movement rate.

A major finding of this study is that differences in movement rate among groups emerged at tone rates above 2 Hz. Results revealed that the PSP and SCA groups moved slower than the intended tone while the PD group moved faster than the intended tone at higher tone rates. However, the negative MRΔ for the PSP and SCA groups may be due to an inability to sustain movement rates above a certain frequency due to incoordination or rigid-bradykinesia. Indeed, participants with PSP incremented movement rate with the tone rate until reaching the tone rate of 2 Hz. At rates above 2 Hz, the PSP group maintained a constant movement rate (2.4 to 2.5 Hz with a standard error of 0.22 to 0.29). In fact, the PSP group did not fall below the intended rate until reaching the tone rate of 2.5 Hz (see Figure 4). Thus, the PSP group demonstrated an inability to increment movement rate above 2.5 Hz. A previous study examining repetitive finger movements in persons with PSP describes the finger tap pattern as "hypokinetic without decrement" [9]. Ling and colleagues [9] further suggest that persons with PSP demonstrate a lack of decrement in movement amplitude during repetitive finger movement compared to persons with PD. Likewise, in the present study, there was no significant change in movement amplitude across tone rates in the PSP group. Taken together, persons with PSP may lock into a steady state performance of repetitive movement, potentially perseverating more, that is unaffected by changing environmental cues (increase in tone rate).

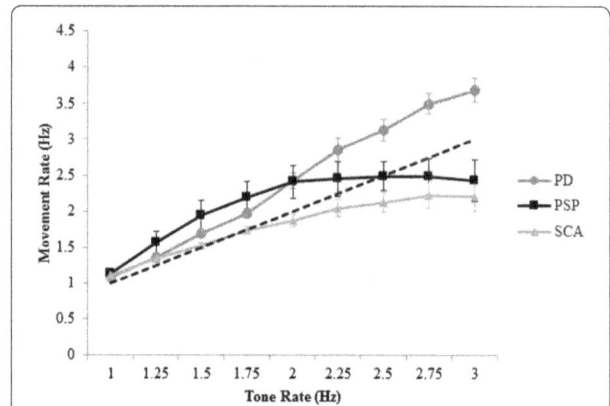

Figure 4 Movement rate. Mean and standard error for movement rate across all tone rates for PD, PSP, and SCA groups.

In contrast to the PSP group, the SCA group remained slower than the intended tone rate beginning at 2 Hz, but were still able to increment movement rate minimally (1.8 to 2.2 Hz with a standard of 0.06 to 0.22) (see Figure 4). This is in keeping with previous studies. Akhlaghi and colleagues [13] demonstrated that persons with Friedreich's ataxia demonstrated a slower finger tapping rate when compared to healthy control participants [13]. Kosaka and colleagues [11] have demonstrated that at rates above 2 Hz, persons with spinocerebellar degeneration demonstrated a decreased movement rate [11]. Interestingly, gait speed has been shown to affect gait variability in persons with cerebellar ataxia, with the highest variability occurring during slow and fast walking [14,15]. In the current study, no significant change in movement amplitude across tone rates was observed, but amplitude variance was significantly increased compared to the PD group. The variance in both movement rate and amplitude in the SCA group did increase, though not significantly, as the tone rate increased. Thus, in this study, we suggest the reduced movement rate in the SCA group may be the result of participants trying to reduce movement variability to allow for a more stable overall movement performance.

Previous research has reported that persons with PD demonstrate impairments in repetitive finger movement performance, characterized by a dramatic increase in movement rate accompanied by hesitations and arrest as well as a loss of movement amplitude, at tone rates near to and above 2 Hz and is not improved with dopaminergic medication [5-8]. This would suggest that non-dopaminergic mechanisms may contribute at least in part to this impairment [5]. In healthy populations, transition in repetitive finger movement performance at rates near to and above 2 Hz is associated with changes in activity over primary and secondary motor areas, as well as changes in motor cortical oscillations [16-18]. This may suggest that a change in motor control of repetitive finger movements, potentially from discrete to continuous movement, occurs at rates near to 2 Hz. The change in motor control may lead to the deterioration of repetitive finger movement performance in persons with PD, as well as, PSP and SCA. In this study, movement rate performance in the PSP and SCA groups diverged from the PD group near 2 Hz. These results indeed support the hypothesis that control of repetitive finger movement performance changes at rates near 2 Hz and may be mediated in part by cerebellar function as cerebellar dysfunction has been previously reported in PD, PSP, and SCA [2-4]. However, given the differences in movement performance across the groups, pathophysiological mechanisms involving cerebellar and basal ganglia function may contribute differentially to the changes in movement performance at high movement rates.

Our study had several limitations. First, as this was a pilot study the sample size was small for each of the three populations studied. Due to the small sample size we were unable to match subjects for age, gender, or disease severity (further difficult given the inherent differences among these disorders), and the individual participant variability may have impacted statistical significance. Second, the SCA group in general was more heterogeneous than the PD or PSP groups and may account in part for the increased variation seen in this group. Third, subjects were evaluated in mid to late disease (average disease duration was at least 5 years for each group). Examining these patients earlier in disease, during the first or second year post-diagnosis, may be more clinically meaningful and could support this approach as a potential diagnostic tool if these findings are validated. There is a possibility that fatigue may have contributed to the decrements in movement performance. Previous research has shown that impairments in repetitive finger movement performance in persons with PD using this same task was not due to fatigue [6]. However, the contribution of fatigue to impairments in persons with PSP or SCA has not been tested. Finally, cognitive impairment is often present in patients with PD, PSP, and SCA, and could potentially affect the variability in the results. No cognitive information was collected in this study to rule this potential confound out. However, the task in this study was rather simple and involved limited cognitive effort.

Conclusion

The results of this study suggest that persons with PD, PSP, and SCA may use different motor control strategies for repetitive finger movement performance at high movement rates. Specifically at movement rates near 2 Hz and above, participants with PD tended to move faster than the intended tone (similar to festination); participants with PSP maintained a constant rate; and participants with SCA moved slower than the intended tone though still minimally incremented movement rate and demonstrated an increase in variance in movement amplitude. Future imaging studies are needed to examine if these differences in movement performance are accounted for by differing pathophysiological mechanisms. However, this study provides initial evidence that quantitatively evaluating repetitive finger movement performance has the potential to differentiate movement disorders that may present similar to PD.

Abbreviations
PD: Parkinson's disease; PSP: Progressive Supranuclear Palsy; SCA: Spinocerebellar ataxia; HZ: Hertz; STN-DBS: Deep brain stimulation of the subthalamic nucleus; CV: Coefficient of variation; MRΔ: Movement rate difference; ANOVA: Analysis of variation.

Competing interest
The authors declare that they have no competing of interest.

Authors' contribution
All authors agree to be accountable for all aspects of the work ensuring accuracy and integrity of the manuscript. ELS - Concept and design, data collection and analysis, drafting and revising manuscript, final approval. JU - Data analysis, revising manuscript. MDT, NRM, SHS, MSO and CJH - Concept and design, revising manuscript, final approval. All authors read and approved the final manuscript.

Acknowledgements
This study was supported in part by the National Institutes of Health (NIH) and National Center for Research Resources (NCRR) CTSA grant 1UL1RR029890.

Author details
[1]Department of Kinesiology, Iowa State University, 235 Forker, Ames, IA 50011, USA. [2]Department of Applied Physiology and Kinesiology, University of Florida, Gainesville, USA. [3]Center for Movement Disorders and Neurorestoration, Department of Neurology, University of Florida, McKnight Brain Institute, Gainesville, USA. [4]Department of Kinesiology and Health Promotion, Troy University, Troy, USA.

References
1. Albin RL, Young AB, Penney JB. The functional anatomy of basal ganglia disorders. Trends Neurosci. 1989;12:366–75.
2. van Gaalen J, Giunti P, van de Warrenburg BP. Movement disorders in spinocerebellar ataxias. Mov Disord. 2011;26:792–800.
3. Tawana K, Ramsden DB. Progressive supranuclear palsy. J Clin Pathol: Mol Pathol. 2001;54:427–34.
4. Giza E, Gotzamani-Psarrakou A, Bostantjopoulou S. Imaging beyond the striatonigral dopaminergic system in Parkinson's disease. Hell J Nucl Med. 2012;15:224–32.
5. Stegemöller EL, Simuni T, MacKinnon C. Effect of movement frequency on repetitive finger movements in patients with Parkinson's disease. Mov Disord. 2009;24:1162–9.
6. Stegemöller EL, Allen DP, Simuni T, MacKinnon CD. Rate-dependent impairments in repetitive finger movements in patients with Parkinson's disease are not due to peripheral fatigue. Neurosci Lett. 2010;182:1–6.
7. Stegemöller EL, Zadikoff C, Rosenow JM, MacKinnon CD. Deep brain stimulation improves movement amplitude but not hastening of repetitive finger movements. Neurosci Lett. 2013;552:135–9.
8. Nakamura R, Nagasaki H, Narabayashi H. Disturbances of rhythm formation in patients with Parkinson's disease: part 1. Characteristics of tapping response to the periodic signals. Percept Mot Skills. 1978;46:63–75.

9. Ling H, Massey LA, Lees AJ, Brown P, Day BL. Hypokinesia without decrement distinguishes progressive supranuclear palsy from Parkinson's disease. Brain. 2012;135:1141–53.

10. Furtado S, Payami H, Lockhart PJ, Hanson M, Nutt JGm Singleton AA, Singletone A, et al. Profile of families with parkinsonism-predominant spinocerebellar ataxia type 2 (SCA2). Mov Disord. 2004;19:622–9.

11. Kosaka K, Nagasaki H, Nakamura R. Finger tapping test as a means to differentiate olivo-ponto-cerebellar atrophy among spinocerebellar degnerations. Tohoku J Exp Med. 1982;136:129–34.

12. Ebersback G, Sojer M, Valldeoriola F, Wissel J, Müller J, Tolosa E, et al. Comparative analysis of gait in Parkinson's disease, cerebellar ataxia and subcortical arteriosclerotic encephalopathy. Brain. 1999;122:1349–55.

13. Akhlaghi H, Corben L, Georgiou-Karistianis N, Bradshaw J, Delatycki MB, Storey E, et al. A functional MRI study of motor dysfunction in Friedreich's ataxia. Brain Res. 2012;1471:138–54.

14. Schniepp R, Wuehr M, Neuhaesser M, Kamenova M, Dimitriadis K, Klopstock T, et al. Locomotion speed determines gait variability in cerebellar ataxia and vestibular failure. Mov Disord. 2012;27:125–31.

15. Wuehr M, Schniepp R, Ilmberger J, Brandt T, Jahn K. Speed-dependent temporospatioal gait variability in long-range correlations in cerebellar ataxia. Gait Posture. 2013;37:214–8.

16. Jantzen KJ, Steinberg FL, Kelso JA. Functional MRI reveals the existence of modality and coordination-dependent timing networks. Neuroimage. 2005;25:1031–42.

17. Mayville JM, Jantzen KJ, Fuchs A, Steinberg FL, Kelso JAS. Cortical and subcortical networks underlying syncopated and synchronized coordination revealed using fMRI. Hum Brain Mapp. 2002;17:214–29.

18. Toma K, Mima T, Matsuoka T, Gerloff C, Ohnishi T, Koshy B, et al. Movement rate effect on activation and functional coupling of motor cortical areas. J Neurophysiol. 2002;88:3377–85.

14

Clinical and programming pattern of patients with impending deep brain stimulation power failure

Raja Mehanna[1*], Kathy M Wilson[2], Scott E Cooper[2], Andre G Machado[2] and Hubert H Fernandez[2]

Abstract

Background: It is important to prevent complications of implanted pulse generators (IPG) depletion by replacing the IPG in time.

Methods: We reviewed the charts of all patients with deep brain stimulation treated movement disorders who were seen at our institution over a period of 6 months. Among these, we retained for analyses those who had undergone IPG replacement within the previous 3 years.

Results: A total of 55 IPG replacements (from 38 patients) were reviewed. Electrodes were implanted in the subthalamic nucleus in all Parkinson's disease patients, in the ventral intermedius nucleus of the thalamus in all essential tremor patients and in the globus pallidus interna in all dystonia patients. Replacements were preceded by a voltage increase due to worsened symptoms in 27.3% (15/55); 25.5% (14/55) had full IPG depletion or had too low IPG reserve to allow for any voltage adjustment; and 21.7% (12/55) did not get a needed voltage increase either for safety reasons (eg: concern for increase in falls with higher voltages) or because the surgery date for IPG replacement was close. Only 25.5% (14/55) remained clinically well-controlled prior to IPG replacement, all of whom had IPG longevity estimates available. Clinical deterioration was noted prior to IPG replacement in 100% of patients without available longevity estimates versus 61% of patients with available longevity estimates (p < 0.001).

Conclusion: Despite best efforts, clinical deterioration prior to IPG replacement can be seen frequently. Routine estimation of IPG life, along with symptom assessment at every follow-up visit may prevent it.

Keywords: Deep brain stimulation, Estimate, Depletion

Background

Deep brain stimulation (DBS) has been approved by the United States Food and Drug Administration (FDA) for the treatment of Parkinson's disease (PD), essential tremor (ET) and dystonia, and is undergoing trials for approval in psychiatric disorders such as depression and obsessive compulsive disorders.

DBS acts through delivering an electrical current in a specific target area of the brain, the target being different according to the disease being treated. This current can be modulated through modification of voltage, frequency and duration of each electrical pulse delivered. The delivered energy creates an electrical field of variable size and shape according to the parameters used for stimulation [1]. The current is generated by an implantable pulse generator (IPG), a small pacemaker-like unit that is implanted under the skin, usually in the chest or less frequently in the abdomen. The current is then delivered through an extension wire and implanted electrode to the target located deep in the brain. Once the IPG is depleted, it has to be replaced so current can continue to be generated and delivered to the brain.

Because IPG depletion can result in worsening of neurological symptoms [2,3], and sometimes lead to medical emergencies [4,5], it is important to prevent it by replacing the IPG in time. This can be done by routinely estimating IPG life and assessing symptoms at every follow-up visit. For the Soletra model, estimate

* Correspondence: raja.mehanna@uth.tmc.edu
[1]University of Texas Health Science Center, 6410 Fannin Street, Suite 1014, Houston, TX 77030, USA
Full list of author information is available at the end of the article

can be done by telephoning Medtronic technical support. Reported DBS settings are entered into a computer software which estimates the longevity of the IPG from the date of implant. A web based application developed by the University of Florida is also available [6]. However, the estimation of IPG life is always an approximation because the actual IPG life depends upon multiple specific DBS treatment parameters, duration of stimulation, lead impedance, as well as many other factors that cannot easily be estimated [7]. While increasing DBS settings correlates inversely with IPG longevity [8], guidelines provided by medical device companies to help approximate the longevity of an IPG cannot take into consideration all possible therapeutic combinations of DBS and are thus far from accurate, especially because DBS treatment parameters change over time with the evolution of the underlying disease. There are many more sources of error that may flaw longevity estimation, including but not limited to device-to-device variation, decreased supplied voltage with battery usage, battery chemistry, impedance fluctuation and battery self-discharge through quiescent current [7].

There is little information in the literature regarding practices when DBS batteries are about to be depleted of power. We reviewed all IPG replacements done at our institution over a period of 42 months to survey our practice patterns, including DBS programming modifications, when DBS batteries are nearing end of life.

Methods

We reviewed the charts of all patients with movement disorders who underwent DBS surgery and who were seen at the Center for Neurological Restoration at Cleveland Clinic between 06/01/2012 and 12/31/2012. We retained for analyses those who had undergone IPG replacement within the previous 3 years. All batteries replaced being of the Soletra model (Medtronic ® Minneapolis, MN, USA), we included all replacements that were done for an IPG voltage of 3.69 or less, or for a drop by 0.3 V or more in the previous 12 months, or for clinical worsening that improved after IPG replacement, or at the family's insistence because the predicted lifespan was reached. We excluded the IPG replacements that were done for other reasons (e.g. replacing the non-depleted contralateral IPG to spare the patient another surgery within a year). The patient's age, gender, diagnosis, duration of disease at time of IPG replacement, IPG model and voltage at the last visit before IPG replacement were noted. The presence of symptoms attributed at the time by the treating clinician to IPG depletion and programming changes to address these symptoms were also recorded, as well as whether the IPG longevity estimate was known at the last visit before replacement, obtained through the Medtronic helpline. This was a minimal risk study utilizing existing data through chart review and not requiring any direct patient evaluation

for the purpose of the study. Data was de-identified, informed consent was waived and the study was submitted to the Cleveland Clinic Foundation Institutional Review Board who exempted it from review.

Results

A total of 55 IPG replacements, involving 38 patients, with 25 (66%) males and a mean age of 67.8 years (range 23 to 90 years), were ultimately included in this survey (Table 1). The diagnoses included PD (44 replacements), ET (5 replacements), primary generalized dystonia with DYT 1 mutation (2 replacements), primary segmental dystonia (1 replacement), secondary generalized dystonia (2 replacements) and secondary segmental dystonia (1 replacement) (Figure 1). All PD patients had their electrodes implanted in the subthalamic nucleus; ET patients had their electrodes implanted in the ventral intermedius nucleus of the thalamus; and all patients with dystonia had theirs implanted in the globus pallidus interna. On average, the batteries were 4.3 years old (range 1.2 – 9 years) and had a mean voltage of 3.39 (range 0 – 3.74 V) when they were replaced (Table 1). When assessing IPG longevity by diagnosis, the mean lifespan was 5.75 years in ET (range 4–6.75 years, SD 1.09, SEM 0.5), 4.4 years in PD (range 1.5-9 years, SD 2.02, SEM 0.3) and 1.9 years in dystonia (range 1.2 to 3 years, SD 0.73, SEM 0.3) (F = 6.451, p = 0.003) (Figure 2).

In 15 of 55 (27.3%) replacements, patients required a voltage increase due to worsened symptoms (mean voltage increase = 0.26 V; SD = 0.1; range: 0.1-0.5 V) (Figure 3). This increase at least partially improved the symptoms until the IPG was replaced. Moreover, for these patients, the side effects noted *after* IPG replacement often required voltage re-adjustment back to their pre-power depletion levels. In 14 (25.5%) additional replacements, a needed voltage adjustment could not be performed because of either full IPG depletion or too low IPG reserve, with the concern that such increase would precipitate depletion before replacement. Additionally, 12 (21.7%) replacements did not get a needed voltage increase either for safety reasons such as concern for increase in falls with higher voltages or because patient declined it as surgery date was close (Figure 3). Only 14 of 55 (25.5%) replacements were clinically well-controlled prior to IPG power depletion (Figure 3). Their IPGs were replaced well ahead

Table 1 Patients characteristics

	Average	Range
Age	67.8 years	23–90 years
M/F ratio	2/1	
Age of battery when replaced	4.3 years	1.2–9 years
Battery voltage when replaced	3.39 V	0-3.74 V

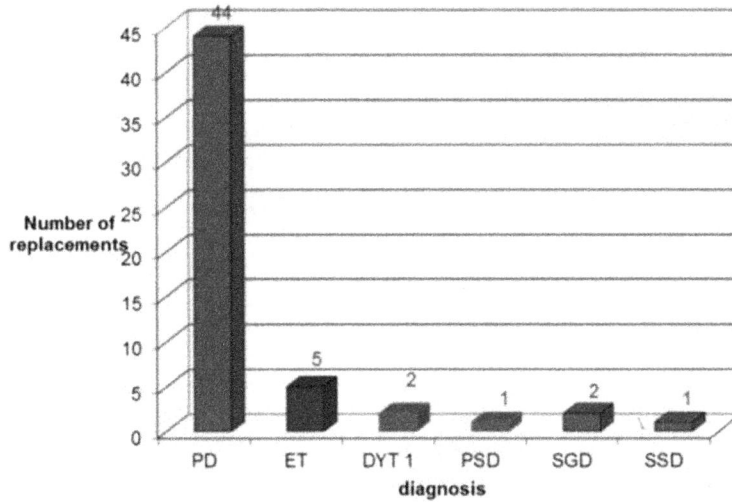

Figure 1 Diagnosis distribution. *Legend:* PD: Parkinson's disease, ET: essential tremor, DYT 1: generalized dystonia with DYT 1 mutation, PSD: primary segmental dystonia, SGD: secondary generalized dystonia, SSD: secondary segmental dystonia.

of full depletion and no programming adjustments were necessary.

In 33 of 55 (60%) of the replacements, the IPG longevity estimate was available. Twenty of these (61%) had motor deterioration before IPG replacement, 5 of which benefited from a voltage increase prior to IPG replacement. 6 replacements were done at the patient's and family insistence based on previous estimates, despite good IPG reserve and the lack of symptoms of IPG depletion. In contrast, all the 22 replacements that did not have estimates available had symptoms of depletion before IPG replacement. The difference in the proportion of patients who experienced worsening of symptoms prior to IPG replacement between the group with estimates available (61%) versus the group without available estimates (100%) was statistically significant using a Chi square test (Chi-square = 11.35; p < 0.001).

Discussion

In our retrospective review of 55 IPG replacements in 38 patients, the most frequent diagnosis was PD (76.3%), followed by dystonia (13.2%) then ET (10.5%). We have found that the average longevity of the Soletra IPG was consistent with previous reports for patients with dystonia at 1.9 years [9-12] and PD at 4.4 years [6,8,13,14]. However, the IPG lasted longer that previous reports in our patients with ET (5.75 vs 2 to 4 years) [6,8,12,13], likely because most of our ET patients turn their IPG off at night precisely to prolong its life. Overall, this was consistent with previously published data that the underlying diagnosis can also affect IPG longevity with the characteristics of the stimulation target as well as the disease pathophysiology likely contributing to battery longevity [6,12,13], with dystonia typically depleting the IPG faster than PD or ET.

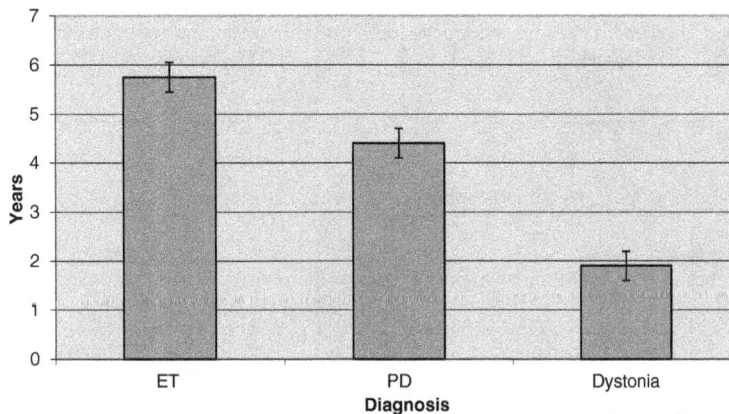

Figure 2 IPG longevity per diagnosis in years. *Legend:* IPG: implantable pulse generator, PD: Parkinson's disease, ET: essential tremor.

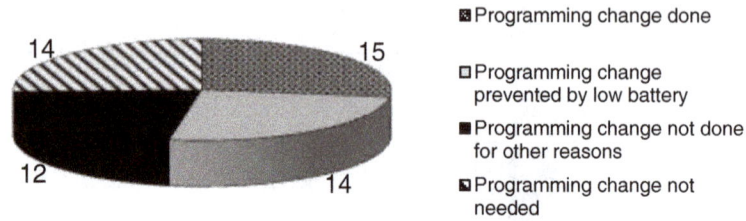

Figure 3 Programming change prior to surgery.

Clinical deterioration prior to IPG replacement occurred frequently. Fifteen of 55 (27.3%) replacements benefited clinically from a voltage increase (mean voltage increase = 0.26 V; SD = 0.1; range: 0.1-0.5 V). Interestingly, side effects noted after IPG replacement often required a voltage re-adjustment to their pre-power depletion levels. In 14 of 55 (25.5%) replacements, patients were clinically worse but could not get a needed voltage increase because of either full IPG depletion or too low IPG reserves. Finally, 14 of 55 (25.5%) IPGs were replaced well ahead of full depletion and no programming adjustments were necessary before or after IPG replacement. All of the latter

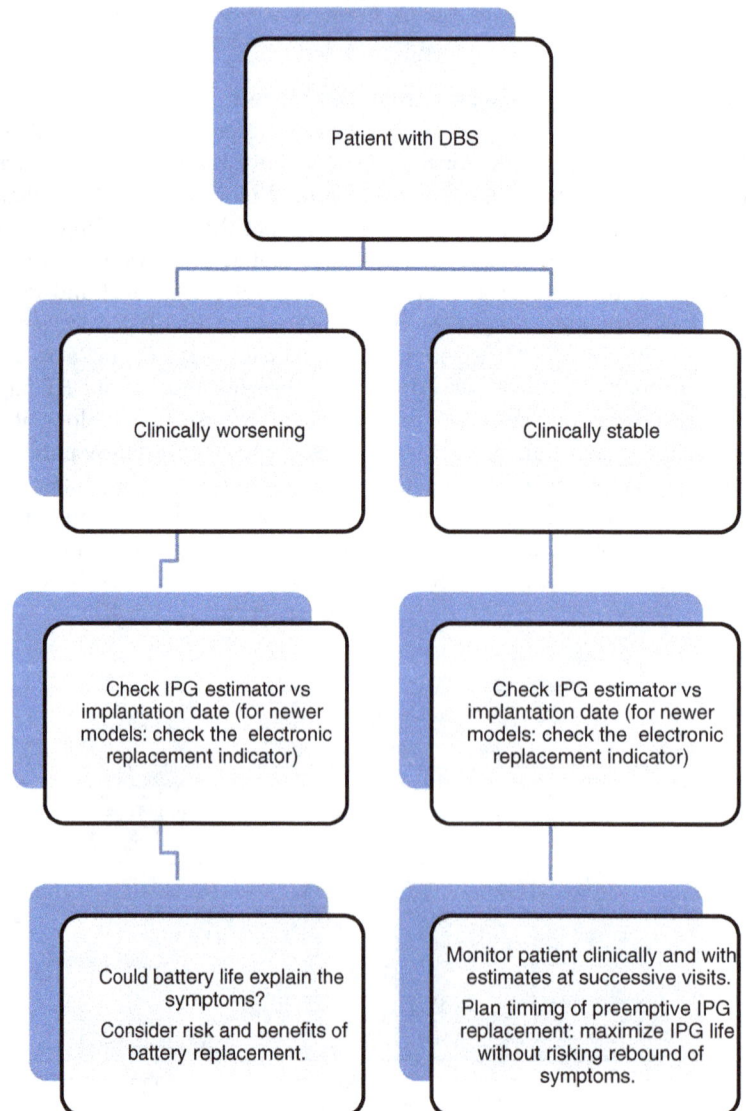

Figure 4 Suggested algorythm for management of IPG life. *Legend*: IPG: implantable pulse generator.

had IPG longevity estimates available. We believe that knowing these longevity estimates prevented clinical deterioration prior to IPG replacements in several patients in our cohort—clinical deterioration was noted in 100% of IPG replacement without longevity estimates, whereas it was seen in 61% of IPG replacements with available longevity estimates (p < 0.001).

Available data regarding the clinical usefulness of longevity estimate are conflicting. In a prospective study on 72 IPG replacements, Stewart and Eljamel [15] demonstrated large differences between the actual longevity and the longevity predicted using a computer-based estimate integrating current DBS parameters. There was no correlation between the 2, and the actual longevity was shorter by a year in some instances. However, in a retrospective review of 320 charts, Fakhar et al. demonstrated that an University of Florida web based estimator/smart phone application (r = .67, p < .001) as well as the Medtronic helpline estimate (r = 0.74, p < 0.001) were correlated with the actual IPG life [6].

Our study replicate the results from Fakhar et al., albeit on a smaller sample and without the use of the University of Florida estimator. These studies actually complement each other with an emphasis on the physical and electrical aspect in Fakhar et al.'s, and on the clinical aspect in ours. The IPG longevity in ET patients was, however, longer in our study (5.75 vs 3.54 years). In our study, knowledge of the estimate was associated with a lower rate of symptomatic IPG depletions. However, because only 4 of the 55 IPGs were totally depleted at the time of surgery, we could not compare the estimated lifetime to the actual lifetime of the IPGs.

While this study has some limitation inherent to its small size and retrospective design such as reliance on recorded data and chart quality, as well as lack of randomization, we believe it is a useful survey of practice patterns at our institution and suggests that IPG longevity estimate is useful in clinical practice. Considering that 6 of 55 (11%) of replacements in our study were done at the patients or family insistence because the predicted lifetime was coming to an end, although there were no clinical or electrical signs of depletion, the question of cost effectiveness of relying solely on longevity estimate should be raised. However, this contrasts with previous reports where the actual life expectancy was typically shorter than estimated [15]. It thus seems that both the estimate as well as the electrical and/or clinical worsening should be taken into consideration when deciding of the best time to replace the IPG, supporting an algorithm previously suggested by Montuno et al. (Figure 4) [7].

Finally, all the patients in this study were found to have the Soletra model of IPG. This specific model is old and has been replaced by newer models such as Activa. The newer models have an elective replacement indicator message that is displayed on patient and clinician programing devices, and suggests that a replacement may be required within approximately three months. The newer models probably predict battery failure more accurately, and the results of our study might not apply to them. However, clinicians taking care of the non-negligible number of patients still carrying Soletra, and until these deplete and get replaced by a newer model, will find our results still useful and clinically relevant.

Conclusions

The patients who had optimal symptom control were those seen well in advance of power depletion, with enough time to have batteries replaced before their symptoms worsened. However, clinical deterioration just prior to end of IPG life was not uncommon. A significant percentage of patients required voltage adjustments prior to IPG placement to improve their worsening clinical state, and often required another voltage readjustment after IPG replacement. Because IPG depletion can lead to worsening of neurological symptoms and even medical emergencies on one hand, and overzealous IPG replacement may not be cost-effective on the other, DBS programming clinicians should routinely estimate IPG life and assess symptoms at every follow-up visit in order to decide when IPGs should be replaced.

Abbreviations
IPG: Implanted pulse generators; DBS: Deep brain stimulation; FDA: Food and Drug Administration; PD: Parkinson's disease; ET: Essential tremor.

Competing interest
R Mehanna has nothing to disclose. KM Wilson is on the Speaker's Bureau for TEVA Pharmaceuticals (Azilect). AG Machado has nothing to disclose. SE Cooper has nothing to disclose. HH Fernandez has received research support from Abbott, Acadia, Biotie Therapeutics, EMD-Serono, Huntington Study Group, Merck, Michael J. Fox Foundation, Merck, Movement Disorders Society, National Parkinson Foundation, NIH/NINDS, Novartis, Parkinson Study Group, Synosia, Teva, but has no owner interest in any pharmaceutical company. HH Fernandez has received honoraria from Advanced Health Media, Cleveland Clinic CME, Medical Communications Media, Movement Disorders Society, Vindico Medical Education as a speaker in CME events. HH Fernandez has received honoraria from Ipsen, Merz Pharmaceuticals, Pfizer, Teva Neuroscience, Zambon Pharmaceuticals, as a speaker and/or consultant. HH Fernandez has received royalty payments from Demos Publishing for serving as a book author/editor. The Cleveland Clinic has contracts with EMD Serono, Abbott and Merz pharmaceuticas for HH Fernandez' role as a member of the Global Steering Committee for Safinamide and LCIG studies; and Head Principal Investigator for the Xeomin Registry Study. HH Fernandez also serves as the Chair of the Publication Committee for Xeomin Studies (Merz Pharmaceuticals); a member of the Publication Committee for Dysport studies (Ipsen Pharmaceuticals); and a consultant for Prostrakan/KyowaHakko, Britannia, Knopp and US WorldMeds but he does not receive any personal compensation for these roles. HH Fernandez has received a stipend from Movement Disorders Society for serving as Medical Editor of the MDS Web Site.

Authors' contributions
RM: data analysis, writing of the first manuscript; KMW: conception and design, data gathering, review and critique; SEC: review and critique; AM: review and critique; HHF: conception and design, review and critique. All authors read and approved the final manuscript.

Author details
[1]University of Texas Health Science Center, 6410 Fannin Street, Suite 1014, Houston, TX 77030, USA. [2]Cleveland Clinic Foundation, Cleveland, Ohio, USA.

References
1. Mehanna R, Lai E: **Deep brain stimulation in Parkinson's disease.** *Transl Neurodegener* 2013, **18**(2):22.
2. Okun MS, Tagliati M, Pourfar M, Fernandez HH, Rodriguez RL, Alterman RL, Foote KD: **Management of referred deep brain stimulation failures: a retrospective analysis from 2 movement disorders centers.** *Arch Neurol* 2005, **62**:1250–1255.
3. Vora AK, Ward H, Foote KD, Goodman WK, Okun MS: **Rebound symptoms followingbattery depletion in the NIH OCD DBS cohort: clinical and reimbursement issues.** *Brain Stimul* 2012, **5**:599–604.
4. Hariz M, Johansson F: **Hardware failure in parkinsonian patients with chronic subthalamic nucleus stimulation is a medical emergency.** *Mov Disord* 2001, **16**:166–168.
5. Alesch F: **Sudden failure of dual channel pulse generators.** *Mov Disord* 2005, **20**:64–66.
6. Fahar K, Hastings E, Butson CR, Foote KD, Zeilman P, Okun MS: **Management of deep brain stimulator IPG failure: IPG estimators, charge density, and importance of clinical symptoms.** *PLoS One* 2013, **8**:e58665.
7. Montuno MA, Kohner AB, Foote KD, Okun MS: **An algorithm for management of deep brain stimulation IPG replacements: devising a web-based IPG estimator and clinical symptom approach.** *Neuromodulation* 2013, **16**:147–153.
8. Ondo W, Meilak C, Vuong K: **Predictors of IPG life for the activa soletra 7426 neurostimulator.** *Parkinsonism Relat Disord* 2007, **13**:240–242.
9. Isaias IU, Alterman RL, Tagliati M: **Deep brain stimulation for primary generalized dystonia: long-term outcomes.** *Arch Neurol* 2009, **66**:465–470.
10. Blahak C, Capelle HH, Baezner H, Kinfe TM, Hennerici MG, Krauss JK: **IPG lifetime in pallidal deep brain stimulation for dystonia.** *Eur J Neurol* 2011, **18**:872–875.
11. Lumsden DE, Kaminska M, Tustin K, Gimeno H, Baker L, Ashkan K, Selway R, Lin JP: **IPG life following pallidal deep brain stimulation (DBS) in children and young people with severe primary and secondary dystonia.** *Childs Nerv Syst* 2012, **28**:1091–1097.
12. Rawal PV, Almeida L, Smelser LB, Huang H, Guthrie BL, Walker HC: **Shorter pulse generator longevity and more frequent stimulator adjustments with pallidal DBS for dystonia versus other movement disorders.** *Brain Stimul* 2014, **7**:345–349.
13. Bin-Mahfoodh M, Hamani C, Sime E, Lozano AM: **Longevity of batteries in internal pulse generators used for deep brain stimulation.** *Stereotact Funct Neurosurg* 2003, **80**:56–60.
14. Halpern CH, McGill KR, Baltuch GH, Jaggi JL: **Longevity analysis of currently available deep brain stimulation devices.** *Stereotact Funct Neurosurg* 2011, **89**:1–5.
15. Stewart CD, Eljamel S: **Prediction of implantable pulse generator longevity in deep brain stimulation: limitations and possible solutions in clinical practice.** *Stereotact Funct Neurosurg* 2011, **89**:299–304.

15

Arrhythmokinesis is evident during unimanual not bimanual finger tapping in Parkinson's disease

Megan H Trager[1], Anca Velisar[1], Mandy Miller Koop[1], Lauren Shreve[1], Emma Quinn[1] and Helen Bronte-Stewart[1,2*]

Abstract

Background: Arrhythmokinesis, the variability in repetitive movements, is a fundamental feature of Parkinson's disease (PD). We hypothesized that unimanual repetitive alternating finger tapping (AFT) would reveal more arrhythmokinesis compared to bimanual single finger alternating hand tapping (SFT), in PD.

Methods: The variability of inter-strike interval (CV_{ISI}) and of amplitude (CV_{AMP}) during AFT and SFT were measured on an engineered, MRI-compatible keyboard in sixteen PD subjects off medication and in twenty-four age-matched controls.

Results: The CV_{ISI} and CV_{AMP} of the more affected (MA) and less affected (LA) sides in PD subjects were greater during AFT than SFT ($P < 0.05$). However, there was no difference between AFT and SFT for controls. Both CV_{ISI} and CV_{AMP} were greater in the MA and LA hands of PD subjects versus controls during AFT ($P < 0.01$). The CV_{ISI} and CV_{AMP} of the MA, but not the LA hand, were greater in PDs versus controls during SFT ($P < 0.05$). Also, AFT, but not SFT, detected a difference between the MA and LA hands of PDs ($P < 0.01$).

Conclusions: Unimanual, repetitive alternating finger tapping brings out more arrhythmokinesis compared to bimanual, single finger tapping in PDs but not in controls. Arrhythmokinesis during unimanual, alternating finger tapping captured a significant difference between both the MA and LA hands of PD subjects and controls, whereas that during a bimanual, single finger tapping task only distinguished between the MA hand and controls. Arrhythmokinesis underlies freezing of gait and may also underlie the freezing behavior documented in fine motor control if studied using a unimanual alternating finger tapping task.

Keywords: Parkinson's disease, Finger tapping, Rhythmicity, Arrhythmokinesis, Quantitative Digitography

Background

Wertham used the term "arrhythmokinesis" to describe the variability in repetitive movements in cerebellar diseases [1]. Arrhythmokinesis has subsequently been revealed in many studies of repetitive movement in Parkinson's disease (PD) and has been shown to be a useful marker of overall disease severity and of the effectiveness of medication and deep brain stimulation [2-10].

Arrhythmokinesis of stride duration during walking and stepping in place tasks has been shown to correlate with self-reported freezing of gait (FOG) severity, and

has been suggested to be a useful marker of FOG [11-13]. Freezing behavior has also been demonstrated in repetitive finger and upper extremity movements [9,14-17]. In studies using single finger flexion-extension movements, alternating between hands, the number of freezing episodes correlated with self-reported (FOG) severity but arrhythmokinesis was not observed during the task [14-17]. The authors concluded that arrhythmokinesis of upper extremity movements may not be a useful marker of freezing behavior as had been reported for FOG. However, other reports have suggested that more complex upper limb tasks may be required to detect arrhythmokinesis in upper limb movements [17]. Using a unimanual alternating finger tapping task we have reported both freezing episodes and arrhythmokinesis

* Correspondence: hbs@stanford.edu

[1]Department of Neurology and Neurological Sciences, Stanford University, 300 Pasteur Drive, Stanford, CA 94305, USA

[2]Department of Neurosurgery, Stanford University, Stanford, CA, USA

[9,10]. This inspired us to investigate whether a more complex task was necessary to reveal arrhythmokinesis in upper extremity movements. In this study, we measure arrhythmokinesis in both amplitude and frequency in a repetitive unimanual alternating finger tapping (AFT) task and compare that to the same measures in a repetitive bimanual single finger tapping, alternating between hands (SFT) task in PD subjects, off medication, and in an age-matched group of healthy subjects.

Methods

Subjects and clinical evaluation

Sixteen subjects (twelve men) with idiopathic Parkinson's disease (PD) were recruited from the Stanford Movement Disorders Clinic and consented to participate in the study, which was approved by the Stanford Institutional Review Board. A fellowship-trained Movement Disorders specialist confirmed the diagnosis in each subject. The age at evaluation was 68.9 ± 9.02 years, and the disease duration from diagnosis was 8.2 ± 5.64 years. Patients reported the body side that was more affected by PD, which was confirmed by the UPDRS III.

Twenty-four age-matched control subjects (57 ± 7.98 years, six men) consented and participated in the study. Control subjects were screened for any coexisting neurological or medical disorder using a comprehensive questionnaire. There were more men in the PD group than in the control group, which would tend to bias the results towards more rhythmic tapping in PD subjects, as men may tap with greater regularity than women [18].

The PD subjects were tested in the off therapy state. Thirteen subjects had not undergone deep brain stimulation (DBS) surgery and three subjects had the DBS system implanted but were tested prior to initial activation of the DBS system. All subjects withheld long- and short-acting dopaminergic medication for >24 and >12 hours respectively prior to testing [10].

Quantitative DigitoGraphy (QDG)

Subjects sat on an armless chair with the elbow flexed at approximately 90 degrees and the wrist resting on a pad at the same level as the keys of a customized engineered, MRI compatible keyboard, which allows for precise measurement of amplitude and timing of finger tapping, Figure 1. We have called this technology Quantitative DigitoGraphy (QDG) [9,10].

Subjects performed the AFT task, Figure 1A and the SFT task, Figure 1B, in a predetermined randomized order. In the AFT task, subjects placed the index and middle finger on each key with the other hand resting

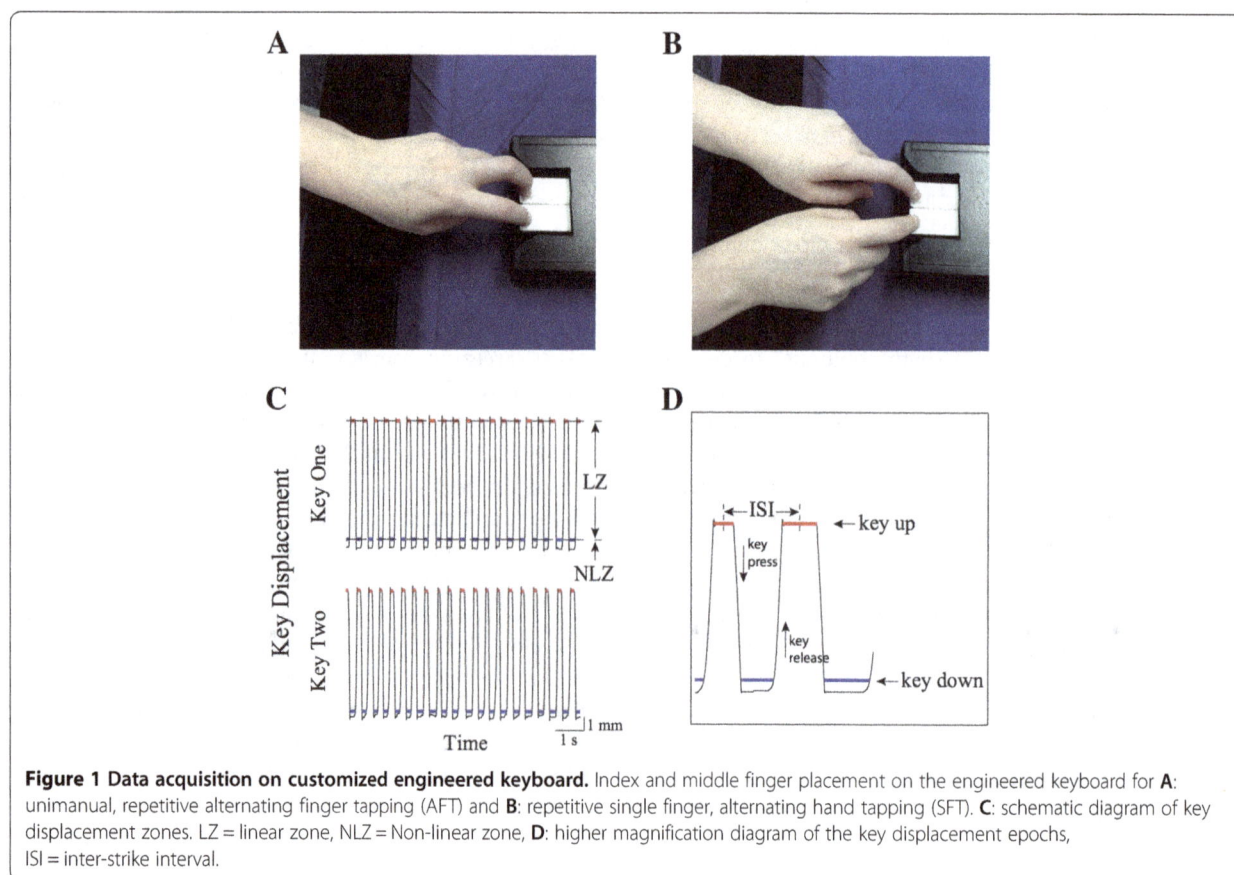

Figure 1 Data acquisition on customized engineered keyboard. Index and middle finger placement on the engineered keyboard for **A**: unimanual, repetitive alternating finger tapping (AFT) and **B**: repetitive single finger, alternating hand tapping (SFT). **C**: schematic diagram of key displacement zones. LZ = linear zone, NLZ = Non-linear zone, **D**: higher magnification diagram of the key displacement epochs, ISI = inter-strike interval.

on the lap. In the SFT task, subjects placed the right and left index finger on each key. The other fingers did not touch the surrounding keyboard or tabletop area. In both tasks, subjects were instructed to tap each key in an alternating pattern as fast and as regularly as possible for 30 seconds, starting and stopping only when they heard an auditory cue, while maintaining the alternating sequence and keeping the wrist stationary. Participants were instructed to attempt to press and release the keys completely. The same instructions were given to each subject.

No external pacing or cueing was provided. Subjects performed the tasks without visual (eyes closed) or auditory feedback. The keys do not produce audible notes and subjects wore headphones through which static "white noise" was transmitted to mask the sound of the finger striking the key. Each subject had a short period of practice before the test began, and all trials were videotaped; the video of the fingers was time-stamped and synchronized with the data.

Data acquisition and analysis: customized engineered keyboard and kinematic algorithm

An engineered keyboard was used to acquire the finger tapping movement, Figure 1. The keyboard was designed to produce an analog output voltage signal proportional to the displacement of the key. The key displacement was linearly related to the output voltage signal with a resolution of 62.5 μm per 40 mV. For key displacements less than 9 mm, the keyboard operated in a linear zone (LZ), Figure 1C. Systematic analysis of the keyboard mechanics revealed that near the base of the key displacement, the key reached a compliant mechanical stop. When the finger pressed down further, the extra displacements were non-linearly related to the output voltage signal. We defined this range of the key displacement as the "nonlinear zone" (NLZ), Figure 1C.

A customized detection algorithm, written in MATLAB (version 8.2, The Mathworks, Inc., Natick, MA, USA), was used to determine specific states in the cycle of finger tapping movement. Each cycle of finger tapping was divided into four epochs, Figure 1D. The "key up" epoch was defined as the period during which the finger changed direction from an upward movement to a downward movement. The "key down" epoch was the time when the finger changed direction from a downward movement to an upward one. The "key press" epoch was the period during which the finger was moving downwards. Finally, the "key release" epoch was the period during which the finger traveled upwards.

The inter-strike interval (ISI), the time to complete one cycle of finger tapping, was calculated from the midpoint of one key up epoch to the midpoint of the following key up epoch, Figure 1D. The variability of key tapping frequency was measured using the coefficient of variation (the standard deviation (SD) divided by the mean) of the inter-strike interval (CV_{ISI}) and was reported as a percentage.

The key strike amplitude was calculated for key displacements in the linear zone of the keyboard. The amplitude of a key press or release was defined as the distance (mm) the key travelled during key press or release epochs respectively. The maximum amplitude for a complete key press or release in the linear zone of the keyboard was 9 mm. For each subject, the average of all the key press and key release epochs was used as the amplitude outcome metric. The variability of amplitude was calculated using the coefficient of variation (CV_{AMP}).

Statistics

The statistical software R (R Core Team, 2013) and lme4 (Bates, Maechler & Bolker, 2012) were used to perform a linear mixed effects analysis of the relationship between group type and test type. Group type (PD-most affected hand, PD- less affected hand, Control- dominant hand, and Control- non-dominant hand) and test type (AFT, SFT) with all interaction terms were fixed effects, and subject number was a random effect. The model included an intercept term. Visual inspection of residual plots did not reveal any obvious deviations from assumptions of homoscedasticity or normality. P values were obtained using the multcomp package in R (Bretz, Hothom, Westfall, 2010) with a Tukey correction for multiple comparisons.

Results

The group's off medication UPDRS III (motor) score ± SD was 35.5 ± 11.34, and the lateralized upper extremity scores (rest tremor, postural tremor, rigidity, finger tapping, hand movements, pronation-supination of the hands) were 10.19 ± 4.74 and 6.2 ± 3.16 in the more affected (MA) and less affected (LA) sides, respectively. Figure 2 demonstrates the QDG data from seven seconds of index finger tapping in the unimanual AFT and bimanual SFT, alternating between hands, tasks from a control subject's non-dominant hand (NDH), Figure 2A and C respectively, and from the MA hand of a PD subject off medication, Figure 2B and D respectively.

The control subject performed the AFT task with fast, regular, and mostly full amplitude key presses, while the PD subject performed AFT with arrhythmic partial key presses, Figure 2A and B, respectively. In contrast, both subjects performed SFT with a regular rhythm and amplitude, although the PD subject tapped more slowly than the control, Figure 2C and D, respectively.

PD subjects, but not controls, exhibited more irregular tapping during the AFT task compared to the SFT task, Table 1 and Figure 3.

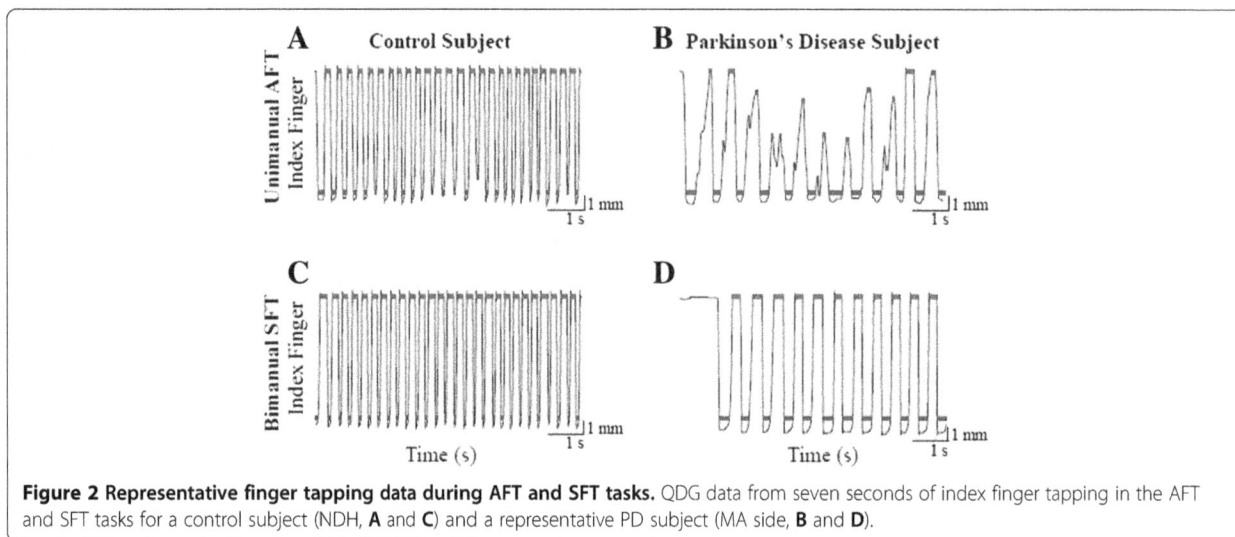

Figure 2 Representative finger tapping data during AFT and SFT tasks. QDG data from seven seconds of index finger tapping in the AFT and SFT tasks for a control subject (NDH, **A** and **C**) and a representative PD subject (MA side, **B** and **D**).

This was evident for both the amplitude and timing (frequency) of tapping among PD subjects in the MA and LA hands, Table 1. There was no difference in variability of amplitude or timing during AFT versus SFT in the DH and NDH of controls. Tapping of the MA hand was more irregular than that of the LA hand in PDs during AFT ($P < 0.01$ for CV_{ISI}, $P < 0.001$ for CV_{AMP}) but not SFT. There was no difference in variability of amplitude or timing between the DH and NDH of controls in either task.

The performance of unimanual AFT was more irregular in both the PD MA and LA hands compared to control DH and NDH for both amplitude (CV_{AMP}, $P < 0.001$, for all) and frequency (CV_{ISI}, $P = 0.01$ for LA vs. NDH, $P < 0.001$ for all others, Figure 3). Comparing the performance of bimanual SFT between PD subjects and controls: CV_{AMP} was greater in the PD MA hand compared to both control DH and NDH ($P < 0.01$ for both) and CV_{ISI} was greater in the PD MA hand compared to the control DH ($P < 0.05$). The CV_{AMP} and CV_{ISI} of

bimanual SFT were not different between the PD LA hand and control DH or NDH.

Discussion

This study has shown that arrhythmokinesis was worse during a repetitive unimanual alternating finger tapping (AFT) task than during a repetitive bimanual single finger tapping, alternating hand (SFT) task in both the more affected and less affected hands in PD subjects, off medication. There was no difference in the regularity of the amplitude or the frequency of tapping between tasks in control subjects. Arrhythmokinesis in PD MA and LA hands was worse in the unimanual AFT compared to the performance of controls DH and NDH, whereas only the PD MA hand was more irregular than the control NDH (amplitude) and DH (amplitude and frequency) in the bimanual SFT task.

Arrhythmokinesis in upper extremity movements in Parkinson's disease has been shown to be a useful marker of overall disease severity and of the effectiveness

Table 1 AFT captures greater arrhythmokinesis than SFT in PDs but not controls

	Unimanual AFT	Bimanual SFT	P Value
	CV_{Amp}(25-75% range) or (SD)	CV_{Amp} (25-75% range) or (SD)	
PD MA	38.6 (16.9)	14.5 (14.3)	P < 0.001
PD LA	25.5 (10.7)	8.55 (9.20)	P < 0.001
Control DH	7.21 (6.76)	2.31 (3.75)	NS
Control NDH	10.5 (8.94)	2.94 (3.82)	NS
	CV_{ISI} (25-75% range) or (SD)	CV_{ISI} (25-75% range) or (SD)	
PD MA	37.0 (12.5)	18.6 (11.4)	P < 0.001
PD LA	26.1 (15.9-30.3)	12.6 (9.15-18.5)	P < 0.05
Control DH	13.8 (5.4)	9.79 (4.21)	NS
Control NDH	14.28 (10.04-17.98)	10.45 (7.61-16.21)	NS

Values are reported as percentages.

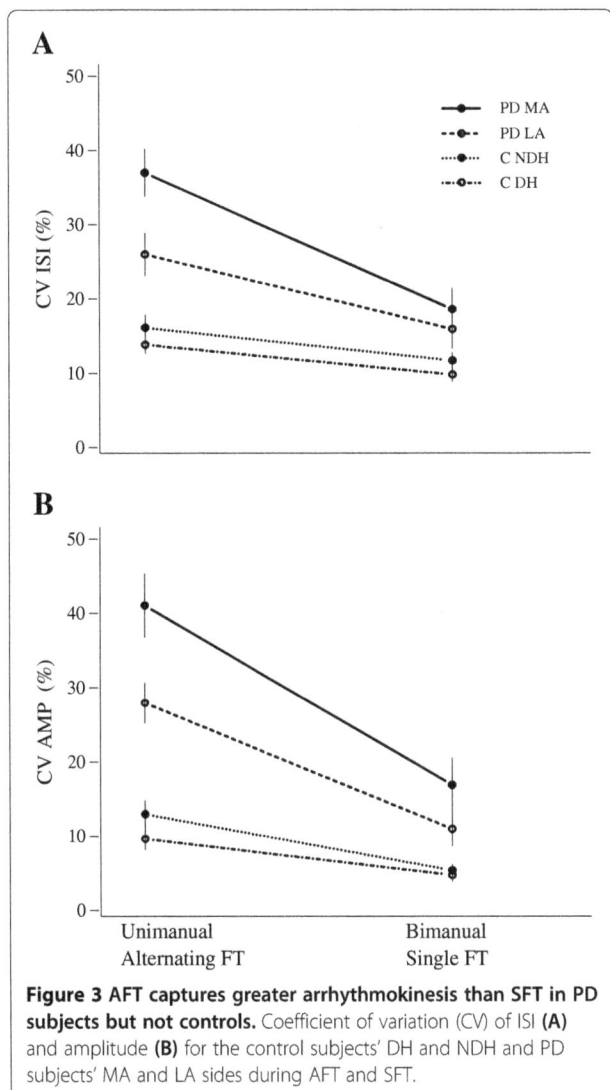

Figure 3 AFT captures greater arrhythmokinesis than SFT in PD subjects but not controls. Coefficient of variation (CV) of ISI **(A)** and amplitude **(B)** for the control subjects' DH and NDH and PD subjects' MA and LA sides during AFT and SFT.

bihemispheric motor network was activated during bimanual and unimanual finger movements in normal subjects [25]. However, there was increased activation in several regions during the unimanual alternating finger movement compared to the bimanual single finger movement. In a study comparing unimanual single and alternating finger tapping in PD, only alternating finger tapping with activation of the contralateral limb correlated with the striatal 6-Fluoro-L-dopa PET uptake [26]. Thus, it may be more challenging for the impaired sensorimotor network in PD to maintain the regularity of an alternating, adjacent finger tapping task of one hand than to maintain regularity in an alternating hand movement with single finger tapping.

Previous studies have shown that the basal ganglia is involved in motor and perceptual timing, and that PD subjects are impaired in repetitive motor timing [27]. In addition, tasks with increased cognitive demands show greater impairment in PD subjects [28]. Therefore, it is possible that the unimanual AFT task captured greater arrhythmokinesis as it involves increased cognitive load compared to single finger tapping. It has also been proposed that the bihemispheric activation of motor circuits during bimanual tasks may facilitate movement of the more affected side [29]. Thus during bimanual SFT, it is possible that the less affected limb is able to maintain a more normal rhythm and "drive" the more affected limb to keep time.

The actual value of the CV that is used to differentiate regular from irregular behavior differs among motor tasks in PD and control subjects, and this may have biological significance. In several studies of FOG, the CVs reported for stride length or duration during walking and stepping tasks were consistently around 3% for non-freezers and controls and 6% for freezers [11-13,21,30]. In this study of unimanual AFT the CVs were greater than 7% for control subjects and greater than 25% for PD subjects and are consistent with our previous AFT studies using a MIDI-interfaced keyboard [10].

The explanation for the difference in CVs of unimanual alternating finger tapping versus those of stride duration may be similar to the explanation for the difference in variability between stride length and duration (2-5%) versus stride width and double support time in healthy subjects (17-27%) [31]. It was postulated that stride length and duration reflect gait patterning, which requires a high degree of consistency, while stride width and double support time are balance control mechanisms well-suite for fine control with a larger degree of variability. Thus higher values of the CVs in unimanual AFT in both control and PD subjects support a motor control mechanism more suited for variability and fine-tuning than for consistency.

of medication and deep brain stimulation [2,7-9]. Arrhythmokinesis of stride duration and amplitude is a reliable marker of freezing of gait (FOG) and is related to cognitive deficits, which may also contribute to FOG [11,12,14,19-23]. However, a study comparing freezing behavior in repetitive upper extremity movements to FOG failed to reveal evidence of arrhythmokinesis even though they did demonstrate freezing episodes that correlated with FOG [14,17,24]. The findings of the current study support the hypothesis that a more complex task than single finger tapping, alternating between hands may be necessary to demonstrate arrhythmokinesis in upper extremity and specifically finger movements.

Coordination of alternating movements of adjacent digits on one hand appears to be more challenging to the brain than the coordination of a simple movement of one digit per hand, alternating between hands. Functional imaging (fMRI) has demonstrated that a similar

Conclusions

Arrhythmokinesis, the variability in repetitive movements, may be regarded as a cardinal motor sign in Parkinson's disease. In this study, unimanual AFT captured greater arrhythmokinesis than bimanual SFT, in PD subjects. This difference was not seen in control subjects. Unimanual AFT also captured a significant difference in arrhythmokinesis between the PD MA and LA hands and controls' DH and NDH whereas bimanual SFT only distinguished between PD MA hand and controls' NDH (amplitude) and DH (amplitude and frequency). Arrhythmokinesis of stride duration is widely used as a marker of FOG. A study of bimanual single finger movements alternating between hands demonstrated freezing episodes, but not arrhythmokinesis, leading to the conclusion that arrhythmokinesis is not a marker of freezing behavior in upper extremity movements. The results of this study demonstrate that arrhythmokinesis in fine motor control may be evident if investigated during more complex finger movement tasks, such as a unimanual alternating adjacent finger tapping task. It remains to be seen if this correlates with FOG metrics.

Abbreviations

PD: Parkinson's disease; AFT: Alternating finger tapping; SFT: Single finger tapping; MA: More affected side; LA: Less affected side; UPDRS: Unified Parkinson's Disease Rating Scale; FOG: Freezing of gait; QDG: Quantitative digitography; LZ: Linear zone; NLZ: Non-linear zone; ISI: Inter-strike interval; NDH: Non-dominant hand; DH: Dominant hand.

Competing interests

The authors declare that they have no competing interests.

Authors' contributions

MHT- study design, subject recruitment, data acquisition, data analysis, manuscript preparation and editing. AV- data analysis, MATLAB script, keyboard technology, manuscript editing and critique. MMK- data analysis, manuscript preparation, editing and critique. LS- subject recruitment, data collection, manuscript preparation editing and critique. EQ- subject recruitment, data collection, manuscript editing and critique. HBS- study design and oversight, data analysis, manuscript preparation and editing. All authors read and approved the final manuscript.

Acknowledgements

We thank Julie Nantel for helpful comments on the study design, Zack Blumenfeld, Bruce Hill, and Tom Prieto for comments during data analysis and manuscript preparation, and Leanel Luciano-Liwanag for coordination of subject scheduling and testing.

Funding

The Helen and John Cahill Family Foundation, the John A. Blume Foundation, the Robert and Ruth Halperin Foundation, the Parkinson's Disease Foundation (PDF-SFW-1330, MK), the National Academy of Sciences Grant-In-Aid of Research (Sigma Xi, The Scientific Research Society, MK), Irene and Eric Simon Brain Research Foundation.

References

1. Wertham F. A new sign of cerebellar disease. J Nerv Ment Dis. 1929;60:486–93.
2. Shimoyama I, Ninchoji T, Uemura K. The finger-tapping test. A quantitative analysis. Arch Neurol. 1990;47:681–4.
3. Nagasaki H, Itoh H, Maruyama H, Hashizume K. Characteristic difficulty in rhythmic movement with aging and its relation to Parkinson's disease. Exp Aging Res. 1988;14:171–6.
4. Nagasaki H, Nakamura R. Rhythm formation and its disturbances–a study based upon periodic response of a motor output system. J Hum Ergol (Tokyo). 1982;11:127–42.
5. Nakamura R, Nagasaki H, Narabayashi H. Disturbances of rhythm formation in patients with Parkinson's disease: part I. Characteristics of tapping response to the periodic signals. Percept Mot Skills. 1978;46:63–75.
6. Nakamura R, Nagasaki H, Narabayashi H. Arrhythmokinesia in parkinsonism. Hoffmann-La Roche; 1976.
7. Stegemoller EL, Simuni T, MacKinnon C. Effect of movement frequency on repetitive finger movements in patients with Parkinson's disease. Mov Disord. 2009;24:1162–9.
8. Stegemoller EL, Zadikoff C, Rosenow JM, Mackinnon CD. Deep brain stimulation improves movement amplitude but not hastening of repetitive finger movements. Neurosci Lett. 2013;552:135–9.
9. Taylor Tavares AL, Jefferis GS, Koop M, Hill BC, Hastie T, Heit G, et al. Quantitative measurements of alternating finger tapping in Parkinson's disease correlate with UPDRS motor disability and reveal the improvement in fine motor control from medication and deep brain stimulation. Mov Disord. 2005;20:1286–98.
10. Bronte-Stewart HM, Ding L, Alexander C, Zhou Y, Moore GP. Quantitative digitography (QDG): a sensitive measure of digital motor control in idiopathic Parkinson's disease. Mov Disord. 2000;15:36–47.
11. Plotnik M, Hausdorff JM. The role of gait rhythmicity and bilateral coordination of stepping in the pathophysiology of freezing of gait in Parkinson's disease. Mov Disord. 2008;23 Suppl 2:S444–50.
12. Nantel J, de Solages C, Bronte-Stewart H. Repetitive stepping in place identifies and measures freezing episodes in subjects with Parkinson's disease. Gait Posture. 2011;34:329–33.
13. Hausdorff JM, Schaafsma JD, Balash Y, Bartels AL, Gurevich T, Giladi N. Impaired regulation of stride variability in Parkinson's disease subjects with freezing of gait. Exp Brain Res. 2003;149:187–94.
14. Nieuwboer A, Vercruysse S, Feys P, Levin O, Spildooren J, Swinnen S. Upper limb movement interruptions are correlated to freezing of gait in Parkinson's disease. Eur J Neurosci. 2009;29:1422–30.
15. Vercruysse S, Spildooren J, Heremans E, Vandenbossche J, Wenderoth N, Swinnen SP, et al. Abnormalities and cue dependence of rhythmical upper-limb movements in Parkinson patients with freezing of gait. Neurorehabil Neural Repair. 2012;26:636–45.
16. Williams AJ, Peterson DS, Ionno M, Pickett KA, Earhart GM. Upper extremity freezing and dyscoordination in Parkinson's disease: effects of amplitude and cadence manipulations. Parkinsons Dis. 2013;2013:595378.
17. Barbe MT, Amarell M, Snijders AH, Florin E, Quatuor EL, Schonau E, et al. Gait and upper limb variability in Parkinson's disease patients with and without freezing of gait. J Neurol. 2013.
18. Schmidt SL, Oliveira RM, Krahe TE, Filgueiras CC. The effects of hand preference and gender on finger tapping performance asymmetry by the use of an infra-red light measurement device. Neuropsychologia. 2000;38:529–34.
19. Nieuwboer A, Chavret F, Willems A, Desloovere K. Does freezing in Parkinson's disease change limb coordination? A kinematic analysis. J Neurol. 2007;254:1268–77.
20. Nieuwboer A, Dom R, De Weerdt W, Desloovere K, Fieuws S, Broens-Kaucsik E. Abnormalities of the spatiotemporal characteristics of gait at the onset of freezing in Parkinson's disease. Mov Disord. 2001;16:1066–75.
21. Plotnik M, Giladi N, Hausdorff JM. Bilateral coordination of walking and freezing of gait in Parkinson's disease. Eur J Neurosci. 2008;27:1999–2006.
22. Stegemoller EL, Wilson JP, Hazamy A, Shelley MC, Okun MS, Altmann LJ, et al. Associations between cognitive and gait performance during single- and dual-task walking in people with Parkinson disease. Phys Ther. 2014;94:757–66.
23. Walton CC, Shine JM, Mowszowski L, Gilat M, Hall JM, O'Callaghan C, et al. Impaired cognitive control in Parkinson's disease patients with freezing of gait in response to cognitive load. J Neural Transm. 2014. [Epub ahead of print].
24. Vercruysse S, Spildooren J, Heremans E, Vandenbossche J, Levin O, Wenderoth N, et al. Freezing in Parkinson's disease: a spatiotemporal motor disorder beyond gait. Mov Disord. 2012;27:254–63.
25. Koeneke S, Lutz K, Wustenberg T, Jancke L. Bimanual versus unimanual coordination: what makes the difference? Neuroimage. 2004;22:1336–50.

26. Pal PK, Lee CS, Samii A, Schulzer M, Stoessl AJ, Mak EK, et al. Alternating two finger tapping with contralateral activation is an objective measure of clinical severity in Parkinson's disease and correlates with PET. Parkinsonism Relat Disord. 2001;7:305–9.

27. Jones CR, Malone TJ, Dirnberger G, Edwards M, Jahanshahi M. Basal ganglia, dopamine and temporal processing: performance on three timing tasks on and off medication in Parkinson's disease. Brain Cogn. 2008;68:30–41.

28. Brown RG, Marsden CD. Dual task performance and processing resources in normal subjects and patients with Parkinson's disease. Brain. 1991;114(Pt 1A):215–31.

29. Kishore A, Espay AJ, Marras C, Al-Khairalla T, Arenovich T, Asante A, et al. Unilateral versus bilateral tasks in early asymmetric Parkinson's disease: differential effects on bradykinesia. Mov Disord. 2007;22:328–33.

30. Nantel J, Bronte-Stewart H. The effect of medication and the role of postural instability in different components of freezing of gait (FOG). Parkinsonism Relat Disord. 2014;20(4):447–51.

31. Gabell A, Nayak US. The effect of age on variability in gait. J Gerontol. 1984;39:662–6.

16

Prevalence of depression in Parkinson's disease patients in Ethiopia

Dawit Kibru Worku[1*], Yared Mamushet Yifru[2], Douglas G Postels[3] and Fikre Enquselassie Gashe[4]

Abstract

Background: Parkinson's disease (PD) is associated with cognitive and psychiatric disturbances including depression, anxiety, psychotic symptoms and sleep disturbances. These psychiatric manifestations have a negative impact on disease course and the medical management of PD patients. Major depression has a greater negative impact on patients' quality of life than abnormal motor function, and is associated with faster cognitive decline and progression of motor deficits. Thus, the objective of this study was to determine the prevalence and pattern of depression in PD outpatients in Ethiopia. We determined the age range in which depression in PD patients is most common, the most common symptoms of depression, and the epidemiologic confounders associated with depression in PD patients.

Methods: We conducted a cross-sectional point prevalence study of all PD patients attending the follow-up clinics of the departments of neurology at Black Lion Teaching and Zewuditu Memorial Hospitals in Addis Ababa, Ethiopia, from May 2013 to August 2013. We collected information using a structured questionnaire which assessed demographic information, clinical history, and neurologic function.

Result: Of the 101 patients surveyed, the prevalence of depression was 58/101(57.4%). Of these patients, 1 of 58(1.7%) was on antidepressant medications. These low proportions likely indicate a low index of suspicion and under treatment of depression in PD outpatients.

Conclusion: In Ethiopian PD outpatients, depression is under recognized and undertreated. We recommend routine use of screening tools. In those who screen positive for depression, treatment is warranted. Further studies are needed to confirm these findings, and to increase our understanding of specific signs and symptoms of depression in the context of PD.

Keywords: Parkinson's disease, Depression, Non-Motor symptoms

Background

Worldwide, Parkinson's disease (PD) is the most common progressive neurodegenerative disorder of adulthood and is characterized by bradykinesia, resting tremor, muscular rigidity, shuffling gait, and flexed posture. PD may be accompanied by a variety of non-motor symptoms, including autonomic, sensory, sleep, cognitive, and psychiatric disturbances [1-5].

Psycihiatric Co-morbidity in Parkinson's disease

In addition to motor abnormalities, PD is associated with cognitive and psychiatric disturbances including depression, anxiety, psychotic symptoms and sleep disturbances

[6,7]. Psychiatric co-morbidities have a negative impact on the course and management of PD patients. Major depression has a greater negative impact on patients' quality of life than impaired motor function [8-10] and accounts for more rapid cognitive decline and progression of motor deficits [11-14].

Early recognition and treatment of co-morbid depressive disorders is critical for comprehensive patient management. Failure to diagnose psychiatric co-morbidities in PD patients is common. In a study of 101 PD patients done in Baltimore, Maryland, USA, the treating neurologists failed to recognize depression, anxiety and fatigue in more than half of patients [15]. Standardized testing showed depression in 44% of patients, anxiety in 39%, fatigue in 42%, and sleep disturbance in 43%. The prevalence of these conditions as identified by the treating

* Correspondence: davulala@yahoo.com
[1]P.O.Box – 29818, Addis Ababa, Ethiopia
Full list of author information is available at the end of the article

neurologist was lower: 21% with depression, 19% with anxiety, 14% with fatigue and 39% with sleep disturbance. The diagnostic sensitivity for the treating neurologists was 35% for depression, 42% for anxiety, 25% for fatigue, and 60% for sleep disturbance [15].

Depression screening tools

Depression screening tools should be both sensitive but also specific to the broad differential diagnosis of depressed mood in PD. They should differentiate between a major depressive episode, adjustment disorder, mood disorder, dementia, "non-motor fluctuation", and transient mood changes in relation to DBS. Although not a substitute for a diagnostic evaluation, scales should distinguish normal emotional variability from symptoms that reflect major depression or a disabling non-major depressive syndrome. Clinician-rated depression scales include the 24-item and 17-item Hamilton Depression Rating Scale, the Montgomery-Åsberg Depression Rating Scale, and the Unified Parkinson's Disease Rating Scale Depression item. Self-reported scales include the Beck Depression Inventory–Version I, the 30-item and 15-item Geriatric Depression Scale, and Quick Inventory of Depressive Symptomatology. Clinician-Rated scales have been shown to be valid in PD [16]. The GDS-15 and Patient Health Questionnaire-9 have also been investigated as diagnostic instruments in PD [17].

A comparison study of nine scales to detect depression in PD showed the QIDS-C16 scale were among the valid screening when PD-specific cutoff scores are used [18]. To determine if the QIDS-C16 measure depression in a manner consistent with the most widely used assessments, Rush et al. [19] examined the relationship between QIDS scores, and the Hamilton Rating Scale for Depression 17 item version (HRSD17) and Beck Depression Inventory (BDI) scores in a sample of 434 outpatients with major depressive disorder and 103 normal controls. QIDS total score was comparable to those obtained by the HRSD17 and BDI, with Pearson product moment correlations of 0.95 between the IDS-C30 and HRSD17. The correlation between the BDI21 and the IDS-C30 was 0.86. The correlation between the BDI21 and the HRSD17 was 0.85.

Providing evidence that the IDS and QIDS are measuring depressive symptoms in the same manner, Trivedi et al. [20] found robust correlations between the QIDS-C16 and IDS-C30 total scores for out-patients with MDD (c = 0.82, n = 544) and Bipolar Disorder (BD) (c = 0.81, n = 402). As the Quick Inventory of Depressive Symptomatology Clinician-Rated – 16 scale includes the core components of the DSM-IV TR criteria for depression, we have chosen it for use in this research.

Trivedi et. al found that by using the QIDS-C16 and IDS-C30, that within the patient population studied

(drawn from 19 regionally and ethnically diverse clinics as part of the Texas Medication Algorithm Project, Texas, USA) the severity of depression varied greatly: 43(42.6%) had mild, 14(13.9%) had moderate, 1(0.99%) had severe depression, and 43(42.6%) had no depression. There was no patient who was very severely depressed (Figure 1). In other studies co-morbid depression prevalence rates vary, ranging from 7% to 90%, with a general consensus that depression in some form (i.e., either major or non-major depression) appears to occur in approximately 40% of PD patients [14,21].

PD-specific cutoff scores (i.e., >12) increase the ability of QIDS to detect depression in PD to: sensitivity of 0.81, specificity of 0.79, positive predictive value of 0.73, and negative predictive value of 0.86. But it's not a recommendation for this cutoff score to be used in clinical practice [18].

Depression and PD are associated. Patients with PD are at higher risk of developing depression than the general population and patients with depressive disorder are at greater risk of developing PD. Indeed, two population-based retrospective cohort studies have shown that, compared with controls of healthy subjects [22] or medical patients [23], patients with PD were more likely to have experienced a history of depression before their neurological diagnosis was made (odds ratios 2.2 and 2.4, respectively (95% CI = 2.1–2.7)).

There is little information available on the prevalence of depression in PD patients in Ethiopia. A study of existing indexed literature indicates that comparatively little PD-related research has been published from Africa [24]. However, because Africa is experiencing a demographic transition, the population will become much older by 2015 (increase in the percentage of persons aged 65 and over) [25], and diseases predominantly affecting older persons, such as PD are expected to become more common. This is also true for Ethiopia. Therefore, epidemiologic data are needed for effective planning of medical services in African countries including Ethiopia, and to compare genetic, environmental, and clinical aspects of PD in Africa with those of other continents.

Depression in PD often begins late in life, in contrast to primary major depression, which is more likely to appear before the age of 40. Analogous to other neurologic disorders where depression is co-morbid (epilepsy, multiple sclerosis and dementia) mood disturbances can antedate the motor manifestations of disease. This occurs in 12-37% of PD patients [21]. Dysphoric symptoms, including irritability, sadness, and pessimism, are more frequent presenting symptoms in PD patients compared to patients with primary mood disorders. Feelings of failure, guilt, and self-blame are less frequent in those with depression and co-morbid PD. Though suicidal ideation is more frequent in PD patients with co-morbid mood disorders

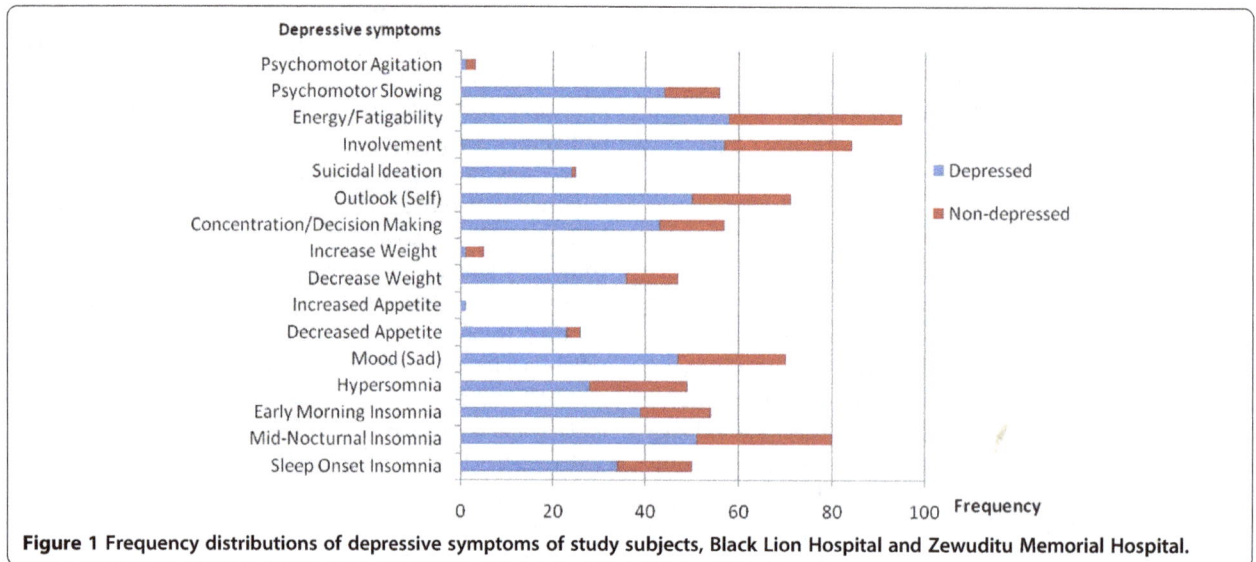

Figure 1 Frequency distributions of depressive symptoms of study subjects, Black Lion Hospital and Zewuditu Memorial Hospital.

compared to patients with primary depression, PD patients are less likely to commit suicide [21].

Depression is also a key determinant of poor health-related quality of life in PD patients and is associated with reduced function, cognitive impairment and increased stress for individuals with PD.

PD patients were significantly more depressed than other disabled patients matched for extent of functional impairment [26]. In studies of the relationship between depression and severity of functional impairment most have identified a modest correlation between mood abnormalities and functional deterioration [21]. Huber et al. reported that depressed patients with PD had a significantly more advanced stage of disability than nondepressed patients with Parkinson's disease [27]. Understanding depression in patients with PD is, therefore, critical to achieve comprehensive care for patients with this disease. Screening and the early identification of depression offer a crucial opportunity to alter the course of the disease and improve quality of life.

The main objective of the study is to determine the prevalence and pattern of depression in PD patients seen in the outpatient clinics of Black Lion and Zewuditu Memorial Hospitals, Addis Ababa, Ethiopia.

Methods

A Cross-sectional point prevalence survey was conducted between June to November 2013 in two governmental referral hospitals; Black Lion Teaching Hospital and Zewuditu Memorial Hospital, Addis Ababa, Ethiopia. All patients diagnosed with PD and attending the Neurology follow-up clinics of Black Lion Hospital or Zewuditu Memorial Hospital were the source population.

Patients were included if they had previous diagnosis of PD, were age ≥18 years old, had clinical symptomatology

in agreement with the UK Parkinson's Disease Society Brain Bank Clinical Diagnostic Criteria for the diagnosis of PD, and informed consent granted for study participation. Patients were excluded if they had Parkinsonism due to other causes or if they were unable to give consent. All patients fulfilling the inclusion criteria from June 2013 to November 2013 in the study area was included.

Clinical data was collected using a structured questionnaire in English. This questionnaire assessed: demographic data; a detailed clinical history including symptoms of PD and their duration; medication history.

A complete clinical and neurologic examination was performed. Nervous system examinations include full assessment of cranial nerves, deep tendon reflexes, Babinski sign, tone, motor and sensory functions, cerebellar signs, postural instability, gait and stance, and abnormal movements.

The 16 item Quick Inventory of Depressive Symptomatology (QIDS-C16) screen was administered and a score for each patient was calculated. Subjects were interviewed by clinicians to complete the QIDS-C16. The symptoms were familiar to clinicians, as the individual items are defined by the constructs represented in the DSM-IV criteria for MDD. Each item is interval-scaled from 0 to 3; 0 indicates absence of the symptom during the last 7 days. The anchors are intended to help raters represent the frequency and intensity associated with each symptom. Total QIDS-C16 total scores range from 0 to 27. The total score was obtained by adding the scores for each of the nine symptom domains of the DSM-IV MDD criteria: depressed mood, loss of interest or pleasure, concentration/decision making, self-outlook, suicidal ideation, energy/fatigability, sleep, weight/appetite change, and psychomotor changes. Sixteen items were used to rate the nine criterion domains of major depression: four for sleep disturbance (early, middle, and late insomnia plus hyper-somnia); two for psychomotor disturbance (agitation and retardation) and four for appetite/weight disturbance. Only one item was used to rate the remaining six domains (depressed mood, decreased interest, decreased energy, worthlessness/guilt, concentration/decision making, and suicidal ideation). Each item was rated 0–3. For symptom domains that require more than one item, the highest score of the item relevant for each domain was taken (e.g. , if early insomnia is 0, middle insomnia is 1, late insomnia is 3, and hypersomnia is 0, the sleep disturbance domain was rated 3). Severity of depression was defined by Total QIDS-C16 score: None for 0 – 5, Mild for 6 – 10, Moderate for 11 – 15, Severe for 16 – 20, and Very Severe for 21 – 27.

Piloting of the questionnaire was done in a sample of ten PD patients attending Black Lion Hospital Neurology Clinic before the starting of data collection for the research. These subjects were not included in the study results. Findings from the pre-test were utilized in modifying questions on the standard questionnaire. Questions that were difficult for subjects to understand were reformulated and repiloted until answers were considered internally valid.

Interviews and data extraction was performed by the principal investigator. Data was checked manually and cleaned. Before processing the data was coded and cross checked for completeness.

Analysis was performed using SPSS/PC version 20.0 software packages for statistical analysis (SPSS, INC, Chicago, IL). Descriptive summaries were employed to describe socio-demographic and clinical characteristics. Appropriate measures of central tendency, frequency distribution and cross tabulation were conducted. Odds ratios and 95% confidence intervals were calculated. A p value less than 0.05 were considered a statistically significant association between assessed variables. Due to the exploratory nature of our study we did not correct for multiple comparisons.

Protocol approvals were obtained from the ethical review Committee of the Department of Neurology and the Institutional Review Board (IRB) and Research and Publication Committee of the College of Health Sciences of Addis Ababa University. Informed patient consent was sought before study enrollment. Patients received standard therapy for PD and co-morbid mood disorders regardless of whether they consented to study enrollment. Patient data was deidentified during subsequent analysis and dissemination.

Results and discussion

One hundred one subjects with PD consented to study participation. Ninety-nine (98%) were right handed and 70/101 (69.3%) were male (Table 1). Depression was diagnosed in 58/101 (57.4%) patients. The prevalence of depression in women was 58.1% and in men 57.1%. Almost half [42/101(41.6%)] of the patients had no formal education. Twelve (20.7%) of depressed patients were employed while 14 (32.7%) of the non-depressed patients were employed. This was not significantly associated (P-value = 0.18, 95% CI = 0.75-4.55).

Forty-five (44.55%) had annual income of <300 USD and only 17(16.83%) of the study patients had a monthly income of >900 USD.

Of the total study population 5(4.95%) had a recent major life event, 2(1.98%) had a previous history of depression, 5(4.95%) had a first degree family history of psychiatric disorder, and 6(5.94%) had a family history of PD.

All subjects had bradykinesia, 94(93.1%) of them had muscular rigidity, and 92(91.1%) had resting tremor. Approximately half [50/101(49.5%)] had postural instability. Almost all subjects [100(99%)] had a progressive disorder and very few [7(6.9%)] had severe levodopa-induced chorea. Most of the subjects 89/101 (88.1%) were taking Levodopa-Carbidopa (250 mg-25 mg) combination, 48 (47.5%) were on Trihexiphendyl, only 3(2.97%) were on antidepressant (Amitriptyline, Flouxitine, and Serteraline each). Thirteen (29.7%) patients had co-morbid medical condition(s) including hypertension, diabetes mellitus, and bronchial asthma. Only 23(22.8%) patients had previous imaging.

Fifteen percent of the study population was classified as having moderate to severe depression (Figure 2). The most common depression symptoms of the screen positive patients were loss of energy, decreased social involvement, and mid-nocturnal insomnia. Increased appetite, increased weight, and psychomotor agitation were among the rare manifestation of depression in the study population.

One third (34.7%) of the patients were diagnosed with PD between the age of 55–64, 27(26.7%) at the age 65 and above, 24(23.8%) at the age 45–54, and only 15(14.9%) at age below 45 years; with mean + SD of 57.10 + 10.84.

Of all the variables evaluated, only annual income was significantly associated (P-Value = 0.01; 95% CI = 0.2 (0.06-0.66)) with having depression in the present study (Table 2).

Depressive symptoms have been recognized to be a major determinant of health-related Quality of life in PD. There is evidence that depression in patients with PD is associated with more severe cognitive and functional impairments, faster progression of illness, worse quality of life and higher burden for caregivers. Several rating scales for screening or assessing the severity of depression are available [28]. A comparison study of nine scales to detect depression in PD showed the QIDS-C16 scale were among the valid screening when PD-specific cutoff scores are used [18].

Table 1 Frequency distributions of sociodemographic characteristics of study subjects, Black Lion Hospital and Zewuditu Memorial Hospital

Variables	Depressed		Not depressed		
	Frequency	Proportion	Frequency	Proportion	P-value
Handedness					
Right	56	96.6%	43	100	
Left	2	3.4%	-	-	0.5
Total	58		43		
Age					
<50	11	19.0%	8	18.6	
50-59	9	15.5%	10	23.3	
60-69	17	29.3%	17	39.5	
70-79	17	29.3%	7	16.3	
80 and above	4	6.9%	1	2.3	
Total	58		43		
Mean ± SD	63.94 ± 12.06		60.13 ± 9.20		0.087
Gender					
Female	18	31.0	13	30.2	1.0
Male	40	69.0	30	69.8	
Total	58		43		
Marital status					
Married	39	67.2	36	83.7	
Separated/divorced	6	10.3	-	-	0.03
Widowed	13	22.4	7	16.3	0.33
Total	58		43		
Employment					
Employed	12	20.7	14	32.6	0.25
Unemployed	46	79.3	29	67.4	
Housewife	10	21.7	7	24.1	1.0
Retired	20	43.5	14	48.3	0.84
Out of job	16	34.8	8	27.6	0.81
Total	58		43		
Education					
No formal education	29	50.0	13	30.2	
Primary	18	31.0	10	23.3	0.80
Secondary	6	10.3	12	27.9	0.02
More than secondary	5	8.6	8	18.6	0.06
Total	58		43		
Monthly income (USD)					
<300	33	56.9	12	27.9	
300-600	14	24.1	13	30.2	0.08
600-900	5	8.6	7	16.3	0.08
>900	6	10.4	11	25.6	0.01
Total	58		43		

Table 1 Frequency distributions of sociodemographic characteristics of study subjects, Black Lion Hospital and Zewuditu Memorial Hospital *(Continued)*

Recent major life events					
Yes	4	6.9	1	2.3	0.40
No	54	93.1	42	97.7	
Total	58		43		
Previous history of depression					
Yes	2	3.4	-	-	1.0
No	56	96.6	43	100	
Total	58		43		
First degree family history of depression					1.0
Yes	3	5.2	2	5.2	
No	55	94.8	41	94.8	
Total	58		43		
Age at onset					
<50	15	25.9	15	34.9	0.44
50-59	20	34.5	12	27.9	
60-69	12	20.7	13	30.2	0.30
>70	11	19.0	3	7.0	0.33
Total	58	100	43	100	
Medication(s) taken/taking					
Carbidopa-Levodopa	54	40.3	35	49.3	0.12
Trihexyphenidyl	29	21.6	19	26.8	0.69
Antidepressant	1	1.7	2	4.7	0.57

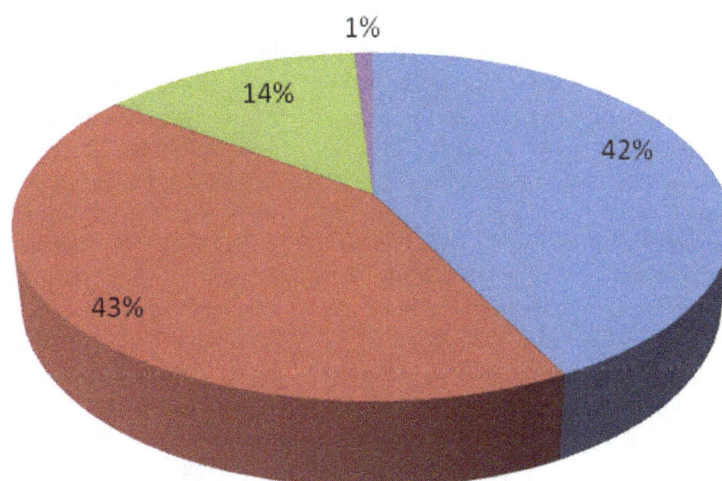

Figure 2 Frequency distributions of severity of depression of study subjects, Black Lion Hospital and Zewuditu Memorial Hospital.

In Tekle-Haimanot's study PD was seen more frequently in males (7:3) and the commonest decade was 61–70 (25/70 cases) which are comparable to our finding, male to female ratio of 7:3 and with an age group of 60–70 respectively. The mean age at onset of symptoms was 54.6 years, which was lesser than our finding, 57.1 years [29]. In Zahodne et al's USA study the male to female ratio was comparable but the age at onset was 59.71 years. These differences may be due to the difference among the life expectancies of the study areas and periods [30].

One third of the patients in the present study were in the age range between 60–69 years. The mean age (years) + SD for depressed patients and non depressed patients were 63.94 + 12.06 and 60.13 + 9.20, respectively (Figure 3). Their mean difference was not significantly associated (t = 1.73, df = 99, P-value = 0.087, 95% CI = −0.56-8.18).

A majority of studies have found no relationship between depression and the patient's current age or the patient's age at onset of the PD [21]. This was true in the present study. The boundary age for early-onset versus late-onset Parkinson's disease has varied among studies, perhaps contributing to the lack of agreement regarding the importance of this variable as a risk factor for depression. Conclusions based on the available data regarding the potential role of age at onset as a contributing factor to the vulnerability to depression would be premature.

The duration of PD might be expected to influence the rate of depression, but most investigators have found no relationship between length of illness and mood changes [21]. It is also in agreement with the present study.

Several studies have found a higher rate of depression among women with PD, but others have failed to identify any relationship between gender and depression [21]. Being female may be a risk factor for depression in PD, but a consensus is lacking and present study also does not show any gender association.

Recent major life events (death of spouse or children, divorce, homelessness, etc), previous history of depression, and family history of depression were among the major risk factor for developing depression [31]. In the present study, 5(4.95%) of them had recent major life event, 2 (1.98%) had previous history of depression, and 5(4.95%) had first degree family history of psychiatric disorder. None of these were significantly associated with increased risk of developing depression in the present study. This may be due to relatively small number of PD patients who had these risk factors. In addition, 30(29.7%) study patients had co-morbid medical condition(s). Different studies show having co-morbid medical conditions predispose to depression which was not significantly associated in the present study [32].

Neuroimaging studies such as CT and MRI are also usually unhelpful in making a diagnosis of PD, because they are generally normal or show only incidental abnormalities. On the other hand neuroimaging abnormalities can be useful in suggesting alternative diagnoses such as Progressive Supranuclear Palsy or Multiple System Atrophy [33]. In our study only 23(22.8%) patients had previous imaging. This may affect the definitive diagnosis of PD since having imaging may exclude alternative causes of Parkinsonism.

Our study population differed from those in previous published evaluations of PD-depression associations. In our study only 25.74% of the study patients were employed which was less than from a W.B.P. Matuja's study. This may be due to the retirement age of the Ethiopian civil servant is currently age >60 which is lesser than our study patients mean(62.33), and also the two studies have different age structure with a mean of 61.50 in W.B.P. Matuja's study [34].

Almost half of our study patients 43(42.57%) have annual income of <300 USD which is less than the national per capita income (410 USD) [35]. Out of the depressed patients 32(56.1%) have annual income <300 USD and over all high annual income is significantly associated with depression in our study with OR of 0.2(0.06-0.66) (Table 2). The association of psychopathology of depression with poverty has been repeatedly demonstrated in other studies [36].

In contrast to the findings in the present study, depression was conspicuously absent in previously published reports of PD patients in W.B.P. Matuja's study. These differences in results may be due to variations in depression screening tools and the small sample sizes of all studies to date [34]. In the Zahodne et al. study, of the 95 patients surveyed, 27 (28%) had depressive episode [30].

Several studies have assessed the intensity of depressive symptoms in Parkinson's disease by using clinical criteria to distinguish between major depressive episodes and dysthymia or by applying rating scales to differentiate mild from moderate-to-severe syndromes. In Cummings review, on average, slightly more than half (54%) of depressed patients with Parkinson's disease met criteria for a major depressive episode (moderate-to-severe symptoms) and slightly less than half (45%) had dysthymia or minor depressions (mild symptoms). These findings are in agreement with the present study, fifteen percent of the study population was classified as having moderate to severe depression (Figure 2). The proportions varied considerably among studies, again suggesting the influence of considerable selection biases in different study populations. Major and minor syndromes differ in several respects in addition to severity: minor depressions are more likely to remit [37] and are more closely related to disability [38].

If PD-specific cutoff scores (i.e., >12) are used to maximize the sum of sensitivity and specificity, the

Table 2 Depression Vs Parkinson's disease characteristics of study subjects, Black Lion Hospital and Zewuditu Memorial Hospital

Variables	Depressed	Non-depressed	Crude OR	P-value
Handedness				
Right	56	43	ref	0.51
Left	2	-	undetermined	
Total	58	43		
Age				
<50	11	8	1.38(0.44-4.27)	0.78
50-59	9	10	0.9(0.30-2.77)	1.0
60-69	17	17	ref	0.18
70-79	17	7	2.43(0.80-7.35)	0.35
80 and above	4	1	4.0(0.40-39.58)	
Total	58	43		
Gender				
Female	18	13	1.04(0.44-2.45)	1.0
Male	40	30	ref	
Total	58	43		
Marital status				
Married	39	36	ref	
Separated/divorced	6	-	undefined	0.03
Widowed	13	7	1.71(0.62-4.78)	0.33
Total	58	43		
Employment				
Employed	12	14	0.54 (0.22-1.33)	0.25
Unemployed	46	29	ref	
Total	58	43		
Education				
No formal education	29	13	ref	
Primary	18	10	0.80(0.29-2.22)	0.80
Secondary	6	12	0.22(0.07-0.73)	0.02
More than secondary	5	8	0.28(0.08-1.02)	0.06
Total	58	43		
Annual income(USD)			ref	
<300	33	12	0.4(0.14-1.07)	0.08
300-600	14	13	0.26(0.07-0.98)	0.08
600-900	5	7		
>900	6	11	0.2(0.06-0.66)	0.01
Total	58	43		
Recent major life events				
Yes	4	1	3.11(0.34-28.88)	0.39
No	54	42	ref	
Total	58	43		

Table 2 Depression Vs Parkinson's disease characteristics of study subjects, Black Lion Hospital and Zewuditu Memorial Hospital (Continued)

Previous history of depression				
Yes	2	-	undefined	0.5
No	56	43	ref	
Total	58	43		
First degree family history of depression				
Yes	3	2	1.12(0.18-7.00)	1.0
No	55	41	ref	
Total	58	43		
Age at onset				
<50	15	15	0.6(0.22-1.65)	0.44
50-59	20	12	ref	
60-69	12	13		
>70	11	3	0.55(0.19-1.60)	0.30
Total	58	43	2.2(0.51-9.51)	0.33
Medication(s) taken/taking				
			ref	0.12
Carbidopa-Levodopa			0.32(0.09-1.16)	
Yes	54	35		
No	4	8		
Trihexyphenidyl				
Yes	29	19	1.26(0.57-2.79)	0.69
No	29	24	ref	
Antidepressant				
Yes	1	2	0.36(0.03-4.10)	0.57
No	57	41	ref	
Co-morbid medical condition(s)				
Yes	21	9	0.19-1.16	0.12
No	37	34	ref	
Total	58	43		

prevalence of depression is 40.59% (41) in our study. This is comparable to Cummings et al's review [21].

In PD patients, depressive symptoms affect all domains, including physical, affective, and cognitive. In a previous study examining the symptom profile of depressed PD patients, depressed mood, tension, loss of interest, and loss of concentration were the most common depressive symptoms. Feelings of guilt, self-blame, appetite disturbance, and suicidal ideation were not as common [39]. Symptoms that are common to both depression and idiopathic PD include motor slowing, bradyphrenia, sleep and appetite disturbance, weight loss, loss of interest and concentration, and reduced libido [40]. Another previous study found that low mood, anhedonia, and lack of interest constituted the most prominent symptoms in depressed PD patients, and that reduced appetite and early morning awakening are two somatic items that discriminate between PD patients with and without depression [41].

Sleep disturbances, among other non-motor symptoms, have been reported in 60–90% PD patients and are unrecognized in over 40% of patients with PD, clinicians should actively and routinely inquire about sleep patterns during consultation [42-44]. It is same in the present study with all the depressed patients had sleep changes.

There are significant difference in the major depressive symptoms (i.e., mood, sleep changes, self outlook, and suicidal ideation) among the depressed PD patients of the present study and Zahodne et al's study (Table 3). These may be due to: 16 of the 27 patients (59.3%) of the depressed PD patients were on antidepressant in Zahodne et al's study while in the present study only 1/58(1.7%) depressed PD patient was on antidepressant [30].

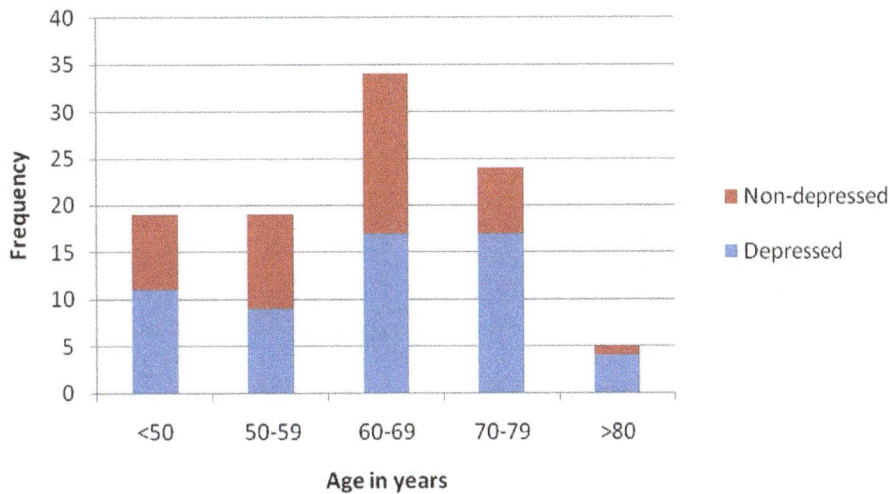

Figure 3 Frequency distributions of different age groups of study subjects, Black Lion Hospital and Zewuditu Memorial Hospital.

Depression is under-recognized in Ethiopian patients with PD. The present study show only one (1.7%) patient out of the 58 depressed PD patients was on antidepressant. This was way lower than in Zahodne et al's study, 16 of the 27 patients (59.3%) of the depressed PD patients were on antidepressant [30]. Even though, not to this extent, diagnosis of depression in PD patients could be missed. In a study of 101 PD patients done in Baltimore, Maryland, USA, the treating neurologists failed to recognize depression. The prevalence of this condition as identified by the treating neurologist was lower: 21% while standardized testing showed depression in 44% of patients [15]. There is also high patient flow in the hospitals since these hospitals are the only teaching and referral hospitals having a Neurology clinics for a country of 80 plus millions peoples [45]. These may reduce patient-doctor interaction time and physicians may not enquire for depressive symptoms. The other main reason may be most of the symptoms of depression are

common manifestation of PD [40]. In general this degree of treatment gap shows low index of suspicion among treating physicians in the two hospitals. Diagnostic evaluations were limited, but treatment was available, although expensive. In spite of the limitations, patients with movement disorders require and seek care in Ethiopia in proportions comparable to developed nations [45].

In the present study, there were no demographic or medical factors except annual income in the PD population that increased the risk of depression in PD patient. This finding may have been due to low study power which increased the risk of a Type II error. Studies to evaluate a larger number of Ethiopian PD outpatients are warranted to identify further risk factors for depression in this patient group.

Conclusion

As depression is one of the most disabling symptoms of PD, the value of regular depression screening and

Table 3 Frequencies of common depressive symptoms among depressed PD patients; study subjects (58) Vs Zahodne et al. study (27), Black Lion Hospital and Zewuditu Memorial Hospital

Common depressive symptoms	Our study		Zahodne et al. study		P value for difference
	Frequency	Proportion	Frequency	Proportion	
Sleep change	58	100%	22	81%	0.003
Sad mood	47	81%	15	56%	0.019
Decreased social involvement	57	98%	25	923%	0.236
Weight/appetite changes	44	76%	16	59%	0.132
Psychomotor agitation/retardation	44	76%	20	74%	1.0
Fatigue	58	100%	25	93%	0.098
Self outlook	50	86%	15	56%	0.003
Concentration difficulties/indecisiveness	43	74%	23	85%	0.283
Suicidal ideation	24	41%	5	19%	0.05

treatment has been repeatedly emphasized [46]. However, very little is known about factors that influence depression severity or the nature of specific depression symptoms in PD. Depression occurred in 58(57.42%) of our patients. Out of these patients only 1/58(1.7%) was on antidepressants. The low index of clinician suspicion and under treatment of depression in PD patients is startling. The QIDS-C16 takes approximately 5 to 7 minutes to complete. It can be used as a screening tool for even busy clinics. Further studies are needed to confirm these findings, and to further increase our understanding of specific signs and symptoms of depression in the context of PD. Routine use of screening tools and subsequent treatment of depression in PD patients are warranted.

Limitations

Co-morbid psychiatric symptoms, particularly anxiety, were not evaluated and may also have been common in this population. Only 23(22.8%) patients had previous imaging. This may affect the definitive diagnosis of PD since having imaging may exclude other causes of Parkinsonism. Another limitation of this study is the absence of a depression control group without PD. Thus, we cannot determine the degree to which the pattern of depressive symptoms discerned in this population is related to co-morbid PD. Although one previous study did not find differences between depressed individuals with PD compared to those without PD, [47] other studies have found differences between depressed patients with PD and those without PD. Another potential limitation is small sample size, which did not provide a strong study power to tell the difference between groups.

Abbreviations

BDI: Beck depression inventory; CT: Computerized tomography; DBS: Deep brain stimulation; DSM-IV: Diagnostic and Statistical Manual of Mental Disorders IV; GDS-15: Geriatric Depression Scale (15); HRSD17: Hamilton Rating Scale for Depression 17 item version; IRB: Institutional Review Board; $IDSC_{30}$: Inventory of Depressive Symptomatology Clinician-Rated(30); MDD: Major Depressive Disorder; MRI: Magnetic Resonant Imaging; PD: Parkinson's Disease; OR: Odds ratio; QIDS-C16: Quick Inventory of Depressive Symptomatology Clinician-Rated (16); REM-Sleep: Rapid Eye movement sleep; UK: United Kingdom.

Competing interests

No competing interest to disclose. The research was fully funded by the primary author.

Authors' contributions

DKW conceived and designed the study, collected the data, performed the statistical analysis and drafted the manuscript. Y MY, DGP and F E G participated in its design and coordination and helped to draft the manuscript. All authors read and approved the final manuscript.

Authors' information

Dawit Kibru Worku, MD is a senior medical specialist (Neurologist) currently works as a University lecturer and clinician, Addis Ababa, Ethiopia
Co-authors:
Yared Mamushet Yifru, MD, Msc is a consultant in Internal medicine and neurology, a subspecialist in Headache medicine at Department of Neurology, Addis Ababa University, Addis Ababa, Ethiopia.

Douglas G. Postels, MD is an Associate Professor of Pediatric Neurology, Michigan State University: 2010-present
Field Volunteer, Médecins Sans Frontières, Lubutu, Democratic Republic of Congo and Port au Prince, Haiti, 2009–2010
Department Head of Neurology, Presbyterian Hospital, Albuquerque, New Mexico, 2003–2009
Staff Pediatric Neurologist, Ochsner Clinic, New Orleans, Louisiana, 1994–2001
Fikre Enquselassie Gashe, PhD is a renowned epidemiologist published more than fifty papers and received many awards for his work. Currently works at Addis Ababa University, Department of Community Health.

Acknowledgements

My thanks to the staffs of the Department of Neurology for their valuable contribution to this work. I am indebted to Yared Mamushet, M.D., Associate Professor of Neurology at the Medical School of Addis Ababa University for his continuous support and supervision.
My special thanks to Fikre Enkuesellassie, PhD, Associate Professor at the Department of Community Health of Addis Ababa University for his invaluable comments and advice. I gratefully acknowledge the patience and the tireless assistance of Douglas Postels, MD., Associate Professor of Pediatric Neurology at the International Neurologic and Psychiatric Epidemiology Program of Michigan State University, East Lansing, Michigan, USA. And I thank Belachew Degefe, MD., Associate Professor of Neurology at the Medical School of Addis Ababa University for his continuous support and advice.
And last, my special thanks to all participating patients for their patience and volunteering for this study.

Author details

[1]P.O.Box – 29818, Addis Ababa, Ethiopia. [2]Department of Neurology, Addis Ababa University, Addis Ababa, Ethiopia. [3]International Neurologic and Psychiatric Epidemiology Program, Michigan State University, Michigan, USA. [4]Department of Community Health, Addis Ababa University, Addis Ababa, Ethiopia.

References

1. Samii A, Nutt JG, Ransom BR: Parkinson's disease. Lancet 2004, 363:1783–1793.
2. de Lau LM, Koudstaal PJ, Hofman A, Breteler MM: Serum cholesterol levels and the risk of Parkinson's disease. Am J Epidemiol 2006, 164(10):998–1002.
3. Aarsland D, Brønnick K, Larsen JP, Tysnes OB, Alves G: Cognitive impairment in incident, untreated Parkinson's disease. Neurology 2009, 72:1121–1126.
4. Racette BA, Simón-Sánchez J, Schulte C: Genome-wide association study reveals genetic risk underlying Parkinson's disease. Nat Genet 2009, 41:1308–1312.
5. Tekele-Haimanot R, Abebe M, Gebre-Mariam A, Forsgren L, Holmgren G, Heijbel J, Ekstedt J: Community-based study of neurological disorders in Ethiopia. Development of a screening instrument. Ethiop Med J 1990, 28:123–137.
6. Levy ML, Cummings JL: Psychiatric management in neurological disease. Washington, DC: American Psychiatric Press; 2000.
7. Marsh L, Berk A: Neuropsychiatric aspects of Parkinson's disease: recent advances. Curr Psychiatry Rep 2003, 5:68–76.
8. Starkstein SE, Mayberg HS, Leiguarda R, Preziosi TJ, Robinson RG: A prospective longitudinal study of depression, cognitive decline, and physical impairments in patients with Parkinson's disease. J Neurol Neurosurg Psychiatry 1992, 33:377–382.
9. Steering GPDS: Committee. Factors Impacting on Quality of Life in Parkinson's Disease: Results From an International Survey. Mov Disord 2002, 17(1):60–67.
10. Weintraub D, Moberg PJ, Duda JE, Katz IR, Stern MB: Effect of psychiatric and other nonmotor symptoms on disability in Parkinson's disease. J Am Geriatr Soc 2004, 52:784–788.
11. Tandberg E, Aarsland D, Laake D, Cummings JL: Risk factors for depression in Parkinson's disease. Arch Neurol 1997, 54:625–630.
12. Starkstein SE, Bolduc PL, Mayberg HS, Preziosi TJ, Robinson RG: Cognitive impairments and depression in Parkinson's disease: a follow up study. J Neurol Neurosurg Psychiatry 1990, 53:597–602.
13. Mayberg HS, Solomon DH: Depression in Parkinson's disease: a biochemical and organic viewpoint. Adv Neurol 1995, 65:49–60.

14. Norman S, Troster AI, Fields JA, Brooks R: Effect of depression and Parkinson's disease on cognitive functioning. *J Neuropsychiatr Clin Neurosci* 2002, **14**:31–36.

15. Shulman LM, Taback RL, Rabinstein AA, Weiner WJ: Non-recognition of depression and other non-motor symptoms in Parkinson's disease. *Parkinsonism Relat Disord* 2002, **8**:193–197.

16. Gotham AM, Brown RG, Marsden CD: Depression in Parkinson's disease: a quantitative and qualitative analysis. *J Neurol Neurosurg Psychiatry* 1986, **49**:381–389.

17. Schuurman AG, van den Akker M, Ensinck KT, Metsemakers JF, Knottnerus JA, Leentjens AF, Buntinx F: Increased risk of Parkinson's disease after depression. *Neurology* 2002, **58**:1501–1504.

18. Williams PESJR, Hirsch MK, Anderson K, Bush AL, Goldstein SR, Grill S, Lehmann S, Little JT, Margolis RL, Palanci J, Pontone G, Weiss H, Rabins P, Marsh L: A comparison of nine scales to detect depression in Parkinson's disease. *Neurology* 2012, **78**:998–1006.

19. Rush AJ, Gullion CM, Basco MR, Jarrett RB, Trivedi MH: The Inventory of Depressive Symptomatology (IDS): Psychometric properties. *Psychol Med* 1996, **26**:477–486.

20. Trivedi MH, Rush AJ, Ibrahim HM, Carmody TJ, Biggs MM, Suppes T, Crismon ML, Shores-Wilson K, Toprac MG, Dennehy EB, Witte B, Kashner TM: The Inventory of Depressive Symptomatology, Clinician Rating (IDS-C) and Self-Report (IDS-SR), the Quick Inventory of Depressive Symtomatology, Clinician Rating (QIDS-C) and Self-Report (QIDS-SR) in public sector patients with mood disorders: a psychometric evaluation. *Psychol Med* 2004, **34**:73–82.

21. Cummings JL: Depression and Parkinson's disease: a review. *Am J Psychiatry* 1992, **149**:443–454.

22. Nilsson FM, Kessing LV, Bowlig TG: Increased risk of developing Parkinson's disease for patients with major affective disorder: a register study. *Acta Psychiatr Scand* 2001, **104**:380–386.

23. Leentjens AF, Van den Akker M, Metsemakers JF, Lousberg R, Verhey FR: Higher Incidence of Depression Preceding the Onset of Parkinson's Disease: A Register Study. *Mov Disord* 2003, **18**(4):414–418.

24. Okubadejo NU, Bower JH, Rocca WA, Demetrius MM: Parkinson's Disease in Africa: A Systematic Review of Epidemiologic and Genetic Studies. *Mov Disord* 2006, **21**(12):2150–2156.

25. Heligman L, Chen N, Babakol O: *Shifts in the structure of population and deaths in less developed regions*. Washington, DC: National Academy Press; 2000.

26. Ehmann TS, Beninger RJ, Gawel M, Riopette R: Depressive symptoms in Parkinson's disease: a comparison with disabled control subjects. *J Geriatr Psychiatry Neurol* 1990, **2**:3–9.

27. Huber SJ, Paulson GW, Shuttleworth EC: Depression in Parkinson's disease. *Neuropsychiatry, Neuropsychology, and Behavioral Neurology* 1988, **1**:47–51.

28. Rodríguez-Violante M, Cervantes-Arriaga A, Berlanga-Flores C, Ruiz-Chow A: Prevalence and determinants of depression in Mexican patients with Parkinson's disease. *Clin Neurol Neurosurg* 2012, **114**(10):1293–1296.

29. Tekle-Haimanot R: Parkinson's disease in Ethiopia: a prospective study of 70 patients. *E Afr Med J* 1985, **62**:571–579.

30. Zahodne LB, Marsiske M, Okun MS, Bowers D: Components of Depression in Parkinson's Disease. *J Geriatr Psychiatry Neurol* 2012, **25**(3):131–137.

31. Klerman GL, Weissman MM: Increasing rates of depression. *JAMA* 1989, **261**(15):2229–2235.

32. World Federation for Mental Health. DEPRESSION: A Global Crisis. World Mental Health Day October 10, 2012 [http://wfmh.com/wp-content/uploads/2013/11/2012_wmhday_english.pdf]

33. Brooks DJ, Seppi K, Neuroimaging Working Group on MSA: Proposed neuroimaging criteria for the diagnosis of multiple system atrophy. *Mov Disord* 2009, **24**(7):949–964.

34. Matuja WBP, Aris EA: Motor and non-motor features of Parkinson's disease. *East Afr Med J* 2008, **85**(1):3–9.

35. Bank W. Ethiopia Overview. Secondary Ethiopia Overview. 2012 [http://www.worldbank.org/en/country/ethiopia/overview]

36. Marmot MG, Bell R: How will the financial crisis affect health? *Br Med J* 2009, **338**:b1314.

37. Mayeux R, Stern Y, Sano M, Williams JB, Cote L: The relation-ship of serotonin to depression in Parkinson's disease. *Mov Disord* 1988, **3**:237–244.

38. Starkstein SE, Preziosi TJ, Bolduc PL, Robinson RG: Depression in Parkinson's disease. *J Nerv Ment Dis* 1990, **178**:27–31.

39. Brown RG, MacCarthy B: Psychiatric morbidity in patients with Parkinson's disease. *Psychol Med* 1990, **20**:77–87.

40. Rickards H: Depression In Neurological Disorders: Parkinson's Disease, Multiple Sclerosis, And Stroke. *J Neurol Neurosurg Psychiatry* 2005, **76**(Suppl I):i48–i52.

41. Leentjens AF, Marinus J, Van Hilten JJ, Lousberg R, Verhey FR: The contribution of somatic symptoms to the diagnosis of depressive disorder in Parkinson's disease: a discriminant analytic approach. *J Neuropsychiatry Clin Neurosci* 2003, **15**:74–77.

42. Trenkwalder C: Sleep dysfunction in Parkinson's disease. *Clin Neurosci* 1998, **5**(2):107–114.

43. Korczyn AD: Management of sleep problems in Parkinson's disease. *J Neurol Sci* 2006, **248**(1–2):163–166.

44. Chaudhuri KR, Prieto-Jurcynska C, Naidu Y, Mitra T, Frades-Payo B, Tluk S, Ruessmann A, Odin P, Macphee G, Stocchi F, Ondo W, Sethi K, Schapira AH, Martinez Castrillo JC, Martinez-Martin P: The nondeclaration of nonmotor symptoms of Parkinson's disease to health care professionals: an international study using the nonmotor symptoms questionnaire. *Mov Disord* 2010, **25**(6):704–709.

45. Bower JH, Teshome M, Melaku Z, Zenebe G: Frequency of movement disorders in an Ethiopian university practice. *Mov Disord* 2005, **20**:1209–1213.

46. Farabaugh AH, Locascio JJ, Yap L, Weintraub D, McDonald WM, Agoston M, Alpert JE, Growdon J, Fava M: Pattern of Depressive Symptoms in Parkinson's disease. *Psychosomatics* 2009, **50**(5):448–454.

47. Merschdorf U, Berg D, Csoti I, Fornadi F, Merz B, Naumann M, Becker G, Supprian T: Psychopathological symptoms of depression in Parkinson's disease compared to depression. *Psychopathology* 2003, **36**:221–225.

17

Agnosia for head tremor in essential tremor: prevalence and clinical correlates

Hatice N. Eken[1] and Elan D. Louis[1,2,3*]

Abstract

Background: Lack of awareness of involuntary movements is a curious phenomenon in patients with certain movement disorders. An interesting anecdotal observation is that patients with essential tremor (ET) often seem unaware of their own head tremor. In the current study, we asked ET patients whether they were aware of head tremor while it was occurring on examination, thereby allowing us to gauge real-time awareness of their involuntary movement.

Methods: ET cases enrolled in an ongoing clinical research study at the Columbia University Medical Center (2009–2014). During a videotaped tremor examination, they were questioned about the presence of head tremor. True positives were cases who exhibited head tremor on examination and were aware of it; false negatives were cases who exhibited head tremor but were unaware of it.

Results: The 126 ET cases had a mean age of 72.6 ± 12.4 years. Nineteen (48.7 %) of 39 cases with head tremor on examination did not report having head tremor at that moment. Even among cases with moderate or severe head tremor on examination, unawareness of head tremor was 45.5 %. We assessed the clinical correlates of unawareness of head tremor, comparing true positives to false negatives, and unawareness was correlated with older age, lower mental status test scores and several other clinical variables.

Conclusions: Nearly one-half of ET cases with head tremor on examination were acutely unaware of their tremor. Whether such agnosia for tremor may be leveraged as a diagnostic feature of ET is a question for future clinical studies.

Keywords: Essential tremor, Clinical, Head tremor, Agnosia

Background

Lack of awareness of involuntary movements is a fascinating and not infrequently observed phenomenon in patients with certain movement disorders. As such, patients with Parkinson's disease are often unaware of their levodopa-induced dyskinesias and patients with Huntington's disease are often not aware of chorea [1, 2]. An interesting anecdotal observation is that essential tremor (ET) patients often seem unaware of their head tremor. In a prior study, we showed that one-third to one-half of ET cases who were observed to have head tremor on neurological examination had not responded "yes" to the question "do you sometimes have head tremor", which

had been asked of them during a previously-administered questionnaire [3]. However, in that study, awareness of head tremor was not assessed in real time (i.e., at the precise instant that tremor was observed on neurological examination); hence, there was a disconnect between the timing of the questionnaire and the timing of the examination. We prospectively designed the current study with this in mind. We asked ET patients whether they were aware of their head tremor while it was occurring on examination, thereby allowing us to gauge real-time awareness of their involuntary movement. In addition to assessing the prevalence of unawareness, we also assessed a broad range of clinical features that we hypothesized could track with greater vs. lesser awareness. The overall goal was to improve our understanding of the clinical phenomenology in ET. As the presence and features of head tremor are often at the center of diagnostic difficulties in ET (e.g., distinguishing ET from dystonia) [4], it is possible

* Correspondence: elan.louis@yale.edu
[1]Department of Neurology, Yale School of Medicine, Yale University, LCI 710, 15 York Street, PO Box 208018, New Haven, CT 06520-8018, USA
[2]Department of Chronic Disease Epidemiology, Yale School of Public Health, Yale University, New Haven, CT, USA
Full list of author information is available at the end of the article

that additional clinical insights could lead to additional diagnostic tools and improved diagnostic accuracy.

Methods

ET cases were enrolled in an ongoing research study of the environmental epidemiology of ET at Columbia University Medical Center (CUMC; 2009–2014) [5]. Cases were derived from two sources: (1) a computerized billing database of ET patients at the Neurological Institute of New York, CUMC, and (2) advertisements to members of the International Essential Tremor Foundation. Cases lived within two hours driving distance of CUMC in New York, New Jersey, and Connecticut. Prior to enrollment, all cases received a diagnosis of ET from their treating neurologist. The CUMC Internal Review Board approved all study procedures, and written informed consent was obtained upon enrollment. Analysis of data was also approved by the Internal Review Board at Yale Medical School.

After enrollment, all ET cases underwent a detailed in-person evaluation conducted by trained research staff, which included the collection of demographic (e.g., age, gender, ethnicity, education) and medical history information. They were asked as variety of questions about their tremor, including, "Does your tremor embarrass you?", "Does your voice almost always tremble when you talk?", "Do you ever have an internal sensation that you are having a head tremor?" and "When you feel your head shaking, do you ever see it in the mirror"? The Center for Epidemiological Studies Depression Scale (CES-D) [6], a self-report ten-item screening questionnaire was used to assess depressive symptoms (range = 0 – 30 [greater depressive symptoms]). The Folstein Mini Mental Status Examination (range = 0 – 30) [7] was used to briefly assess cognition.

A videotaped tremor examination included assessments of arm, head (i.e., neck) and voice tremors. During the assessment of neck tremor, the neck muscles were exposed in order to facilitate the evaluation of any dystonic spasms and/or neck muscle hypertrophy. During the videotape, ET cases were asked "Are you experiencing any head tremor at the moment?" This question was asked at two time points (Time point 1 and Time point 2) when the videographer observed head tremor and at one time point when no head tremor was observed by the videographer.

All videotaped neurological examinations were reviewed by a senior neurologist specializing in movement disorders (E.D.L.). Neck tremor in ET was coded as present or absent and was distinguished from dystonic tremor by the absence of twisting or tilting movements of the neck, jerk-like or sustained neck deviation, or hypertrophy of neck muscles. Head tremor had to be both rhythmic and oscillatory to be ascribed to ET. The severity of the head tremor was assessed using a 0 – 3 scale (0 = absent, 1 = mild, 2 = moderate, 3 = severe) [8]. The total tremor score (range = 0 – 36) was the sum of all 0 – 3 postural and kinetic tremor ratings in the arms [5].

Using the clinical questionnaire and videotape data, the diagnosis of ET was reconfirmed in 126 ET cases using published diagnostic criteria (either moderate or greater amplitude kinetic tremor during at least three activities, or a head tremor in the absence of Parkinson's disease, dystonia, or another neurological disorder) [9].

Awareness of head tremor was indicated using four different groups. *True positives* were cases who exhibited head tremor on examination and who were aware of that tremor when questioned. *True negatives* were cases who did not exhibit head tremor on examination and indicated that they were not experiencing tremor when questioned. *False positives* were cases who did not exhibit head tremor on examination but reported its presence when asked. *False negatives* were patients who exhibited head tremor on examination but were unaware of it. *Unawareness of head tremor* was the number of cases who reported no head tremor over the number of cases who had head tremor on examination (i.e., false negatives/false negatives + true positives). We report unawareness separately at Time points 1 and 2.

We assessed the clinical correlates of awareness of head tremor, comparing true positives to false negatives (Table 1). We carefully chose a range of variables for which we had an *a priori* hypothesis about an association with awareness (e.g., longer duration of tremor and higher education might be associated with greater awareness; similarly being in the workforce might be associated with greater awareness) (Table 1). Given the potential for learning effects by Time 2 (i.e., cueing the patient with a reduction in the number of false negatives), we focused these analyses on Time point 1. These analyses were performed using the statistical software package SPSS (version 21.0; SPSS, Inc., Chicago, Ill., USA). All tests were 2-sided, and significance was accepted at the 5 % level. Using a Kolmogorov-Smirnov test, we determined that several continuous variables were not normally distributed. For these, we compared group differences using a nonparametric (Mann–Whitney U) test rather than a Student's t test. Chi-square (χ^2) tests or Fisher's Exact tests were used to compare categorical variables.

Results

The 126 ET cases had a mean age of 72.6 ± 12.4 years. Nineteen of 39 cases with head tremor on examination at Time point 1 did not report head tremor; i.e., unawareness of head tremor at Time point 1 was 48.7 % (Additional file 1). Even among 22 cases with moderate or severe head tremor on examination, 10 (45.5 %) were unaware of head tremor (Table 1, Additional file 1). At time point 2, unawareness of head tremor was approximately 10 % less (13/34 = 38.2 %).

Table 1 Clinical characteristics of participants

	All participants	True positives[d]	False negatives[e]	p value*
n	126	20	19	
Age (years)	72.6 ± 12.4	73.5 ± 15.0	81.5 ± 6.9	0.04[a]
Female gender	64 (50.8)	15 (75.0)	12 (63.2)	0.50[b]
White ethnicity	117 (92.9)	19 (95.0)	16 (84.2)	0.34[b]
Current smoker	6 (4.8)	0 (0.0)	1 (5.3)	0.49[b]
Education (years)	15.8 ± 2.8	15.6 ± 2.9	14.9 ± 2.5	0.44[a]
Married	69 (54.8)	7 (35.0)	6 (31.6)	0.86[b]
Lives alone	42 (33.3)	12 (60.0)	9 (47.4)	0.43[b]
Currently in work force	26 (20.6)	3 (15.0)	1 (5.3)	0.61[b]
Years since last hospitalization	10.7 ± 14.5 [4.0]	7.6 ± 12.1 [3.0]	12.8 ± 21.8 [4.0]	0.36[c]
Answered "yes" to the question "Does anyone in your family have tremor?"	83 (65.9)	14 (70.0)	10 (52.6)	0.27[b]
Age first noticed tremor (years)	39.5 ± 20.1	41.3 ± 21.5	41.4 ± 16.9	0.98[a]
Duration of tremor (years)	33.2 ± 19.1	32.3 ± 21.9	40.0 ± 17.7	0.25[a]
Answered "yes" to the question "Does your tremor embarrass you?"	67 (53.2)	11 (55.0)	12 (63.2)	0.61[b]
Answered "yes" to "Does your voice almost always tremble when you talk?"	26 (20.6)	9 (50.0)	4 (25.0)	0.13[b]
Reply to "Do you ever have an internal sensation that you are having a head tremor?"				0.016[b]
No	84 (66.7)	5 (25.0)	12 (63.2)	
Yes	42 (33.3)	15 (75.0)	7 (36.8)	
Reply to "When you feel your head shaking, do you ever see it in the mirror"?				0.002[b]
No	87 (69.0)	3 (15.0)	12 (63.2)	
Yes	39 (31.0)	17 (85.0)	7 (36.8)	
Reply to "How often do you feel nervous or anxious?"				0.36[b]
Never/No	48 (38.1)	6 (30.0)	8 (42.1)	
Rarely	17 (13.5)	4 (20.0)	2 (10.5)	
Sometimes	34 (27.0)	6 (30.0)	7 (36.8)	
Frequently	16 (12.7)	1 (5.0)	2 (10.5)	
Always/Yes	11 (8.7)	3 (15.0)	0 (0.0)	
CESD score	9.0 ± 5.7	8.8 ± 5.0	9.0 ± 5.8	0.91[a]
Severity rating of head tremor (examination)[f]				0.81[b]
1 (mild)	17 (13.5)	8 (40.0)	9 (47.4)	
2 (moderate)	19 (15.1)	10 (50.0)	9 (47.4)	
3 (severe)	3 (2.4)	2 (10.0)	1 (5.3)	
Total tremor score (examination)	21.1 ± 6.2	23.9 ± 6.5	21.05 ± 6.7	0.19[a]
Folstein Mini Mental Status Examination Score	28.4 ± 1.9 [29.0]	29.0 ± 1.6 [30.0]	27.6 ± 1.9 [28.0]	0.01[c]

All values represent means ± standard deviations [median] or numbers (percentage)
Center for Epidemiological Studies Depression Scale
*Comparing true positives vs. false negatives
[a]Student's t test
[b]Chi square test or Fisher's Exact test
[c]Mann Whitney test
[d]True positives were cases who exhibited head tremor on examination and who were aware of that tremor when questioned
[e]False negatives were patients who exhibited head tremor on examination but were unaware of it
[f]Based on 39 ET cases with head tremor on examination at Time point 1

We assessed the correlates of awareness, comparing true positives to false negatives (Table 1). True positives were nearly a decade younger than false negatives ($p = 0.04$) and they had higher Folstein Mini Mental Status Examination scores ($p = 0.01$) (Table 1). A larger proportion of true positives than false negatives answered "yes" to the questions "Do you ever have an internal sensation that you are having a head tremor?" ($p = 0.016$) and "When you feel your head shaking, do you ever see it in the mirror?" ($p = 0.002$) (Table 1). A larger percentage of true positives than false negatives were female (75.0 % vs. 63.2 %) and white (95.0 % vs. 84.2 %), were currently in the work force (15.0 % vs. 5.3 %), reported a family history of tremor (70.0 % vs. 52.6 %), and answered "yes" to the question "Does your voice almost always tremble when you talk?" (50.0 % vs. 25.0 %), but not to a statistically significant degree (Table 1). Interestingly, the severity of head tremor on examination was not significantly associated with greater awareness ($p = 0.81$), although two of three ET cases with severe head tremor on examination were aware of it (Table 1).

Discussion

Nearly one-half of ET cases with head tremor on examination were acutely unaware of their tremor. Even among cases with moderate or severe head tremor on examination, unawareness of head tremor was similarly high (45.5 %). In a prior study that used a different design [3], we reported a similar result; however, in that study we did not link the question about head tremor with the observation of head tremor on examination. The current study makes the point that even when asked about tremor at the moment of tremor, one-half of the ET cases were unaware of it.

Agnosia of head tremor could be the result of changes in the regions of the brain that perceive head tremor. Perhaps the brain develops mechanisms to shut down the stimuli caused by these involuntary movements. With some types of oscillatory cranial movements (e.g., patients with congenital nystagmus, who rarely experience oscillopsia), perceptual stability (i.e., the lack of awareness of nystagmus) is achieved through a reduced sensitivity to the motion [3]. Development of such mechanisms in the brain might have had an evolutionary advantage, as it would have allowed individuals to focus their attention on external stimuli that were novel to them, instead of being distracted by a repetitive movement.

The clinical correlates of awareness of head tremor have not been assessed previously in any study. We carefully chose a range of variables for which there was an *a priori* hypothesis about an association with awareness (e.g., longer duration of tremor and higher education might be associated with greater awareness). Cases who were unaware of their head tremor were almost a decade older than those who were aware, and they had lower scores on the Folstein Mini Mental Status Examination (Table 1). This might indicate that unawareness might be a result of cognitive deterioration. Our results were not, however, confounded by the presence of dementia. In a secondary analysis, we assessed the number of cases with Folstein Mini Mental Status Examination scores below <25, an indicator of dementia [10]. We found that only 2 of the cases (one true positive and one false negative) had such scores. A number of other factors correlated with awareness, but not to a significant degree, including education and whether the cases was currently

in the work force. Significantly more of the true positives answered "yes" to the questions "Do you ever have an internal sensation that you are having a head tremor?" and "When you feel your head shaking, do you ever see it in the mirror?" This confirms a greater self-awareness of head tremor in these individuals.

This study assessed awareness of tremor at a precise instant in time. Questionnaires that assess whether tremor is more chronically present (e.g., "do you sometimes have tremor") could result in more true positives. Indeed, in our prior study [3], which asked patients in a similar setting whether they sometimes had tremor, unawareness of head tremor was only 38.7 %, compared to 48.7 % here.

A limitation of this study is that our sample size is relatively small. Although the number of cases studied was 126, there only 39 cases who were true positives or false negatives. As such, some of the associations with non-significant p values could be significant in a larger sample. Hence, they were reported here.

Conclusions

In summary, nearly one-half of ET cases with head tremor on examination were acutely unaware of their tremor. Whether such agnosia for tremor can be leveraged as a diagnostic feature of ET is a question for future studies.

Abbreviations
ET: Essential tremor; CUMC: Columbia University Medical Center; CES-D: Center for epidemiological studies depression scale.

Competing interests
Hatice Eken has no conflicts of interest and no competing financial interests. Elan Louis has no conflicts of interest and no competing financial interests.

Authors' contributions
HNE: Conduct of study, statistical analyses, manuscript preparation. EDL: Design of study, collection of data, obtaining funding, statistical analyses, manuscript preparation. All authors read and approved the final manuscript.

Acknowledgements
None.

Funding
Dr. Louis has received research support from the National Institutes of Health: NINDS R01 NS042859 (principal investigator), NINDS R01 NS39422 (principal investigator), NINDS R01 NS086736 (principal investigator), NINDS R01 NS073872 (principal investigator), NINDS R01 NS085136 (principal investigator) and NINDS R01 NS088257 (principal investigator).

Author details
[1]Department of Neurology, Yale School of Medicine, Yale University, LCI 710, 15 York Street, PO Box 208018, New Haven, CT 06520-8018, USA. [2]Department of Chronic Disease Epidemiology, Yale School of Public Health, Yale University, New Haven, CT, USA. [3]Center for Neuroepidemiology and Clinical Neurological Research, Yale School of Medicine, Yale University, New Haven, CT, USA.

References

1. Vitale C, Pellecchia MT, Grossi D, Fragassi N, Cuomo T, Di Maio L, et al. Unawareness of dyskinesias in Parkinson's and Huntington's diseases. Neurol Sci. 2001;22:105–6.

2. Snowden JS, Craufurd D, Griffiths HL, Neary D. Awareness of involuntary movements in Huntington disease. Arch Neurol. 1998;55:801–5.

3. Louis ED, Pellegrino KM, Rios E. Unawareness of head tremor in essential tremor: a study of three samples of essential tremor patients. Mov Disord. 2008;23:2423–4.

4. Jain S, Lo SE, Louis ED. Common misdiagnosis of a common neurological disorder: how are we misdiagnosing essential tremor? Arch Neurol. 2006;63:1100–4.

5. Louis ED, Jiang W, Gerbin M, Viner AS, Factor-Litvak P, Zheng W. Blood harmane (1-methyl-9H-pyrido[3,4-b]indole) concentrations in essential tremor: repeat observation in cases and controls in New York. J Toxicol Environ Health A. 2012;75:673–83.

6. Andresen EM, Malmgren JA, Carter WB, Patrick DL. Screening for depression in well older adults: evaluation of a short form of the CES-D (Center for Epidemiologic Studies Depression Scale). Am J Prev Med. 1994;10:77–84.

7. Folstein MF, Folstein SE, McHugh PR. "Mini-mental state": a practical method for grading the cognitive state of patients for the clinician. J Psychiatr Res. 1975;12:189–98.

8. Herndon RM. Handbook of neurologic rating scales. 2nd ed. New York: Demos Medical Publishing; 1997.

9. Louis ED, Ottman R, Ford B, Pullman S, Martinez M, Fahn S, et al. The Washington Heights-Inwood genetic study of essential tremor: methodologic issues in essential tremor research. Neuroepidemiology. 1997;16:124–33.

10. Roalf DR, Moberg PJ, Xie SX, Wolk DA. Comparative accuracies of two common screening instruments for classification of Alzheimer's disease, mild cognitive impairment, and healthy aging. Alzheimers Dement. 2013;9:529–37.

18

Adductor focal laryngeal Dystonia: correlation between clinicians' ratings and subjects' perception of Dysphonia

Celia Faye Stewart[1*], Catherine F. Sinclair[2], Irene F. Kling[3,4], Beverly E. Diamond[5] and Andrew Blitzer[6]

Abstract

Background: Although considerable research has focused on the etiology and symptomology of adductor focal laryngeal dystonia (AD-FLD), little is known about the correlation between clinicians' ratings and patients' perception of this voice disturbance. This study has five objectives: first, to determine if there is a relationship between subjects' symptom-severity and its impact on their quality of life; to compare clinicians' ratings with subjects' perception of the individual characteristics and severity of AD-FLD; to document the subjects' perception of changes in dysphonia since diagnosis; to record the frequency of voice arrest during connected speech; and, finally, to calculate inter-clinician reliability based on results from the Unified Spasmodic Dysphonia Rating Scale (USDRS) (Stewart et al, J Voice 1195-10, 1997).

Methods: Sixty subjects with AD-FLD who were receiving ongoing injections of BoNT participated in this study. Subjects' mean age was 60.78 years and their mean duration of symptoms was 16.1 years. Subjects completed the Disease Symptom Questionnaire (DSQ) (specifically designed for this study) and the Voice Handicap Index-10 (VHI-10) (Jacobson et al, Am J Speech Lang Pathol 6:66–70, 1997) to measure the symptoms of their dysphonia and the impact of the disease on their quality of life.
Two speech-language pathologists and two laryngologists used the Voice Arrest Measure (VAM) (specifically designed for this study) and the USDRS to independently rate voice recordings of 56/60 subjects.

Results: The mean VHI-10 score was 21.3 which is clinically significant. The results of the DSQ and the USDRS were highly correlated. The most severe symptoms identified by both subjects and clinicians were roughness, strain-strangled voice quality, and increased expiratory effort. Voice arrest, aphonia, and tremor were uncommon. Subjects rated their current voice quality at the time of reinjection (i.e., at the time of the study) as significantly better than at the time of their initial AD-FLD diagnosis ($p < 0.0001$). Inter-clinician reliability on the USDRS was significant at the 0.001 level.

Conclusions: The findings from the VHI-10 suggest that AD-FLD has a profound impact on quality of life. The results of the DSQ and the USDRS suggest that there is a strong correlation between subjects' perception and clinicians' assessment of the individual symptoms and the severity of the dysphonia. The findings from the VAM suggest that voice arrests are infrequent in subjects with AD-FLD who are receiving ongoing BoNT injections. The strong inter-clinician reliability on the USDRS suggests that it is an appropriate measure for identifying symptoms and severity of AD-FLD.

Keywords: Dystonia, Voice, Quality of life, Botulinum toxin, Adductor focal laryngeal dystonia

* Correspondence: cs8@nyu.edu
[1]New York University, Steinhardt School of Culture, Education, and Human Development, 665 Broadway, Suite 900, New York NY 10012, USA
Full list of author information is available at the end of the article

Background

Patients with AD-FLD whose management involves on-going injections of BoNT schedule reinjection based on the reemergence of their symptoms. [1] In addition to the patient's report of symptoms, clinicians rely on medical history, visualization of the vocal folds, and the vocal phenomena associated with AD-FLD (e.g., strained-strangled voice quality, roughness, and increased expiratory effort) to determine the severity of the dysphonia and make treatment decisions. [2–4] The reliability of perceptual ratings between laryngologists and speech-language pathologists, however, is not well documented. Further, the literature related to AD-FLD has not compared clinicians' ratings and subjects' perception of these voice symptoms.

It is well accepted that voice problems may impede the development of social relationships as well as negatively affect educational, and vocational growth [5–10]. Although the VHI-10 [5] has been used to measure the impact of AD-FLD on quality of life, it does not chronicle the patient's perception of specific vocal symptoms or the severity of the dysphonia associated with this complex, neurological disorder. [5–8] To this end, the investigators developed The Disease Symptom Questionnaire (DSQ) (see Additional file 1), a self-rating instrument on which subjects identify the specific symptoms associated with AD-FLD and rate their severity. We can then examine the relationship between patients' perception documented on the DSQ with clinicians' ratings from the USDRS [11].

Historically, voice arrest has been described as a central phenomenon and a necessary component in the diagnosis of AD-FLD. [12–15] Nevertheless, in our clinical experience voice arrest has been relatively infrequent. The Voice Arrest Measure (VAM) was developed to document the frequency and duration of voice arrest during connected speech.

As is the case with many medications, BoNT washes out of the system over time requiring ongoing reinjection in order to maintain the patient's improvement in voice production. The expected duration of benefit from injections is three to four months, with subjects requiring ongoing reinjections to maintain an easy, efficient manner of phonation. [16–20] The patient determines when it is time to seek reinjection, but the criteria for their decision remain unclear. Thus far, no studies have compared the subjects' rating of symptoms at baseline with those ratings just prior to reinjection to determine whether BoNT treatment may alter the disease process.

This study has five aims: first, to ascertain the relationship between the VHI-10 and the DSQ; to compare clinicians' ratings from the USDRS to the subjects' perceptual ratings from the DSQ; to identify the subjects' perception of changes in their dysphonia since diagnosis as measured by the DSQ; to determine the frequency of voice arrests based on the (VAM); and, finally, to measure the inter-clinician (i.e., two laryngologists and two speech-language pathologists) reliability from the ratings on the USDRS.

Methods

Subjects

Between March 20 and July 17, 2012, sixty adults (forty-two females 70% and 18 males 30%) suffering from AD-FLD presented to a single clinical research center for continuing treatment with injections of BoNT. Subjects mean age was 60.78 years (SD 14.13) and the mean time between diagnosis of AD-FLD and participation in the study was 16.8 years (SD 9) with a mean age at the onset of symptoms of 46.05 years (SD 14.28). Data were collected just prior to reinjection when subjects self-determined that the symptoms had deteriorated to the point when reinjection was necessary. The mean interval between the previous injection of BoNT and participation in the study was 20 weeks (SD 12.04), with 49/52 (94%) having received between five and forty injections.

The inclusion criteria for this study were based on a previous diagnosis of AD-FLD, participation in ongoing laryngeal injections of botulinum toxin (BoNT) to minimize symptoms, and the subjects reported benefit from BoNT injections. Subjects had self-selected to return for continuing BoNT management of their voice symptoms when the benefits of the BoNT injections had diminished. Exclusion criteria included co-existing upper respiratory tract infection, concomitant neurological disorders, and non-neurological laryngeal pathologies. Although 100% of the subjects were known to the laryngologists, only 5% of the subjects were known to the speech-language pathologists.

The subjects gave informed consent to participate in a video recording of a voice assessment and to complete self-evaluation questionnaires (Voice Handicap Index-10[4] and Disease Symptom Questionnaire) as part of the study. This study was approved by the Institutional Review Board (IRB) at New York University School of Medicine.

Self-rating scales

VHI-10

The Voice Handicap Index-10 (VHI-10) [5] measures the impact of the voice disorder on the patients' quality of life.

DSQ

The Disease Symptom Questionnaire (DSQ) (see Additional file 1) was designed as part of this study to ascertain the subjects' perception of the individual characteristics and severity of the voice problem at the time of initial diagnosis and at the time of the study. Subjects were asked to document their current age, medical comorbidities, age at diagnosis, and time since initial diagnosis, and since last injection. The authors designed the DSQ to parallel the symptoms rated on the Unified Spasmodic Dysphonia Rating Scale (USDRS) ensuring that the subjects would rate the same symptoms as the otolaryngologists and speech-language pathologists (e.g., severity of dysphonia, hoarse-rough-husky voice quality, strain-strangled, increased expiratory effort).

The DSQ rates the severity of the current symptoms and the symptoms at diagnosis using a 5-point interval scale (i.e., mild, mild-moderate, moderate, moderate-severe or severe). One question asks subjects to compare the severity of their symptoms at diagnosis to their symptoms at the time of participation in the study using a 3-point interval scale (i.e., less severe than before treatment, the same as before treatment, and worse than before treatment).

Clinician-rating scales
USDRS
The Unified Spasmodic Dysphonia Rating Scale (USDRS) [11] provides a framework for clinicians to rate the individual characteristics and the severity of a subject's dysphonia using a 7-point Likert scale.

VAM
The Voice Arrest Measure (VAM) (see Additional file 2) was designed as part of this study for clinicians to identify the occurrence and duration of each voice arrest during the oral reading of the first paragraph of the Rainbow Passage. [21] This scale is based on the Stuttering Severity Index (SSI). [22] The duration of each voice arrest identified on the VAM ranges from momentary (< 1 s), brief (1–2 s), or long (>2 s in duration).

Procedures
A student intern recorded voice samples in a quiet room on a Kay/Pentax VLS 1190 STK distal chip camera system with an Audio-Technica Pro 8HEmW head-mounted microphone placed 4 in. from the subjects' mouth. The subjects read the first paragraph of the Rainbow Passage aloud, described the Cookie Theft picture [23], and counted from eighty to eighty-nine. Two laryngologists and two speech-language-pathologists independently reviewed the video/audio recordings in a quiet room and rated the severity of the voice symptoms on the USDRS. The mean of the severity of dysphonia rated by the four clinicians was calculated and compared to each subject's ratings on the DSQ. The clinicians reviewed the Rainbow Passage a second time and used the VAM to identify the occurrence and duration of voice arrest.

Information pertaining to age at data collection and symptom onset, number of years since initial diagnosis of AD-FLD, time since first BoNT injection, number of BoNT injections, and time since most recent BoNT injection was obtained on the DSQ and analyzed with descriptive statistics.

Inter-clinician reliability for the severity of dysphonia and individual voice symptoms evaluated on the USDRS was calculated using SPSS version 23 interclass correlation coefficient. Paired sample T-tests were used to compare the subject's ratings (DSQ) of the severity of symptoms with the clinicians' ratings (USDRS). The relationship between the DSQ and the USDRS was calculated with a two-tailed correlation. Due to the comparative infrequency of voice arrest identified by the clinicians on the VAM, only descriptive statistics were used to describe these data.

Results
The impact of AD-FLD on quality of life
The mean VHI-10 score was 21.3 (+/−9.6) with 86.7% of subjects scoring greater than 11, which indicates a voice handicap that substantially affects quality of life. Subjects identified symptoms across all three domains included on the VHI-10 (i.e., functional, physical, and emotional). The VHI-10 scores were positively correlated with the overall severity of dysphonia on the DSQ and negatively correlated with age at the time of diagnosis such that those subjects who were younger at the time of diagnosis reported higher VHI-10 scores. The VHI-10 was not correlated with number of injections, time since diagnosis, or time since previous BoNT injection. See Table 1.

Correlations between the Subject's ratings of the current severity of the Dysphonia and the individual voice symptoms
Pearson analysis revealed a strong positive correlation (see Table 2) between the subjects' ratings on the DSQ of severity of dysphonia and the individual symptoms of strain-strangled, roughness, voice tremor, and voice arrest.

Relationship between the VHI-10 and the DSQ
Correlations between subjects' ratings on the VHI-10 and the individual DSQ items were significant for severity of dysphonia, strain-strangled voice quality, roughness, voice tremor, and voice arrest (see Table 3). These positive correlations suggest that more severe voice (e.g., roughness) and sensory (e.g., increased expiratory effort) symptoms are associated with greater handicap as assessed on the VHI-10.

Relationship between USDRS and DSQ
The similarity between the findings on the subjects' DSQ and the clinicians' USDRS was highly correlated

Table 1 Correlation of VHI-10 with DSQ N = 60

	VHI-10	
	Pearson Correlation	Significance
Overall Severity of Dysphonia on the DSQ	0.536	.000*
Age at Time of Diagnosis	−0.328	.011*
Number of Injections	10.162	.25
Time Since Diagnosis	−0.049	.71
Duration Since Previous BoNT Injection	−0.09	.94

*Finding was statistically significant at the .01 level

for current severity of dysphonia, strain-strangled voice quality, roughness, voice arrest, and increased expiratory effort, but not for voice tremor (see Table 4).

Subject's perception of changes in voice symptoms since original diagnosis

All subjects reported that at the time of their original diagnosis of AD-FLD their voice symptoms were worse than at the time of this study. This perceived reduction in symptom severity was statistically significant for all symptoms except roughness. See Table 5.

Clinician ratings on the USDRS

Due to technical errors on four of the recordings, only 56/60 of the voice recordings were analyzed by four clinicians. Two speech-language pathologists and two laryngologists listened independently to the recording of each subject's first paragraph of the Rainbow Passage (fifty-one words), description of the Cooke Theft Picture, and counting from eighty to eighty-nine. They then identified and rated the severity of the individual symptoms and overall severity of the dysphonia using the USDRS. The mean score for the severity of dysphonia was 4.2 (moderate impairment). The mean for roughness,

Table 2 Correlations Between the Subjects' Ratings of the Current Severity of the Dysphonia and the Individual Voice Symptoms N = 56

	Subjects' Ratings of Severity of Dysphonia	
	Pearson Correlation	Significance (2-tailed)
Subjects' Ratings Strain-Strangled	0.673	0.000*
Subjects' Ratings Roughness	0.549	0.000*
Subjects' Ratings Increased Expiratory Effort	0.187	0.000*
Subjects' Ratings Voice Tremor	0.477	0.000*
Subjects' Ratings Voice Arrest	0.564	0.000*

*All findings were statistically significant at the 0.01 level

Table 3 Correlations Between Ratings on the VHI-10 and Severity of Current Symptoms on DSQ N = 56

	Subjects' Ratings on the VHI-10	
	Pearson Correlation	Significance (2-tailed)
Subjects' Ratings of Severity of Dysphonia	0.474	0.000*
Subjects' Ratings Strain-Strangled	0.417	0.001*
Subjects' Ratings Roughness	0.490	0.000*
Subjects' Ratings Increased Expiratory Effort	0.275	0.039
Subjects' Ratings Voice Tremor	0.539	0.000*
Subjects' Ratings Voice Arrest	0.458	0.000*

*Findings was statistically significant at the .01 level

strain-strangled, and increased expiratory effort was 4 indicating that these were the most remarkable symptoms. Symptoms of voice arrest, aphonia, and breathiness were mild with a mean of 1.

During a second evaluation of the recordings of the first paragraph of the Rainbow Passage, voice arrest was identified and timed by the four clinicians, and only 21/56 subjects, (38.1%) exhibited this symptom. Of those twenty-one individuals, 16 (28.6%) exhibited infrequent voice arrest (i.e., one or two instances of voice arrest), three (.05%) had occasional voice arrest (i.e., three to 10 occurrences of voice arrest), and just two (.03%) had more than 10 voice arrests. Eighteen (32%) of these subjects demonstrated momentary voice arrest (< 1 s), three (.05%) had brief voice arrest (1–2 s), but none had long voice arrest (> 2 s). Due to the infrequency of voice arrest, only descriptive statistics were performed.

Inter-clinician reliability for rating vocal Symptomatology on USDRS

Four clinicians independently rated the severity of the dysphonia and the individual vocal symptoms on the USDRS for 56/60 subjects. Assessment of inter-clinician reliability for the clinician ratings was statistically

Table 4 Correlation Between Subjects' and Clinicians' Ratings of Voice Symptoms N = 56

Voice Symptom	Pearson Correlation	Sig (2-tailed)
Dysphonia	0.353	0.008*
Strain-Strangled Voice Quality	0.389	0.003*
Roughness	0.466	0.000*
Voice Arrest	0.502	0.000*
Increased Expiratory Effort	0.454	0.000*
Voice Tremor	0.216	0.109

Note: All clinician ratings were made during review of the video recording of the Rainbow Passage and description of the Cookie Theft picture
*Findings were statistically significant at the .01 level

Table 5 Comparison of Severity of Current Symptoms with Severity at Diagnosis*

Vocal symptom N = 60	Corresponding DSQ Questions	Mean severity at initial diagnosis (SD)	Mean current severity (SD)	P
Severity of dysphonia	Q1, Q2	4.47 (0.68)	3.19 (0.89)	<0.00001*
Strain-Strangled Voice Quality (effortful phonation)	Q8, Q9	4.21 (0.86)	3.02 (1.00)	<0.00001*
Voice arrest (voice cuts off)	Q3, Q4	4.20 (0.97)	2.89 (1.02)	<0.00001*
Roughness (hoarse / husky)	Q5, Q7	3.41 (1.40)	3.01 (1.18)	0.10000
Voice tremor (shaking voice)	Q10, Q11	3.76 (1.31)	2.71 (1.19)	0.00002*
Increased expiratory effort	Q12, Q13	4.21 (0.90)	3.07 (1.11)	<0.00001*

Note: The DSQ symptom severity rating scale is a 5-point scale (i.e., 1 = mild, 2 = mild-to-moderate, 3 = moderate, 4 = moderate-to-severe, and 5 = severe). Q = question
*Findings were statistically significant at the .01 level

significant, yielding a Cronbach Alpha of .905 for all parameters (see Table 6). The interclass correlations were significant for all symptoms on the USDRS except aphonia. See Tables 6 and 7. This high inter-clinician reliability may be associated with the clinician's access to visual as well as audio information, which parallels the clinical assessment protocol.

Discussion

The VHI-10 is frequently used to measure the impact of a voice problem on a patient's quality of life. The present study asked whether the subjects' perception of handicap as identified on the VHI-10 is correlated with the severity of voice symptoms associated with AD-FLD and selective medical history as identified on the DSQ (i.e., time since initial diagnosis, time since last injection, age at diagnosis, current age, total number of BoNT injections). The subjects' perception of handicap as identified on the VHI-10 was positively correlated with the severity of the voice symptoms and negatively correlated with subjects' age at the time of diagnosis. The strong positive correlation between the subjects' ratings on the VHI-10 and the DSQ (e.g., dysphonia, strain-strangled, roughness, increased expiratory effort) suggests that the handicap associated with AD-FLD is related, not only to the severity of the dysphonia, but to the severity of the individual symptoms. Furthermore, subjects who were younger at the age of diagnosis (16–30 years) indicated greater handicap on the VHI-10 than those who were older when the symptoms began. This finding suggests that the psychosocial aspects of AD-FLD are not only relevant to the effectiveness of long-term management

but require additional research to better understand their impact on quality of life.

Prerequisite to the effective management of patients with AD-FLD is agreement between the laryngologist and the speech-language pathologist with respect to the manifestations of the disease and its severity. Robust inter-clinician reliability ratings on the USDRS suggests that these clinicians are rating similar phenomena. Further, the strong correlation between the clinicians' ratings on the USDRS and the subjects' ratings on the DSQ suggests that clinicians and patients are identifying similar features and estimating the severity in an analogous way.

To date there has been little research investigating subjects' perception of changes in their symptoms since the time of diagnosis. To that end, the current study asked subjects to compare the severity of their dysphonia as well as the individual characteristics at the time of the original diagnosis and then at the time of the study. All subjects rated the severity of their symptoms (with the exception of

Table 6 Inter Clinician Reliability on the USDRS N = 56

	Cronbach's Alpha	Interclass Correlation Coefficient F-Test
Reliability across all parameters on USDRS	0.905	<0.001*

*The reliability of clinician ratings of all perceptual symptoms was significant

Table 7 Inter-Clinician Reliability of Symptoms on the USDRS

Perceptual Rating	Interclass Correlation Coefficient	F Test Significance
Severity of Dysphonia	0.939	<0.001*
Roughness	0.840	<0.001*
Breathiness	0.444	0.003*
Strain-Strangled Quality	0.849	<0.001*
Abrupt Voice Initiation	0.755	<0.001*
Voice Arrest	0.413	0.007*
Aphonia	0.241	0.098
Voice Tremor	0.903	<0.001*
Increased Expiratory Effort	0.809	<0.001*
Speech Rate	0.694	<0.001*
Intelligibility	0.688	<0.001*

Note: All clinician ratings were made during review of the video recording of the Rainbow Passage and description of the Cookie Theft picture
*The reliability of clinician ratings of perceptual symptoms was statistically significant at the .01 level

roughness) to be significantly more serious at the time of initial AD-FLD diagnosis than at the time of the study. Tremor and voice arrest were the two symptoms that were identified as having the greatest continuing improvement. At the time of diagnosis of AD-FLD, the mean severity of tremor and voice arrest was 4 on the DSQ (i.e., moderate-to-severe), but at the time of the study the mean rating on the DSQ was 2 (i.e., mild-to-moderate). This perceived reduction in severity raises questions as to whether the occurrence of voice arrest is potentially more responsive to treatment with BoNT than are other symptoms (e.g., roughness). Alternatively, do subjects develop adaptive behavioral strategies to minimize the frequency of voice arrest during connected speech, or is it the case that subjects overestimate the incidence of voice arrest at onset due to recall bias? If so, why was the severity of voice arrest and tremor overestimated more frequently than other symptoms (e.g., roughness) at the time of diagnosis?

Further research is necessary to explore whether voice arrest is more responsive to BoNT injections or behavioral control than other symptoms. Moreover, the improvement of AD-FLD symptoms since onset may result from an alteration in sensory feedback. The effect of BoNT injections on sensory pathways is an area of active research. It is hypothesized that BoNT alters sensory feedback in dystonia, resulting in improvement in symptoms long after the BoNT has dissipated. Individuals with oromandibular dystonia (OMD) and blepharospasm, for example, have noted improvement in their OMD symptoms following injection of BoNT into the orbicularis oculi alone. [24]

The VAM was used to identify voice arrests in first paragraph of the Rainbow Passage. Clinicians identified voice arrest in only 21/56 (38%) subjects. Several possible explanations may account for the infrequent occurrence of voice arrest in this subject population: voice arrest may not be a predominant characteristic of AD-FLD; voice arrest may continue to diminish following BoNT treatment; or subjects may learn to compensate for voice arrest more easily than for other symptoms. On the surface, it would be expected that clinicians familiar with spasmodic dysphonia would be as effective at documenting the incidence of voice arrest as with the occurrence of other voice symptoms. Further research is necessary to explore these alternative hypotheses.

Conclusions

The diagnosis of AD-FLD is based on clinical symptoms and medical history. The high inter-clinician reliability of perceptual ratings by laryngologists and speech-language pathologists based on the USDRS, and the high correlation of clinician ratings with subjects' ratings from the DSQ suggest that clinicians and subjects are rating similar phenomena using comparable criteria. The ratings

of severity of dysphonia for both clinicians and subjects are related to the interaction of the symptoms and not to any single symptom. For subjects and clinicians alike, the most severe and frequently identified symptoms at the time of assessment were roughness, strain-strangled voice quality, and increased expiratory effort. Subjects and clinicians judged aphonia and voice tremor to be infrequent and less severe than other symptoms. The occurrence and duration of voice arrest as measured by the VAM were infrequent and relatively brief.

The severity of the handicap identified on the VHI-10 was strongly correlated, not only with greater severity of voice symptoms, but with a younger of age of onset of AD-FLD. These findings suggest that future research that addresses the psychosocial impact of AD-FLD in younger individuals may provide information that will enhance treatment and the quality of life for individuals suffering from adductor focal laryngeal dystonia.

Abbreviations

AD-FLD: Adductor focal laryngeal dystonia; BoNT: Botulinum toxin; DSQ: Disease Symptom Questionnaire; FLD: Focal laryngeal dystonia; USDRS: Unified Spasmodic Dysphonia Rating Scale; VAM: Voice Arrest Measure; VHI-10: Voice Handicap Index-10

Acknowledgements

The authors wish to thank Ashish Ankola, MS, for his assistance with data collection.

Funding

Not applicable.

Authors' contributions

CFS, CFS, AB - all made substantial contributions to conception, design, acquisition of data, analysis and interpretation of data, drafting the manuscript and gave final approval of the version to be published. Each author has participated sufficiently in the work to take public responsibility for appropriate portions of the content; and agreed to be accountable for all aspects of the work in ensuring that questions related to the accuracy or integrity of any part of the work are appropriately investigated and resolved. IFK - made substantial contributions to acquisition of data, analysis and interpretation of data; been involved in drafting the manuscript or revising it critically for important intellectual content; given final approval of the version to be published. IFK has participated sufficiently in the work to take public responsibility for appropriate portions of the content; and agreed to be accountable for all aspects of the work in ensuring that questions related to the accuracy or integrity of any part of the work are appropriately investigated and resolved. BED - made substantial contributions to analysis and interpretation of data; has been involved in drafting the manuscript or revising it critically for important intellectual content; given final approval of the version to be published. Each author should have participated sufficiently in the work to take public responsibility for appropriate portions of the content; and agreed to be accountable for all aspects of the work in ensuring that questions related to the accuracy or integrity of any part of the work are appropriately investigated and resolved. All authors read and approved the final manuscript.

Competing interests

The authors declare that they have no competing interests.

Author details

[1]New York University, Steinhardt School of Culture, Education, and Human Development, 665 Broadway, Suite 900, New York NY 10012, USA. [2]Icahn School of Medicine at Mount Sinai, 425 West 59th Street, New York NY 10019, USA. [3]Mannes College the New School for Music, 55 West 13th St, New York 10011, USA. [4]Adelphi University, 75 Varick St, New York 10013, USA. [5]Clinical Endocrinology and Metabolism, Endocrine Society, 2055 L Street NW, Suite 600, Washington, DC 20036, USA. [6]Columbia University College of Physicians and Surgeons, Neurology, Icahn School of Medicine at Mt. Sinai, Center for Voice and Swallowing Disorders, 425 West 59th Street, New York NY 10019, USA.

References

1. Novakovic D, Waters HH, D'Elia JB, et al. Botulinum toxin treatment of adductor spasmodic dysphonia: longitudinal functional outcomes. Laryngoscope. 2011;121(3):606–12.

2. Aronson AE, Brown JR, Litin EM. Pearson. Spastic dysphonia. II. Comparison with essential (voice) tremor and other neurologic and psychogenic dysphonias. Speech Hear Disord. 1968;33:219–31.

3. Blitzer A, Brin MF, Fahn S. Lovelace. Localized injections of botulinum toxin for the treatment of focal laryngeal dystonia (spastic dysphonia). Laryngoscope. 1988;98(2):193–7.

4. Langeveld TP, Drost HA, Frijns JH. Zwinderman, Baatenburg de Jong. Perceptual characteristics of adductor spasmodic dysphonia. Ann Otol Rhinol Laryngol. 2000;109(8 Pt 1):741–8.

5. Jacobson BH, Johnson A, Grywalski C, et al. The voice handicap index (VHI): development and validation. Am J Speech Lang Pathol. 1997;6(3):66–70.

6. Rosen CA, Lee AS, Osborne J. Zullo, Murry. Development and validation of the voice handicap index-10. Laryngoscope. 2004;114(9):1549–56.

7. Hogikyan ND, Sethuraman G. Validation of an instrument to measure voice-related quality of life (V-RQOL). J Voice. 1999;13(4):557–69.

8. Morzaria S, Damrose EJ. A comparison of the VHI, VHI-10, and V-RQOL for measuring the effect of botox therapy in adductor spasmodic dysphonia. J Voice. 2012;26(3):378–80.

9. Dejonckere PH, Neumann KJ, Moerman MB, et al. Tridimensional assessment of adductor spasmodic dysphonia pre- and post-treatment with Botulinum toxin. Eur Arch Otorhinolaryngol. 2012;269(4):1195–203.

10. Tanner K, Roy N, Merrill RM, et al. Spasmodic dysphonia: onset, course, socioemotional effects, and treatment response. Ann Otol Rhinol Laryngol. 2011;120(7):465–73.

11. Stewart CF, Allen EL, Tureen P, et al. Adductor spasmodic dysphonia: standard evaluation of symptoms and severity. J Voice. 1997;11(1):95–10.

12. Braden MN, Hapner ER. Listening: the key to diagnosing spasmodic dysphonia. ORL Head Neck Nurs. 2008;26(1):8–12.

13. Patel RR, Liu L, Galatsanos N. Galatsanos. Differential vibratory characteristics of adductor spasmodic dysphonia and muscle tension dysphonia on high-speed digital imaging. Ann Otol Rhinol Laryngol. 2011;120(1):21–32.

14. Roy N. Differential diagnosis of muscle tension dysphonia and spasmodic dysphonia. Curr Opin Otolaryngol Head Neck Surg. 2010;18(3):165–70.

15. Sapienza CM, Cannito MP, Murry T, Branski R, Woodson G. Acoustic variations in reading produced by speakers with spasmodic dysphonia pre-botox injection and within early stages of post-botox injection. J Speech Lang Hear Res. 2002;45(5):830–43.

16. Jankovic J, Schwartz K, Donovan DT. Botulinum toxin treatment of cranial-cervical dystonia, spasmodic dysphonia, other focal dystonias and hemifacial spasm. J Neurol Neurosurg Psythiatry. 1990;53:633–9.

17. Liu TC, Irish JC, Adams SG. Durkin, hunt. Prospective study of patients' subjective responses to botulinum toxin injection for spasmodic dysphonia. J Otolaryngol. 1996;25(2):66–74.

18. Courey MS, Garrett CG, Billante CR. Outcomes assessment following treatment of spasmodic dysphonia with botulinum toxin. Ann Otol Rhinol Laryngol. 2000;109(9):819–22.

19. Brin, M.F., Blitzer, A., Fahn, S, Gould, Lovelace. Adductor laryngeal dystonia (spastic dysphonia): treatment with local injections of botulinum toxin (Botox). Mov Disord. 1989;198 4(4):287-296.

20. Blitzer A, Brin MF, Stewart CF. Botulinum toxin management of spasmodic dysphonia (laryngeal dystonia): a 12-year experience in more than 900 patients. Laryngoscope. 1998;08(10):1435–41.

21. Fairbanks G. Voice and articulation drillbook. New York: Harper & Row; 1960.

22. Riley GD. A stuttering severity instrument for children and adults. J Speech Hearing Dis. 1972;37:314–22.

23. Goodglass H, Kaplan E, Barresi B. The assessment of aphasia and related disorders ed 3. Philadelphia: Lea Febiger; 2001.

24. Grandaas P, Elston J, Quinn N, et al. Blepharospasm: a review of 264 patients. J Neurol Neurosurg Psych. 1988;51:767–72.

19

The phenomenology and treatment of idiopathic adult-onset truncal dystonia: a retrospective review

Debra J. Ehrlich[*] and Steven J. Frucht

Abstract

Background: Focal dystonia is the most common type of adult-onset dystonia; however, it infrequently affects truncal musculature. Although commonly attributed to secondary etiologies such as a neurodegenerative illness or tardive syndromes, the entity of idiopathic adult-onset truncal dystonia has only been previously described in a few case reports and small case series. Here we characterize seven cases of adult-onset primary truncal dystonia and present them within the scope of the existing literature.

Methods: Retrospective chart review of medical records and patient videos of seven adult patients with idiopathic truncal dystonia evaluated by the senior movement disorder neurologists in an urban outpatient clinic.

Results: The mean age of onset of idiopathic truncal dystonia was 47.6 years old and the majority of patients were male. Truncal flexion was the most common direction of dystonic movement and the dystonia was most frequently induced by action and could be improved by use of a sensory trick. The majority of patients were refractory to 3 or more oral treatments and only two patients exhibited significant functional improvement with botulinum toxin injections. One patient enjoyed significant benefit with bilateral internal globus pallidus deep brain stimulation.

Conclusions: Although a relatively rare presentation, patients with idiopathic adult-onset truncal dystonia can be identified by a common phenomenology. Diagnosis of this highly disabling condition is important because these patients are frequently refractory to multiple oral treatments and may benefit from early treatment with botulinum toxin or deep brain stimulation.

Keywords: Truncal, Axial, Dystonia, Adult

Background

Focal dystonia is the most common type of adult-onset dystonia, and dystonia may affect the face, voice, hand or leg. Aside from the neck, dystonia rarely affects axial musculature unless associated with exposure to a dopamine receptor blocker or as a feature of a neurodegenerative illness. Truncal dystonia is characterized by involuntary contractions and postures of the paraspinal, abdominal or chest muscles. Idiopathic truncal dystonia of adult onset has only been previously described in a few case reports and small case series.

Here we report seven cases of adult-onset dystonia involving primarily the axial musculature. We also compare the current case series to previous reports of idiopathic adult-onset truncal dystonia and review the challenges of designing effective treatments for this condition.

Methods

We conducted a retrospective review of medical records and patient videos of patients with the diagnosis of idiopathic truncal dystonia, evaluated by senior movement disorder physicians in the outpatient clinic of an urban academic center between 1/2009 and 1/2016. Patients were included if symptom onset occurred over 18 years of age and they exhibited primary dystonia of the trunk or axial muscles. Cases of secondary dystonia or tardive syndromes were excluded. The study was approved by the Institutional Review Board of the Mount Sinai

* Correspondence: Debra.ehrlich@mountsinai.org
Icahn School of Medicine at Mount Sinai, 5 East 98th Street, 1st Floor, Box 1637, New York, NY 10029, USA

School of Medicine. Written informed consent for videotaping and use of videos in research and publication was obtained prior to video recording.

Results

Seven patients with a primary diagnosis of idiopathic truncal dystonia were evaluated in the movement disorders clinic between 1/2009 and 1/2016. Within this group of patients, the mean age of onset of truncal dystonia was 47.6 years (SD 9.2). Six patients were male (85.7 %). Patients were symptomatic for an average of 4.7 years (SD 4.8) before their initial visit. Most patients presented with a chief complaint of pulling or tightness of the muscles in the back, abdomen or trunk. There was no history of neuroleptic exposure and no known family history of dystonia in any of the patients. All patients had a spinal MRI (see Table 1) and two patients (28.6 %) had a history of spinal surgery, though symptom onset preceded the operative procedure in one patient (Table 1, case 6). There were no myopathic findings in any of the patients. Additionally, examination of the abdomen did not reveal evidence of involuntary movements consistent with belly dancer dyskinesia. Anterior flexion of the trunk was the predominant direction of dystonic movement in four patients (57.1 %) while lateral flexion was seen in one patient (14.3 %) and truncal extension was the primary direction of involuntary movement in two patients (28.6 %). In most patients the dystonic movements were isolated to the musculature of the trunk; however, associated movements of a shoulder were seen in 2 patients. In more than half of patients (57.2 %), dystonia was present only with specific voluntary movements or action, while dystonia was present at rest though worsened by action in the remainder. In most patients, standing or walking provoked dystonic movements. Additionally, most patients (71.4 %) were aware of a specific sensory trick that suppressed the dystonic movement. Common sensory tricks included running, placing hands in the pants pockets, or tucking hands in the posterior pants waistband. Video 1 (Additional file 1) includes short samples demonstrating the characteristic dystonic truncal movements seen in each patient in this case series.

Most patients proved refractory to multiple oral medications. In fact, five patients (71.4 %) were tried on three or more oral treatments (see Table 1) with minimal to no benefit. All seven patients were treated with trihexyphenidyl; however only two patients exhibited mild improvement in their dystonia while the other five had no benefit. Poor tolerability to low dose trihexyphenidyl limited dose escalation in three of the patients who showed no benefit (see Table 1 for maximum dose of trihexyphenidyl used in each patient). Similar findings were observed in the five patients treated with baclofen, with

a mild benefit seen in 40 % and no benefit in the other 60 %. Botulinum toxin injections were attempted in all seven patients, with two patients (28.5 %) who exhibited at least 50 % functional improvement after injections. In both patients who exhibited significant functional improvement after injections, each received a total of 700U of onabotuliumtoxinA divided between multiple sites in the bilateral rectus abdominis muscles with continuing benefit for at least 1 year. All patients who showed functional benefit after botulinum toxin injections exhibited flexion as the primary direction of axial movement while no improvement was seen in the two patients with the extensor phenotype. One patient (Table 1, case 5) had deep brain stimulation (DBS) to the bilateral internal globus pallidus (GPi) with significant functional improvement sustained for at least 3 months (at the time of writing this paper).

Discussion

We summarize the clinical features and phenomenology of previously published case reports and case series in Table 2. The largest such series was reported by Bhatia et al, who described a group of 18 patients with primarily axial dystonia with adult or late adolescent onset. Our results are similar to Bhatia's in that dystonia most commonly affected men in the fifth decade of life and flexion was the most common direction of involuntary truncal movements [1]. Other reports of idiopathic truncal dystonia are much smaller, although all prior published reports support an onset in the forth to sixth decades of life [1–5]. Also consistent with our findings, truncal flexion was the most common direction of dystonic movement while truncal extension and lateral bending were relatively rare [1–5]. When occurrence at rest compared to action was considered, our results are consistent with prior reports in that dystonia was precipitated or worsened by action [1, 2]. Also consistent with our findings, most patients employed a sensory trick to ameliorate their dystonia [1, 2].

Similar to our case series, most prior reports found that patients with adult onset truncal dystonia were refractory to multiple oral medications [1–5]. While two patients in our case series benefited from botulinum toxin injections, few prior studies report response to botulinum toxin in idiopathic truncal dystonia. One patient with flexion dystonia of the trunk did enjoy transient relief of the dystonia of his upper thoracic region with type A botulinum toxin injections, however he ultimately developed resistance and injections were no longer effective [3]. Although pain relief was reported in some patients, other publications report no benefit with botulinum toxin [1, 2, 5]. Interestingly, in our case series, only patients with

Table 1 Summary of demographics and clinical features in case series

Case #	Sex	Age of onset	Presenting complaint	Family history of dystonia/ genetic testing	Spine imaging or history of trauma	Exposure to dopamine depleting/ blocking agents	Primary axial movement	Secondary axial movement	Involvement of other body regions	Action vs rest	Provoking positions or actions	Sensory trick	Treatment response
1	M	64	Pulling sensation of lower abdominal muscles	No/negative 14 gene dystonia-dyskinesia panel	MRI T/L spine: left L4/L5 herniated disc, exaggerated kyphosis of thoracic spine	No	Flexion	Slight right lateral tilt	No	Action	Standing, walking	Running, dancing, hands in posterior waistband of pants	BAC-small improvement THP (max dose unknown), CARB/LEVO, BTX-no benefit
2	M	44	Tightness and pulling in left lower back	No/no	MRI C/T/L spine: mild disc herniation and osteophytic changes, no cord pathology	No	Left lateral flexion	None	Downward left shoulder movement	Action	Walking or turning	Running	THP (6 mg/day), BTX-small improvement
3	M	43	Abdominal contractions	No/no	L4/L5 fusion for degenerative disc disease, 6 months post-op developed involuntary abdominal contractions	No	Flexion	None	Anterior right shoulder movement	Rest, worse with action	Sitting, worsened by standing or walking	None	BTX-50 % benefit CNZ, CARB/LEVO-no benefit THP (9 mg/day)-small benefit OXC, GBP, PGB-transient benefit
4	M	54	Muscle spasms in chest	No/no	MRI C/T/L spine: mild DJD, no cord pathology	No	Extension	None	No	Rest, worse with action	Supine, reclining, walking	None	BAC, THP (4 mg/day), CNZ, BTX-no benefit
5	M	47	Abnormal pelvic movements and gluteal clenching while standing	No/no	MRI C/T/L spine: no pathology	No	Flexion	Left lateral tilt	No	Action	Standing	Marching, running	CNZ-modest benefit THP (2 mg/day)-no benefit BAC, BTX-small benefit
6	M	46	Forward flexion of trunk when walking	No/no	MRI L spine: L4/L5 stenosis and mild-moderate disc herniation/ after symptom onset had L3-L5 laminectomy and L4/L5 disc micro-dissection with improvement in pain but no change in dystonia	No	Flexion	None	No	Action	Walking, running, going up/down stairs	Hands in pockets, holds hands against torso with mild pressure	BTX-70 % improvement THP (10 mg/day), BAC-no benefit

Table 1 Summary of demographics and clinical features in case series (Continued)

							Extension	Right lateral tilt	No	Rest, worse with action	Writing, worsened by standing or walking	Running, leaning against wall, lying on stomach, voluntary inversion of right leg while walking	DBS-excellent benefit THP (12 mg/day), BAC, CARB/LEVO, LEV, BTX, HYZ-no benefit
7	F	35	Pulling of the trunk backwards and to the right	No/no	MRI L spine: DJD at L4/L5 and L5/S1, no cord pathology	No							

Abbreviations: C cervical, T thoracic, L lumbar, DJD degenerative disc disease, FHx family history, BAC baclofen, THP trihexyphenidyl (the maximal daily dose of THP tried in each patient is noted in parentheses), BTX botulinum toxin, CNZ clonazepam, CARB/LEVO carbidopa/levodopa, OXC oxcarbazepine, HYZ hydroxyzine, LEV levetiracetam, GBP gabapentin, PGB pregabalin, DBS deep brain stimulation

Table 2 Comparison of prior published reports of idiopathic truncal dystonia

Case series/ report	Year	No. of cases	Mean age of onset	Male %	Predominant truncal movement- flexion (%)	Predominant truncal movement- extension (%)	Predominant truncal movement- lateral (%)	Precipitated or worsened by action	Sensory trick
Bhatia et al. [1]	1997	18	41	55.6	55.6	22.2	5.6	In the majority	In some
Zittel et al. [2]	2009	1	36	0	100	0	100	Yes	————
Sobstyl et al. [3]	2012	1	43	100	100	0	0	————	————
Shaikh et al. [4]	2014	4	55.5	50	50	50	0	————	————
Voos et al. [5]	2014	1	33	0	0	100	0	————	————
Current case series	2016	7	46.7	85.7	57.1	28.6	14.3	100 %	71.4 %

truncal flexion showed improvement after botulinum toxin injections while no benefit was seen in patients with truncal extension.

Bilateral GPi DBS has been previously shown to improve axial symptoms in patients with primary generalized dystonia [6] in addition to patients with truncal dystonia occurring as a result of secondary etiologies [7–10]. However, there are only a few case reports of the use of DBS in the treatment of primary truncal dystonia. Shaikh et al report a series of 4 patients with adult-onset axial dystonia who were treated with bilateral GPi DBS. All patients exhibited a substantial functional improvement in truncal dystonia with percent improvement in the Burke-Fahn-Marsden dystonia rating scale (BFMDRS) ranging from 72.4 to 100 % [4]. Another case of predominately adult-onset axial dystonia, although also with later spread to the neck and shoulders, demonstrated complete improvement in axial symptoms after 12 months of treatment with bilateral GPi stimulation. A similar patient with adult onset truncal dystonia exhibited a substantial improvement in axial dystonia with unilateral GPi stimulation (BFMDRS motor score decreased from 33 to 6 after 6 months) [3]. Our patient who was treated with bilateral GPi DBS stimulation showed a similar excellent response to GPi stimulation after 3 months.

Limitations of our case series include the fact that genetic testing was not completed on most patients. Additionally, while all patients denied prior exposure to neuroleptics, it is possible that a tardive case may have been inadvertently included. Given that this was a retrospective chart review, the treatments tried in each patient were not standardized, complicating direct comparisons. Similarly, botulinum toxin injections were not standardized, and different injectors employed different techniques, injected different muscle groups, and used different doses. We also do not have long-term data available on some patients, including the long-term response to DBS. Nevertheless, we believe that our patients add to the growing recognition of this syndrome.

Conclusions

Identification of this highly disabling condition is important, as most patients are refractory to the typical oral treatments for dystonia. Early treatment with botulinum toxin or DBS might be considered to reduce the degree of functional impairment.

Abbreviations
BFMDRS: Burke-Fahn-Marsden dystonia rating scale; DBS: Deep brain stimulation; GPi: Internal globus pallidus

Acknowledgements
None.

Funding
This study has no sponsors or funding support.

Authors' contributions
DJE contributed to data collection and analysis, video editing, creation of figures, and manuscript preparation and revision. SJF contributed to the study design, evaluated and identified appropriate cases, supervised the collection of study data and data analysis, and manuscript preparation and revision. Both authors read and approved the final manuscript.

Competing interests
The authors declare that they have no competing interests.

References

1. Bhatia KP, Quinn NP, Marsden CD. Clinical features and natural history of axial predominant adult onset primary dystonia. J Neurol Neurosurg Psychiatry. 1997;63(6):788–91.
2. Zittel S, Moll CK, Hamel W, Buhmann C, Engel AK, Gerloff C, et al. Successful GPi deep brain stimulation in a patient with adult onset primary axial dystonia. J Neurol Neurosurg Psychiatry. 2009;80(7):811–2.
3. Sobstyl M, Zabek M, Dzierzecki S, Gorecki W. Unilateral pallidal stimulation in a patient with truncal dystonia. Clin Neurol Neurosurg. 2012;114(10):1320–1.
4. Shaikh AG, Mewes K, Jinnah HA, DeLong MR, Gross RE, Triche S, et al. Globus pallidus deep brain stimulation for adult-onset axial dystonia. Parkinsonism Relat Disord. 2014;20(11):1279–82.
5. Voos MC, Oliveira Tde P, Piemonte ME, Barbosa ER. Case report: Physical therapy management of axial dystonia. Physiother Theory Pract. 2014;30(1): 56–61.
6. Vidailhet M, Vercueil L, Houeto JL, Krystkowiak P, Lagrange C, Yelnik J, et al. Bilateral, pallidal, deep-brain stimulation in primary generalised dystonia: a prospective 3 year follow-up study. Lancet Neurol. 2007;6(3):223–9.
7. Micheli F, Cersosimo MG, Piedimonte F. Camptocormia in a patient with Parkinson disease: beneficial effects of pallidal deep brain stimulation. Case report. J Neurosurg. 2005;103(6):1081–3.
8. Thani NB, Bala A, Kimber TE, Lind CR. High-frequency pallidal stimulation for camptocormia in Parkinson disease: case report. Neurosurgery. 2011;68(5): E1501–5.
9. Trinh B, Ha AD, Mahant N, Kim SD, Owler B, Fung VS. Dramatic improvement of truncal tardive dystonia following globus pallidus pars interna deep brain stimulation. J Clin Neurosci. 2014;21(3):515–7.
10. Franzini A, Marras C, Ferroli P, Zorzi G, Bugiani O, Romito L, et al. Long-term high-frequency bilateral pallidal stimulation for neuroleptic-induced tardive dystonia. Report of two cases. J Neurosurg. 2005;102(4):721–5.

20

Effects of a sensory-motor orthotic on postural instability rehabilitation in Parkinson's disease

Daniele Volpe[1*], Elisa Pelosin[2], Leila Bakdounes[1], Stefano Masiero[3], Giannettore Bertagnoni[4], Chiara Sorbera[1] and Maria Giulia Giantin[1]

Abstract

Background: Proprioceptive deficits have been largely documented in PD patients, thus external sensory signals (peripheral sensory feedback) are often used to compensate the abnormalities of proprioceptive integration. This pilot study aims to evaluate the feasibility and the effectiveness of a rehabilitation-training program, combined with the use of a sensory-motor orthotic in improving balance in a small sample of PD patients.

Methods: Twenty PD patients were randomly allocated into two groups: (i) *the Experimental group*, where participants were asked to wear a sensory-motor orthotic during the balance training program and (ii) *the Control group*, where subjects performed an identical training program without wearing any kind of orthotics. In all, the training program lasted 10 sessions (5 days a week for 2 weeks) and the clinical and instrumental assessments were performed at baseline, immediately after the end of the training and 4 weeks after the rehabilitative program was stopped.

Results: All clinical outcome measures tested improved significantly at post and follow-up evaluations in both groups. Interestingly, at the end of the training, only the experimental group obtained a significant improvement in the functional reaching test (sway area - eyes closed) measured by means of stabilometric platform and this result was maintained in the follow-up evaluation.

Conclusions: Our preliminary results suggested that the use of a sensory-motor orthotic, in combination with a tailored balance training, is feasible and it seems to positively impact on balance performance in Parkinson's disease.

Keywords: Parkinson's disease, Sensory-motor orthotic, Postural instability, Rehabilitation

Background

Parkinson's disease (PD) is a neurological progressive disorder characterized by balance dysfunctions, often associated with the high risk of falling [1] that negatively impacts on the quality of life [2]. In PD, most of the falls occur during a sudden change of posture or during walking [3] in various circumstances (i.e., gait initiation, dual task conditions). Balance problems, in PD patients, are probably due to the overlapping of different factors, such as stopped posture, deficits in postural responses [4], reduced limit of stability [5] and impaired executive function (i.e., deficit in selective attention) [6]. Although much is known about the multifactorial nature of gait disturbances and falls in PD, the pathophysiology of postural instability is still unclear. It seems to depend on a complex interactions between the impairment caused by the disease at different levels of the nervous system and compensatory strategies [7, 8]. It is well-known that postural control in PD patients mainly relies on visual information, which is possibly used for compensating proprioceptive impairments [9, 10]. Indeed, PD patients seem to have somatosensory abnormalities with abnormal proprioceptive (kinesthetic) processing that produces a reduced perception of passive motion limb position [11, 12] and space orientation [13]. Therefore, abnormalities in sensory processing have been suggested

* Correspondence: dott.dvolpe@libero.it
[1]Department of Physical Medicine and Rehabilitation, Neurorehabilitation Unit "Villa Margherita,", Via Costacolonna n.6 Arcugnano, Vicenza, Italy
Full list of author information is available at the end of the article

to play a major role in the pathogenesis of sensory dysfunctions in PD [14]. Some authors demonstrated that in a gravity environment, healthy subjects mainly rely on somatosensory information in order to maintain an upright posture [15] and that artificially impairing proprioception worsens postural stability, particularly reducing the COP displacements in response to external perturbations during visual deprivation [16]. In fact, in PD, a defective scaling and habituation of postural reactions during either neck or leg vibration has been revealed [17, 18].

Beside the poor effect of dopaminergic treatment in improving balance problems, the effects of physical activity and exercise programs on improving balance [19–21] and quality of life [21] have been extensively proven in patients with PD. However, the possibility of enhancing training effects, by combining intervention with proprioceptive orthotic, has never been tested.

Proprioceptive rehabilitation aims to improve or enhance the perception of proprioceptive signals and their central integration, thus possibly compensating the impaired "gating" function of the basal ganglia [22]. Furthermore, external sensory signals (peripheral sensory feedback) can be used to compensate the abnormal sensorimotor integration in PD patients [23]. Moreover, muscle spindle endings respond to proprioceptive stimulations with an increased muscular activation, thus producing a tonic contraction on the stimulated muscle [24, 25].

In detail, the sensory-motor (SM) orthotic [Fig. 1] used in this study, combines biomechanical and sensory-motor input on the plantar surface of the feet by modulating through function activation of specific muscle groups. In fact, it has been demonstrated that tendon stimulation has an influence on muscular tone with increased voluntary activation and improved muscle velocity and strength [26, 27]. The proposed novel orthotic is composed of four spots, which through muscle

tendon stimulation exerts a compression which activates anticipated muscle contractions: a) the medial spot which activates the medial muscular kinetic chain (tibia, adductor, paraspinal muscles); b) the lateral spot which activates the lateral muscular kinetic chain (peroneal, abductor, iliotibial, paraspinal muscles muscles); c) the metatarsal and under digital spots which stimulate the extensor muscular kinetic chain (fingers flexors, triceps, femoris biceps s, gluteus and paraspinal muscles). No prior study of SM orthosis on balance dysfunctions in PD has been published before. We have no evidence to support this hypothetical mechanism of function.

The present study aims (i) to explore the feasibility and the safety of using a Sensory-Motor orthotic as a tool of increasing plantar proprioceptive information and (ii) investigating if the combination of the SM orthotic, with a balance training, might enhance postural control, balance and gait in a small group of PD patients.

Methods
Participants
A total of 30 patients with idiopathic PD, according to the United Kingdom Parkinson's Disease Society Brain Bank criteria [28], were recruited from the Department of Neurorehabilitation in Villa Margherita, Arcugnano (Vicenza), Italy.

Participants were enrolled in the study if they met the following inclusion criteria: stage 3 of the Hoehn and Yahr (H&Y) scale, Mini Mental State Examination (MMSE) [29] with score > 24, ability to walk independently without a walking aid and to attend a physiotherapy venue, the absence of serious co-morbidities (cardiac, pulmonary or orthopaedic diseases) that could impact gait or balance. Patients were excluded if they suffered from major depression (diagnosed by means of a Diagnostic and Statistical Manual of Mental Disorders - DSM V criteria), had Deep

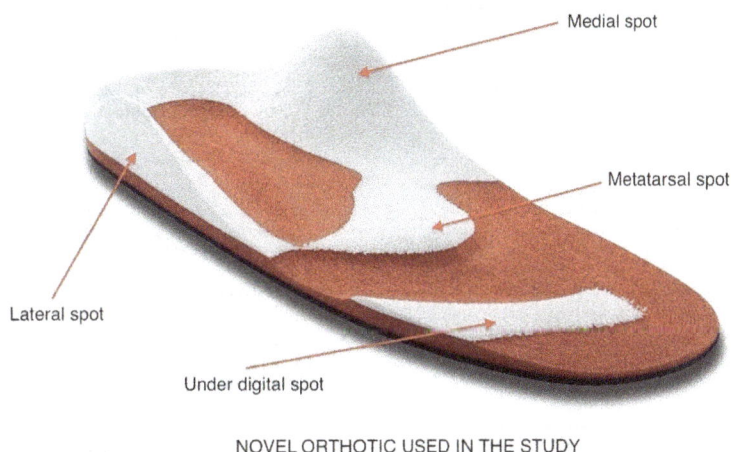

Medial spot

Metatarsal spot

Lateral spot

Under digital spot

NOVEL ORTHOTIC USED IN THE STUDY

Fig. 1 Example of the sensory-motor orthotic

Brain Stimulation implants, were medically unstable or had medication induced (dyskinesias), had an history of other conditions affecting stability (e.g., poor visual acuity or vestibular dysfunction, neuropathy or sensory ataxia). In this pilot study, we recruited patients in stage 3 of H&Y scale exclusively. Thus, all patients were in a moderate stage of PD and had balance problems probably due to abnormal sensory motor integration. In addition, as this was a pilot study, we selected only PD in H&Y = 3 because we wanted to limit, as much as possible, the heterogeneity amongst the patients recruited. At the end of the screening phase, twenty patients with PD were enrolled in the study and ten patients were excluded because six participants did not meet the inclusion criteria ($n = 1$ had MMSE > 24; $n = 2$ needed assistance during walking; $n = 2$ had DBS and $n = 1$ had severe dyskinesia) and four patients were unable to attend the physiotherapy program due to personal reasons.

Study design (Fig. 2)

In this pilot study, after the initial screening procedures, participants were randomly allocated into two groups: (i) *The Experimental group*, in which participants were asked to wear a SM orthotic before and after the training program or (ii) *The Control group*, where subjects performed an identical training program without wearing any kind of orthotics.

All the clinical and instrumental assessments were performed at baseline (PRE - within 1 week before the beginning of the intervention), after the end of the training (POST - within two days after the last training session) and 4 weeks after the completion of the rehabilitative program (FU - follow-up assessment). Randomization procedure, conducted by a third party, was used to allocate participants to one of the two treatment groups (i.e., experimental or control groups). The assessors were blinded to the group allocation during the whole duration of the study. The study coordinator responsible for the SM orthotics supervision was not blinded to the group allocation, but he was not involved in rehabilitation procedures or outcome assessments. The physiotherapists providing the training program were blinded and not involved in other aspects of the trial (i.e., aims, hypothesis or predictions of the study were not disclosed).

Interventions

All PD subjects underwent a training balance program composed by 10 sessions (5 days a week for 2 weeks). Each session lasted 50 min and the exercises were identical for both groups. Table 1 details the type of daily balance training program provided by the hospital physiotherapists in accordance to the Koninklijk Nederlands Genootschap voor Fysiotherapie - KNGF Guidelines for Physiotherapy. At the beginning of each session, participants were

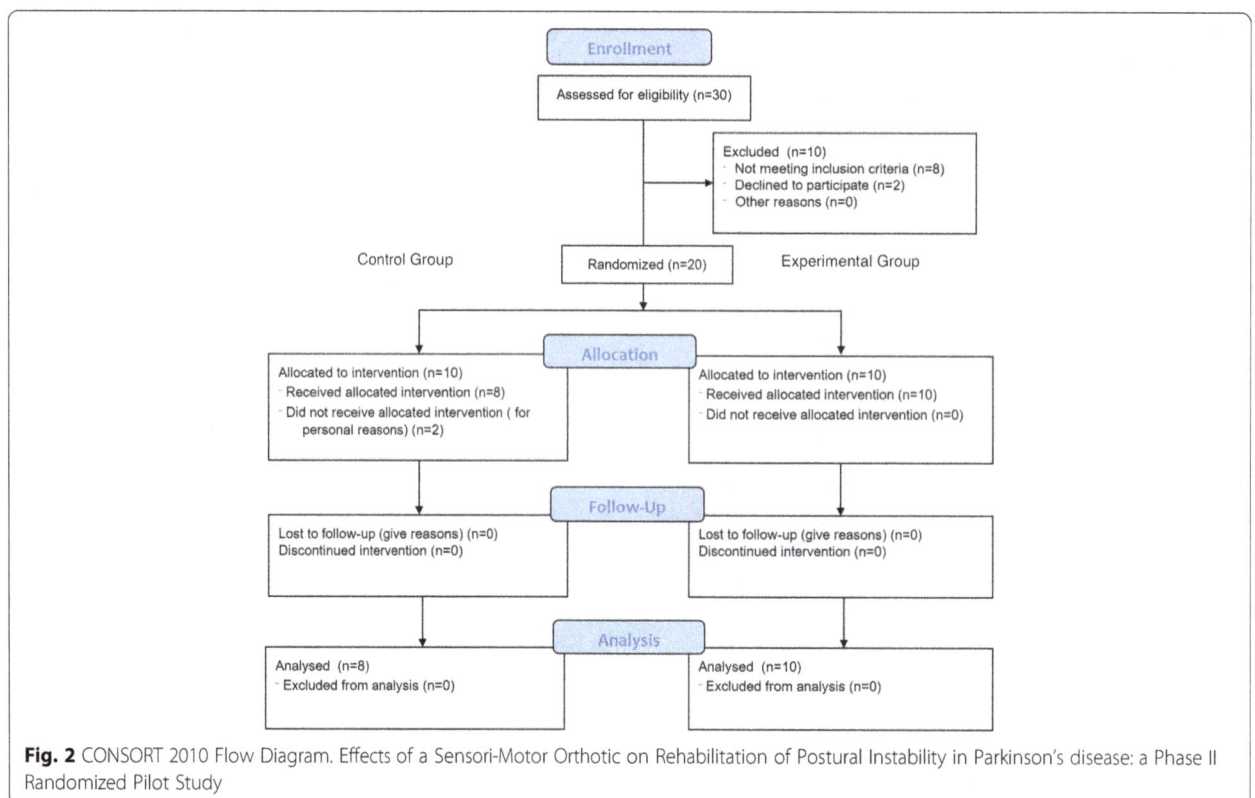

Fig. 2 CONSORT 2010 Flow Diagram. Effects of a Sensori-Motor Orthotic on Rehabilitation of Postural Instability in Parkinson's disease: a Phase II Randomized Pilot Study

Table 1 KNGF Guidelines: physiotherapy program for balance training

Improvement of physical capacity	To maintain or to improve physical capacity with training of aerobic muscle strength (with the emphasis on the muscles of the trunk and legs), joint mobility (among others, axial) and muscle length (among others, muscles of the calf and the hamstrings, flexor and extensor of the knee)
Improvement of the transfers	To train transfers by applying cognitive improvement strategies and cues to initiate and continue movements
Normalizing body posture	To prevent or treat postural deformities with exercises for postural alignment and coordinated movements
Training balance	To optimize balance during the performance of activities in static and dynamic conditions with exercises for training strength and perturbation-based balance training with emphasis of functional reaching test in protected condition and how to activate postural responses to perturbation. Falls prevention strategies.
Gait training	To walk safely and to increase (comfortable) walking speed with exercise walking with the use of cues and cognitive movement strategies and to train muscle strength and mobility of the trunk and upper and lower limbs.

required to sign a form in order to attest their attendance. The physiotherapy protocol included 30 min of exercises designed to improve balance. Precisely, intervention included a perturbation-based balance-training program, where patients were asked to voluntarily reach their limit of stability. During these exercises, participants were required to concentrate and activate the appropriate postural responses in order to react to the external perturbations. Balance training was preceded by warming up and stretching exercises and followed by a cooling down period. Each phase lasted approximately 10 min. Subjects who enrolled in the Experimental group were required for the entire duration of the study (2 weeks) to wear the SM orthotics all day long except during the training balance sessions.

Clinical and instrumental tests

Clinical assessments

Motor impairment was assessed during the III section (motor examination) of the Unified Parkinson's disease Rating Scale (UPDRS) [30], the Berg Balance Scale (BBS) [31], the Timed Up and Go (TUG) [32], and the Six-minute Walking Test (6mWT) [33]. We also quantified the health-related quality of life in all participants using the Parkinson's Disease Questionnaire (PDQ-39) [34]. All adverse events such as injuries, distress and hospital admissions were verified by phone interviews and recordings taken during the pilot study period.

Posturography assessments

Static posturography was assessed in keeping with current guidelines [35]. The Center of Pressure (CoP) excursion was recorded by means of a force platform (Milletrix model 2.0–Rome, Italy). All data were collected with a 50 Hz sampling frequency. The CoP was recorded during an upright stance in a quiet room. Participants were instructed to stand erect, with their arms alongside their body. Their feet were kept at an angle of about 30° opened to the front and with the heels approximately 3 cm apart. Furthermore, an instrumental version of the functional reaching test (FRT) [36] was executed by asking the subject to elevate their arm to shoulder's height and then to perform a maximum

forward reach, while maintaining the heel on the platform with their feet planted in a standing position.

In all the tasks, data was collected for 51.2 s, in both eyes opened (EO) and eyes closed (EC) conditions. The following parameters were taken into account: the sway area (mm^2), measured as the 95th percentile of an ellipse fitted to the overall CoP trace; COP velocity (mm/s) and the Romberg index. These parameters were chosen as a tool to evaluate CoM displacement during sway as a response to perturbation.

Statistical analysis

Demographic and clinical characteristics between the two intervention groups of PD (Experimental and Control) were tested by means of Chi-square (χ^2) test (gender) and t-test (age, UPDRS - Part III Motor, and disease duration) statistics. All clinical and instrumental variables were examined for normality (Shapiro-Wilk W test), and mean and standard deviation (SD) were calculated. For the analysis a Repeated Measures (RM) Analysis of Variance (ANOVA) was used with Group (Experimental, Control) as between-subjects factor and Time (Baseline, Post and Follow-up) as within-subjects factor. The pre-defined level of significance was set at $p < 0.05$. Post hoc analysis of significant interactions was performed by means of -tests applying the Bonferroni correction for multiple comparisons when necessary. All statistical analyses were performed with SPSS 22.0.

Results

At the end of the study, two patients were excluded from the analysis because they dropped out from the training protocol due to personal reasons. Patients with PD enrolled into two groups, did not differ for demographic, clinical characteristics (Table 2) and clinical assessment (p always > 0.05) recorded at the baseline. For the sample as a whole, 100% of intervention sessions were delivered across study arms. No major adverse event or death was recorded during the study period.

Table 2 Baseline demographic and clinical variables of the two groups enrolled in the study

	EXP Group mean ± SD	CTRL Group mean ± SD	Statistics Baseline
Gender (M/F)	7/3	5/3	
Age (yr)	69.18 ± 7.61	63.37 ± 6.89	p = 0.24
Height (cm)	160.91 ± 9.58	160.62 ± 14.74	p = 0.96
Weight (kg)	69.54 ± 13.33	67.62 ± 8.31	p = 0.72
Disease duration (yr)	7.82 ± 4.00	8.12 ± 2.90	p = 0.86
Falls (n)	1.45 ± 2.16	0.87 ± 0.99	p = 0.07
Levodopa (mg/day)	455.32 ± 355.49	409.19 ± 340.68	p = 0.74
• *Dopamine agonist (LEDD mg)*			
Pramipexole E.R.	n = 2	n = 3	N.A.
Ropirinole E.R.	n = 3	n = 3	N.A.
Rotigotine (n = 1)	n = 1	n = 1	N.A.
Rasagiline (n = 1)	n = 2	n = 1	N.A.
• *Other drugs (LEDD mg)*			
Entacapone	n = 1	n = 2	N.A.
Selegiline	n = 1	n = 2	N.A.
Amantadine	n = 2	n = 2	N.A.

Exp, Experimental; CTRL, Control; M, Male; F, Female; Yr, Years; Cm, centimeters; Kg, Kilograms; Mg = Milligrams; N, number; ER = Extended Released; N.A., Not Applicable

Clinical assessments

All data [mean ± standard deviation (SD)] collected at baseline, post and follow-up examinations are reported in Table 3. Statistical analysis showed a positive effect of the balance-training program with no differences between groups in all the variables considered. Precisely, the mean score of UPDRS-III was significantly reduced in the Experimental as well as in the Control groups. RM-ANOVA revealed a significant effect of TIME ($p < 0.01$), without any significant Time X Group interaction ($p = 0.41$). Interestingly, improvements were seen both immediately after the training and at the FU examination (p always < 0.01).

For the tests assessing dynamic balance performance (BBS and TUG), RM-ANOVA showed a main effect of TIME (BBS: $p < 0.01$ and TUG: $p < 0.01$) with no Time X Group interaction. In details, for BBS a significant increase of the total score was seen at Post ($p < 0.01$) and at the FU ($p < 0.01$) evaluations as well as for TUG, where a significant decrease of time in performing the test was seen immediately after the training ($p = 0.01$) and 1 month later (FU: $p < 0.01$). No Time X Group interaction was revealed by the statistical analysis. Similar results were also found in gait resistance performance. Indeed, the analysis of 6MWT data showed a significant effect of Time ($p = 0.02$) with no differences between the two groups. Thus, an overall improvement

was seen immediately after the training (Post: $p = 0.03$) and it was maintained at the FU examination ($p = 0.01$). Balance and gait improvements were also confirmed by a significant decrease of fall rate. Indeed, RM-ANOVA showed a main effect of Time ($p < 0.01$) with an improvement at post ($p = 0.01$). However, no significant Time X Interaction was recorded by the statistical analysis ($p = 0.55$). Finally, positive changes on participants' QoL recorded by means of PDQ-39 questionnaire were seen at the end of the training (Post: $p = 0.03$) as well as the following testing time (FU: $p = 0.02$). Indeed, RM-ANOVA revealed a significant effect of TIME ($p = 0.02$) with no significant Time X Group interaction.

Posturography

Statistical analysis did not reveal significant changes for sway area recorded in the quiet stance test (p always >0.05) in both conditions (EC and EO). However, RM ANOVA showed a significant main effect of Group ($p = 0.04$) and a significant Group x Time interaction ($p = 0.03$) for 95% confidence ellipse area data obtained during the FRT test in the EC condition. Furthermore, post-hoc analysis revealed that only the experimental group obtained a significant improvement at the end of the training period ($p = 0.02$) and this result was maintained at the follow-up examination (Fig. 3). Similar results were also found for the values obtained for the Romberg index. Indeed, statistical analysis (RM-ANOVA) revealed a significance of the factor Group ($p = 0.04$) as well as a significant Group x Time interaction. Post-hoc analysis showed that only in the experimental group, velocity increased at the end of the training ($p = 0.03$) and at the follow-up evaluation ($p = 0.04$) (Fig. 4). No significant changes were detected during static and dynamic (FRT) evaluation under EO condition. Finally, no significant changes were found for CoP velocity in any experimental condition (EC and EO).

Discussion

The aim of the present study was to explore the feasibility and the safety of using a Sensory-Motor orthotic as a tool for increasing plantar proprioceptive information. Furthermore, it was carried out to verify if the combination of the SM orthotic, with a rehabilitative intervention, could enhance postural control, balance and gait in a group of subjects with PD.

The rehabilitative program was delivered successfully, with a good level of adherence rate confirmed by the patient's participation and involvement. On the whole, our results demonstrated that combining balance training with a sensory-motor orthotics in a rehabilitation setting is feasible and might lead to some clinically meaningful effect in PD patients with postural instability. However, only subjects enrolled in the experimental protocol

Table 3 Clinical variables of the two groups enrolled in the study and their comparisons at each time point

	PSM Group	CTRL Group	Statistic post-hoc TIME
Motor UPDRS section III at T0-Baseline	40.87 ± 6.01	39.00 ± 11.89	
Motor UPDRS section III at T1-Discharge	37.12 ± 6.66	36.90 ± 12.02	$p < 0.01$
Motor UPDRS section III at T2-Follow up	35.55 ± 6.57	36.80 ± 11.80	$p < 0.01$
Berg Balance Scale T0-Baseline	45.63 ± 5.92	45.12 ± 4.58	
Berg Balance Scale T1-Discharge	49.3 ± 3.15	47.12 ± 5.05	$p < 0.01$
Berg Balance Scale T2-Follow up	50.1 ± 2.72	49.37 ± 5.35	$p < 0.01$
Falls T0-Baseline	1.45 ± 2.16	0.87 ± 0.99	
Falls T1-Discharge	0.45 ± 1.03	0.12 ± 0.31	$p < 0.01$
Falls T2-Follow up	0.00 ± 0.00	0.00 ± 0.00	N.A.
Timed Up and Go T0-Baseline	13.08 ± 2.17	13.8 ± 3.43	
Timed Up and Go T1-Discharge	12.13 ± 1.35	12.8 ± 2.81	$p = 0.01$
Timed Up and Go T2-Follow up	10.81 ± 1.07	13.2 ± 2.75	$p < 0.01$
6MWT T0-Baseline	305.64 ± 48.89	319.8 ± 48.59	
6MWT T1-Discharge	335.64 ± 44.09	332.5 ± 66.00	$p = 0.03$
6MWT T2-Follow up	342.2 ± 59.99	328.38 ± 70.18	$p = 0.01$
PDQ-39 T0-Baseline	57.7 ± 22.93	59 ± 14.38	
PDQ-39 T1-Discharge	54.36 ± 24.47	49.5 ± 20.52	$p = 0.03$
PDQ-39 T2-Follow up	52.1 ± 27.44	51.25 ± 19.46	$p = 0.02$

Exp, Experimental, *CTRL* Control, *UPDRS* Unified Parkinson Disease Rating Scale, *6MWT* Six Meters Walking Test, *PDQ-39* Parkinson's Disease Questionnaire-39 items. N.A., not applicable

P values represent the post hoc analysis (T0 vs T1 and T0 vs T2) when a main effect of TIME was detected with Repeated Measures ANOVA

significantly improved their limit of stability measured by a stabilometric platform. Precisely, an increase of sway area values, obtained during the instrumental functional reaching test, and an improvement of the Romberg index were seen only in the experimental group immediately after the training and follow-up evaluation. As stated in the introduction, PD-related abnormality in proprioception might manifest itself as alteration of kinesthesia (for a review see [13]. Indeed, PD patients have an impaired sense of the timing [37] and discrimination [38] of

proprioceptive inputs, which can also lead to deficient compensation of mechanical perturbations, especially during the activation of anticipatory postural adjustments [39]. The enhancement of the proprioceptive inflow, as that induced by the sensory-motor orthotic used in this study, might overcome the subtle impairment in kinesthesia, as previously argued [37]. PD patients used to have a reduced limit of stability particularly during dynamic conditions, thus pointing to dynamic posturography as a better instrument of capturing improvements in

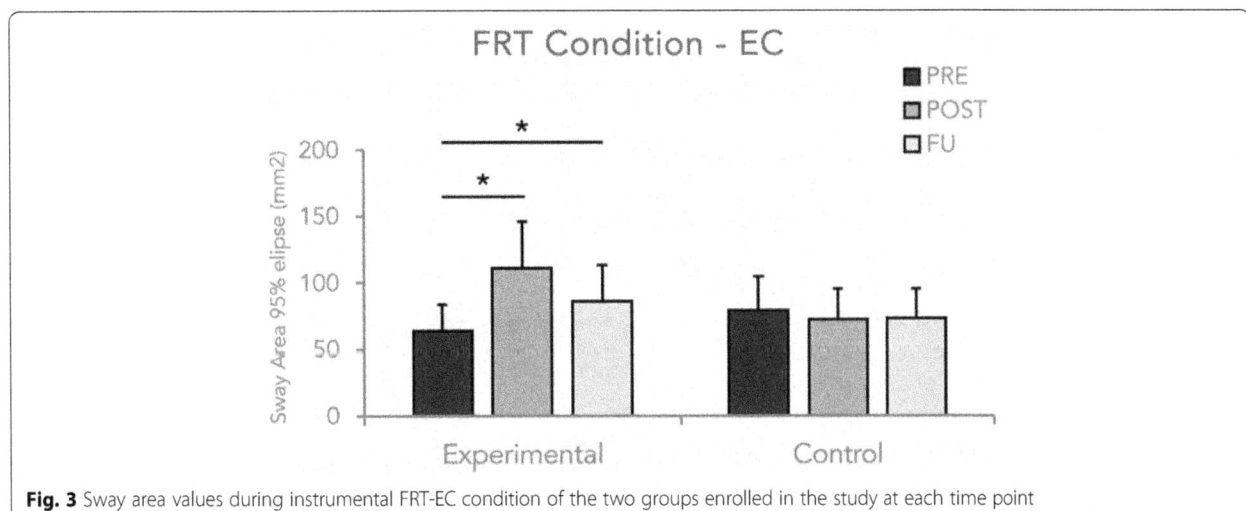

Fig. 3 Sway area values during instrumental FRT-EC condition of the two groups enrolled in the study at each time point

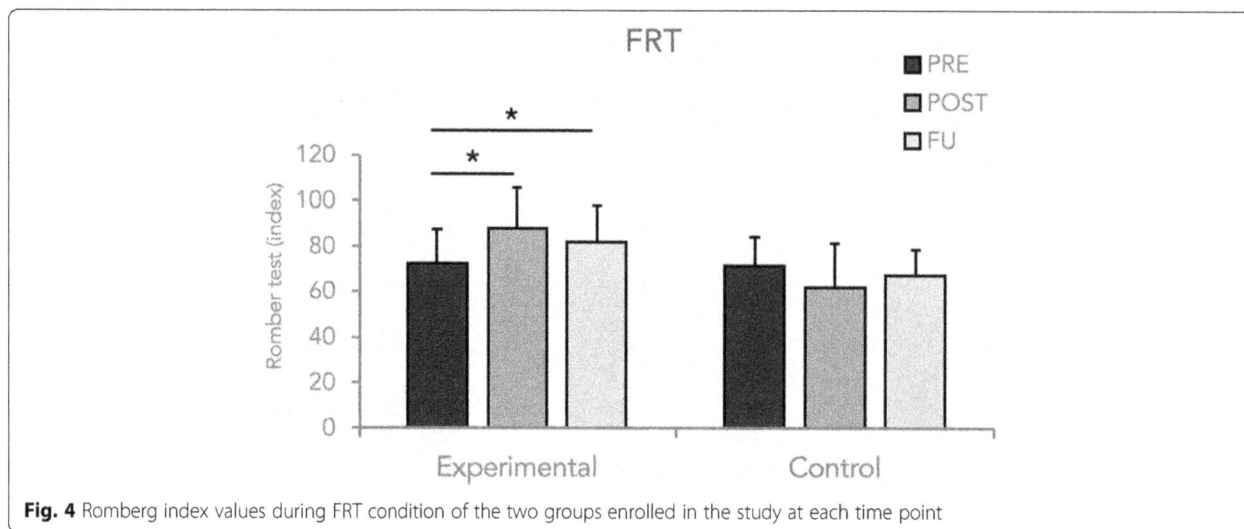

Fig. 4 Romberg index values during FRT condition of the two groups enrolled in the study at each time point

balance [5, 35]. It is well-known that anticipatory postural adjustments and reactive postural reactions in PD are compromised, in the sense that they are reduced in amplitude and velocity [39]. So another possible mechanism of action could be related to the influence on muscles of proprioceptive stimulation exerted by the SM orthotic, since tendon stimulation [40, 41] seems to increase muscular tone and velocity promoting the activation of anticipatory postural adjustments and reactive postural reactions. Finally, it is important to notice that significant changes in the posturographic data during the FRT in the experimental group were seen only when patients were required to execute the test with their eyes closed, a set-up relying on proprioceptive information. This fact might suggest an improvement of proprioceptive signals derived from the effect of the SM orthotic.

This pilot study has a number of limitations. Firstly, even if testing occurred at the peak dose of the morning medications, we cannot rule out the bias introduced by fluctuations in levodopa plasmatic concentration. Secondly, even though the sample size allowed the detection of significant changes, here we reported results obtained in a small group of patients, thus our results have to be replicated by larger trials. Thirdly, due to the shortness of training and the follow-up examination, we did not evaluate changes in fall rates. Further study should have to include episode supervision of falls. Fourthly, even if the physiotherapy program for balance training was conducted in accordance with published guidelines, the execution of exercises were influenced by therapists expertise and patients' motivation, meaning that our protocol does not necessarily reflect the clinical practice in other parts of the world. Fifthly, we did not include in this pilot study, an aged matched control group for evaluating changes in balance related to basal ganglia dysfunction, so we cannot conclusively ascribe our findings to basal ganglia malfunction in PD.

Finally, we want to underline that postural control measured by dynamic posturography might give more information about mechanisms of postural instability in PD than static posturography. Performing the FRT might not be as good as a test measured by dynamic posturography.

Conclusions

This pilot study shows that a tailored balance training, in association with the sensory-motor orthotic, appears to be safe and feasible and is able to positively impact on mobility, balance, gait and quality of life. This preliminary study provides promising data on the feasibility and safety of our protocol, thus supporting the development of a large scale Randomized Control Trial. Future studies are certainly needed and will expand our knowledge on the mechanisms of action of SM orthotic, on the time needed to achieve a meaningful improvement and its long-term duration.

Abbreviations
6mWT: Six minutes walking test; ANOVA: Analysis of Variance; BBS: Berg Balance Scale; CoP: Center of Pressure; DSM: Diagnostic and Statistical Manual of Mental Disorders; EC: Eyes closed; EO: Eyes open; FRT: Functional Reaching Test; H&Y: Hoehn and Yahr; KNGF: Koninklijk Nederlands Genootschap voor Fysiotherapie; MMSE: Mini Mental State Examination; PD: Parkinson's disease; PDQ-39: Parkinson's Disease Questionnaire; RM: Repeated Measures; SD: Standard Deviation; SM: Sensory motor; TUG: Time Up and Go; UPDRS: Unified Parkinson's Disease Rating Scale

Acknowledgements
We acknowledge Sanitaria Elena Ortopedia for providing the SM orthotics used in the study and also the PD patients that gently participated in this trial.

Funding
This pilot study was unfunded. The research was performed in the course of the author's clinical duties at the Department of Neurorehabilitation, Villa Margherita (VI).

Authors' contributions

DV conceived the study, participated in the design, oversaw data collection, contributed to data interpretation and results analysis, and drafted the manuscript. EP was responsible of statistical analysis, contributed to data interpretation, results analysis and drafted the manuscript. LB participated in data collection, was responsible for assessments, contributed in manuscript preparation. SM oversaw data collection, contributed to data interpretation and results analysis. GB oversaw data collection, contributed to data interpretation and results analysis. CS participated in data collection, was responsible for assessments, contributed to manuscript preparation. MGG participated in data collection, was responsible for assessments, contributed in manuscript preparation. All authors read and approved the final manuscript.

Competing interests

The authors declare that they have no competing interests.

Author details

[1]Department of Physical Medicine and Rehabilitation, Neurorehabilitation Unit "Villa Margherita", Via Costacolonna n.6 Arcugnano, Vicenza, Italy. [2]Department of Neuroscience, University of Genoa, Genoa, Italy. [3]School of Physical Medicine and Rehabilitation, University of Padua, Padua, Italy. [4]Department of Physical Medicine and Rehabilitation, S. Bortolo Hospital, Vicenza, Italy.

References

1. Grimbergen YA, Munneke M, Bloem BR. Falls in Parkinson's disease. Curr Opin Neurol. 2004;17(4):405–15.
2. Soh SE, Morris ME, McGinley JL. Determinants of health-related quality of life in Parkinson's disease: a systematic review. Parkinsonism Relat Disord. 2011;17:1–9.
3. Stack E, Jupp K, Ashburn A. Developing methods to evaluate how people with Parkinson's disease turn 180 degrees: an activity frequently associated with falls. Disabil Rehabil. 2004;26:478–84.
4. Lee RG, Tonolli I, Viallet F, Aurenty R, Massion J. Preparatory postural adjustments in parkinsonian patients with postural instability. Can J Neurol Sci. 1995;22:126–35.
5. Schieppati M, Hugon M, Grasso M, Nardone A, Galante M. The limits of equilibrium in young and elderly normal subjects and in parkinsonians. Electroencephalogr Clin Neurophysiol. 1994;93:286–98.
6. Hausdorff JM, Balash J, Giladi N. Effects of cognitive challenge on gait variability in patients with Parkinson's disease. J Geriatr Psychiatry Neurol. 2003;16:53–8.
7. Fasano A, Plotnik M, Bove F, Berardelli A. The neurobiology of falls. Neurol Sci. 2012;33:1215–23.
8. Benatru I, Vaugoyeau M, Azulay JP. Postural disorders in Parkinson's disease. Neurophysiol Clin. 2008;38:459–65.
9. Demirci M, Grill S, McShane L, Hallett M. A mismatch between kinesthetic and visual perception in Parkinson's disease. Ann Neurol. 1997;41:781–8.
10. Carpenter MG, Bloem BR. Postural control in Parkinson patients: a proprioceptive problem? Exp Neurol. 2011;227(1):26–30.
11. Zia S, Cody F, O'Boyle D. Joint position sense is impaired by Parkinson's disease. Ann Neuro. 2000;47:218–28.
12. Konczak J, Krawczewski K, Tuite P, Maschke M. The perception of passive motion in Parkinson's disease. J Neurol. 2007;254:655–63.
13. Conte A, Khan N, Defazio G, Rothwell JC, Berardelli A. Pathophysiology of somatosensory abnormalities in Parkinson disease. Nat Rev Neurol. 2013;9:687–97.
14. Nolano M, Provitera V, Estraneo A, Selim MM, Caporaso G, Stancanelli A, Saltalamacchia AM, Lanzillo B, Santoro L. Sensory deficit in Parkinson's disease: evidence of a cutaneous denervation. Brain. 2008;131:1903–11.
15. Peterka RJ. Sensorimotor integration in human postural control. J Neurophysiol. 2002;88:1097–118.
16. Mohapatra S, Krishnan V, Aruin AS. Postural control in response to an external perturbation: effect of altered proprioceptive information. Exp Brain Res. 2012;217:197–208.
17. Valkovic P, Krafczyk S, Saling M, Benetin J, Botzel K. Postural reactions to neck vibration in Parkinson's disease. Mov Disord. 2006;21:59 65.
18. in Parkinson's disease: scaling deteriorates as disease progresses. Neurosci Lett. 2006;401:92–6.
19. Hirsch MA, Toole T, Maitland CG, Rider RA. The effects of balance training and high-intensity resistance training on persons with idiopathic Parkinson's disease. Arch Phys Med Rehabil. 2003;84:1109–17.
20. Allen NE, Sherrington C, Paul SS, Canning CG. Balance and falls in Parkinson's disease: a meta-analysis of the effect of exercise and motor training. Mov Disord. 2011;26:1605–15.
21. Goodwin VA, Richards SH, Henley W, Ewings P, Taylor AH, et al. An exercise intervention to prevent falls in people with Parkinson's disease: a pragmatic randomised controlled trial. J Neurol Neurosurg Psychiatry. 2011;82:1232–8.
22. Abbruzzese G, Trompetto C, Mori L, Pelosin E. Proprioceptive rehabilitation of upper limb dysfunction in movement disorders: a clinical perspective. Front Hum Neurosci. 2014;8:961.
23. Abbruzzese G, Berardelli A. Sensorimotor integration in movement disorders. Mov Disord. 2003;18:231–24060.
24. Roll JP, Vedel JP. Kinaesthetic role of muscle afferents in man, studied by tendon vibration and microneurography. Exp Brain Res. 1982;47:177–90.
25. Marsden CD, Meadows JC, Hodgson HJ. Observations on the reflex response to muscle vibration in man and its voluntary control. Brain. 1969;92:829–46.
26. Cordo P, Gurfinkel VS, Bevan L, Kerr GK. Proprioceptive consequences of tendon vibration during movement. J Neurophysiol. 1995;74:1675–88.
27. Bosco C, Colli R, Introini E, Cardinale M, Tsarpela O, et al. Adaptive responses of human skeletal muscle to vibration exposure. Clin Physiol. 1999;19:183–7.
28. Hughes AJ, Daniel SE, Kilford L, Lees AJ. Accuracy of clinical diagnosis of idiopathic Parkinson's disease: a clinico-pathological study of 100 cases. J Neurol Neurosurg Psychiatry. 1992;55:181–4.
29. Folstein MF, Folstein SE, McHugh PR. "Mini-mental state". A practical method for grading the cognitive state of patients for the clinician. J Psychiatr Res. 1975;12:189–98.
30. Fahn S, Elton R, et al. Recent developments in Parkinson's disease. Folorham Park: Macmillan Health Care Information; 1987. p. 153–63. 293–304.
31. Berg K, Wood-Dauphinee S, Williams JI. The Balance Scale: reliability assessment with elderly residents and patients with an acute stroke. Scand J Rehabil Med. 1995;27:27–36.
32. Podsiadlo D, Richardson S. The timed "Up & Go": a test of basic functional mobility for frail elderly persons. J Am Geriatr Soc. 1991;39:142–8.
33. Casanova C, Celli BR, Casas A, Cote C et al. The 6-min walk distance in healthy subjects: reference standards from seven countries. Eur Respir J. 2011;37:137–56.
34. Peto V, Jenkinson C, Fitzpatrick R, Greenhall R. The development and validation of a short measure of functioning and well being for individuals with Parkinson's disease. Qual Life Res. 1995;4:241–8.
35. Scoppa F, Capra R, Gallamini M, Shiffer R. Clinical stabilometry standardization: basic definitions-acquisition interval–sampling frequency. Gait Posture. 2013;37:290–2.
36. Duncan PW, Weiner DK, Chandler J, Studenski S. Functional reach: a new clinical measure of balance. J Gerontol. 1990;45:M192–7.
37. Fiorio M, Stanzani C, Rothwell JC, Bhatia KP, Moretto G, et al. Defective temporal discrimination of passive movements in Parkinson's disease. Neurosci Lett. 2007;417:312–5.
38. Jacobs JV, Horak FB. Abnormal proprioceptive-motor integration contributes to hypometric postural responses of subjects with Parkinson's disease. Neuroscience. 2006;141:999–1009.
39. Horak FB, Dimitrova D, Nutt JG. Direction-specific postural instability in subjects with Parkinson's disease. Exp Neurol. 2005;193(2):504–21.
40. De Nunzio AM, Nardone A, Picco D, Nilsson J, Schieppati M. Alternate trains of postural muscle vibration promote cyclic body displacement in standing parkinsonian patients. Mov Disord. 2008;23:2186–93.
41. Nonnekes J, de Kam D, Geurts A, Weerdesteyn V, Bloem BR. Unraveling the mechanisms underlying postural instability in Parkinson's disease using dynamic posturography. Expert Rev Neurother. 2013;13:1303–8.

21

Pathophysiology of writer's cramp: an exploratory study on task-specificity and non-motor symptoms using an extended fine-motor testing battery

Ali Amouzandeh[1], Michael Grossbach[1], Joachim Hermsdörfer[2] and Eckart Altenmüller[1*]

Abstract

Background: Writer's cramp (WC) is a task-specific focal dystonia which manifests itself as abnormal postures interfering with motor performance. As the spread of motor symptoms remains controversial and non-motor symptoms are widely discussed, in this exploratory study, we explore the pathophysiology of WC, focusing on task-specificity and the psychological profiles of WC patients.

Methods: In 14 right-handed WC patients and matched controls, we assessed motor control by applying motor performance tests (Vienna Test Series), as well as using writing analysis and grip-force measurements. Moreover, detailed psychological factors were assessed. Classification trees were used to distinguish patients from controls.

Results: The total duration of writing and the vertical writing frequency of the pen are the most important variables to split the data set successfully into patients and controls. No other variables concerning motor performance tests, grip-force measurements or psychological factors correctly separated patients and controls.

Conclusions: Only variables from the writing tasks successfully separated patients and controls, indicating a strong task-specificity of WC in our patient group. Future research should be performed with larger samples of untreated WC patients in early stages of impairment, without any secondary motor disturbances, to verify our findings.

Background

Writer's Cramp (WC) is a task-specific movement disorder that manifests itself as abnormal postures and unwanted muscle spasms that interfere with motor performance while writing [1]. According to the new classification, WC is considered a sporadic focal dystonia (FD) with late adult onset between the ages of 30 and 50 years [2].

One symptom of WC, typically during the initial stage, is a tight grip on the pen. Hand–wrist flexors are more commonly involved than extensors, though hyperextension of the distal phalanges or even the fingers may occur [3]. Slowly, handwriting becomes less legible. About half of the patients with simple cramps progress to having dystonia with other activities. Remissions are uncommon,

and symptoms can progress to the other hand in about 5% of cases [4].

Symptoms appear at a mean age of 38 years [3]. Generally, FD of the limb is rare, and prevalence has been estimated in a more recent meta-analysis to be 15 per 100,000 people [5]. The prevalence rate of WC was reported to be 6.9 per 100,000 persons, whereas the incidence was 0.27 per 100,000 in one year [6].

It is still under debate whether WC is task-specific or not. Task-specificity in general remains a fascinating topic in focal dystonia, and it is still not completely understood (see Pirio Richardson et al. 2017 for an actual discussion [7]). Brain imaging studies revealed that the connectivity between the parietal and premotor areas was weaker. It appears that a specific parietal-premotor pathway is malfunctioning in WC [8]. In clinical practice, an initial classification divided the patients into two groups, those with simple and those with dystonic WC, on the basis of the absence or presence of dystonia while

* Correspondence: eckart.altenmueller@hmtm-hannover.de
[1]Institute of Music Physiology and Musicians' Medicine (IMMM), University of Music, Drama and Media, Emmichplatz 1, 30175 Hannover, Germany
Full list of author information is available at the end of the article

performing other tasks [9]. However, this simple classification seems inappropriate, as there may be transitions from highly specific deficits, which only affect the writing of specific letters [10], to simple and then to dystonic WC, and eventually to multifocal dystonias. Moreover, even patients with simple WC frequently report discomfort in other daily activities, like typing on a computer keyboard [11] or using a spoon [12]. Marsden et al. noted frequent association of other features of segmental and generalized dystonia in patients with dystonic WC over 30 years ago [7] and, nowadays, even the spread of motor symptoms to the opposite hand are reported [13]. Secondary motor disturbances with reduced range of motion in other task than writing have also been described in patients suffering from WC [14]. These were related to the severity and duration of the disorder and explained by biomechanical abnormalities of the hand, possibly as a consequence of a combination of innate factors and long-term effects of treatment with botulinum toxin. Indeed, in other focal dystonias, biomechanical abnormalities might contribute to the development. Wilson et al. [15] showed increased stiffness and reduced range of motion in fingers in 10 out of 14 musicians suffering from musician's dystonia (MD), interestingly also in the unaffected hand. This was also impressively demonstrated in a guitarist with MD [16]. Such biomechanical abnormalities might affect other fine motor tasks, if they are similar to the dystonic task. In keeping with this, such secondary motor disturbances were present in 53% of MD patients [17] when movements were very similar to the main affected task; for example, playing piano and typing on a computer keyboard. However, in a previous study applying the same methodology as in the present paper, Hofmann and colleagues (2015) could not find such spread of symptoms [18]. Similarly, Schneider et al. [19] investigated grip force in patients with WC and did not find a spread of symptoms to other sensorimotor tasks [19].

The primary goal of the present study was to clarify whether a spread of symptoms to other fine motor task could be demonstrated. We applied an extensive fine motor test battery, targeted at writing movements, other controlled guided fine motor movements, ballistic targeting movements and grip force. The test battery applied is the largest one represented in the literature and exceeds the one applied by Schneider and colleagues [19].

An additional goal of this study was related to assess psychological factors related to the triggering of WC. In a recent study on MD, Ioannou and Altenmuller demonstrated that 56% of musicians with dystonia were suffering from psychological symptoms, such as increased trait anxiety and obsessive-compulsive behavior [20]. These premorbid psychological factors seem to play a role in triggering task-specific dystonia, since, on

average, symptoms of dystonia occurred 10 years earlier in musicians with psychological issues as opposed to MD patients with no elevated levels of stress and anxiety [21]. Here, we wanted to address the question, whether anxiety, perfectionism and other psychological symptoms might also contribute to triggering WC.

Methods

A total of 15 WC patients participated in the study. As we intended to investigate a homogeneous population, one of the patients was excluded from further analyses because of being left-handed, according to the Edinburgh Handedness Inventory [22]. All patients (7 females, 8 males) had been diagnosed with WC by a movement disorders specialist (senior author EA) and were recruited from the outpatient clinic at the Institute of Music Physiology and Musicians' Medicine at the Hanover University of Music, Drama and Media. The institute is registered with the German health board, and offers treatment for non-musician patients suffering from task-specific movement disorders. None of the patients in the present study were professional musicians. Patients did not suffer from any other neurological deficit; in particular, musicians' dystonia was excluded. The mean age of the subjects was 47.20 years (SD: 12.99; range: 26.67 to 69.67). Of 14 patients, 13 were affected in the right (dominant) hand or arm, while one was suffering from symptoms in both hands or arms, though mainly in the right hand or arm. No patient had symptoms in the left hand or arm exclusively. Eight of the 14 patients were amateur musicians, who had played their instrument for an average of 19.83 years (SD: 14.39; range: 8 to 40). Even though some discomfort, e.g. perceived tension after prolonged playing was reported by 5 of the 8 amateur musicians, patients did not suffer from MD with involuntary flexion or extension of fingers etc. The duration of WC amounted to a mean of 9.52 years (SD: 5.48; range: 0.5 to 19).

Ten patients had been treated with Botulinum Toxin (BT), partly combined with trihexyphenidyl (THX) or an additional retraining/physiotherapy to reduce symptoms of WC. In all cases, the last treatment of BT had taken place more than 6 months before the study. As several studies have shown that the effect of BT lasts about 12 weeks [23], a clinical effect of the medication on the results can most likely be excluded. Three patients were treated with a combination of THX and retraining/physiotherapy, whereas one was exclusively treated with retraining/physiotherapy in a training program targeting at improving WC. All patients had benefitted from treatment and were considered in a stable state of WC. Clinical data of the patients are displayed in Table 1.

Table 1 Overview of clinical data of examined WC patients

Gender	Age (in years)	Duration of FD (in years)	Handedness	Dystonic hand	Therapy
F	32.75	0.5	R	R	BT
F	66.75	0.75	R	R	BT
F	49.67	4	R	R	BT
F	56.25	10	R	R	Physical therapy, BT, Retraining
F	30.92	6	R	R	Physical therapy, BT, Retraining
F	33.33	12	R	B	BT, THX
F	26.67	14	R	R	Physical Training, Retraining
M	54.08	10	R	R	BT
M	44.33	12	R	R	BT
M	48.92	16	R	R	BT
M	42.83	13	R	R	Physical therapy, BT, Retraining
M	51.67	6	R	R	Physical Training, Retraining
M	69.67	19	R	R	Physical therapy, THX, Retraining
M	53	10	R	R	Physical therapy, THX, Retraining

Fourteen healthy controls without any neurological deficits were matched in gender, age and handedness. Mean age of the controls was 48.05 (SD: 13.88; range: 28.67 to 71.17).

Participants were asked to fill in a psychological questionnaire to assess the most important personality factors (the Big Five personality traits, NEO-FFI [24]). Furthermore, we assessed the impairment of daily tasks and symptoms of loss of control (Arm Dystonia Disability Scale, ADDS [25]). To distinguish temporary state anxiety from sustained trait anxiety, the State-Trait Anxiety Inventory, STAI [26], was used. Additionally, we asked to report accumulated lifetime practice of fine motor activities. Since all participants' first language was German, standardized translations of the questionnaires were used [27].

Motor abilities were examined using 3 different test batteries. All participants began with the computer-assisted Motor Performance Test series, Vienna Test Series (https://www.schuhfried.com/test/MLS). This battery sub-divides into several fine motor manipulation tasks, including everyday life-like activities. Motor performance in handwriting and drawing was analyzed with the aid of a digitizing tablet, which has been used in a WC study by Zeuner and colleagues [28]. Finally we examined the grip force, as introduced by Hermsdörfer and colleagues [29].

Motor Performance Tests (MPT) and Grip Force Tasks (GFT) were carried out with both hands. Patients began these tests with their dystonic hand, and controls started with the hand corresponding to the affected hand of the respective matched patient. The Writing Task (WT) test was performed with the dominant hand exclusively.Patients started with the MPT, which requires the most steadiness, concentration and precision. Secondly, the WT was conducted, demanding less precision than the MP task. Furthermore, WT requires high activation of arm muscles, unlike MPT. Finally, GFT was conducted, predominantly registering grip force during lifting, holding, and moving an object, with less movement precision.Informed consent was obtained from all participants before study participation. The study was approved by the local ethics committee of the Hannover Medical University.

All variables obtained and analyzed in this study are displayed in Table 2.

Motor performance tests

To assess general fine motor skills, we used the MPT series (Schuhfried GmbH, Mödling, Austria, version 6.34.001). The work panel (see Fig. 1: the MPT work panel (https://www.schuhfried.com/test/MLS), W × H × D: 300 × 300 × 15 mm.) contained holes, grooves and contact surfaces. To perform most of the sub-tests, 2 metal rods (each 150 mm long, containing a 30 mm long contact pin) were used as a "pointing device" by the subjects. Nearly all tasks were performed with the dominant hand first and then with the non-dominant hand (see below for exceptions).

We applied the test form according to Schoppe & Hamster (https://www.schuhfried.com/test/MLS), which contains seventeen sub-tests. In the sub-test "Steadiness", participants were required to steadily hold one of the metal rods with one hand in a hole (5 mm diameter), without touching the walls or the bottom, for a duration of 32 s. Number and duration of touches were recorded as errors in this sub-test, which can be considered as a test for tremor or involuntary shaking of the hand.

The "Line tracking" test required leading one of the metal rods through a 5 mm wide and 5 mm deep groove without touching the walls or the bottom. The required

Table 2 Overview of clinical data of examined WC patients

Biographical Variables		
Age	[years]	
Sex		
Main Musical Instrument, Instrumental Group	strings, woodwind, none etc.	
Musical Level	professional, amateur, non-musician	
Level of Education	secondary modern school, grammar school final exams (comparable to UK A levels), vocational school, university degree	
Previous Health Conditions		
Affected Hand in patients and respective hand in controls		
Handedness		
Lifetime Cumulative Fine Motor Activity: Handwriting, Keyboard Typing, Instrumental Music, Other, Summed; all: [yrs]	[years]	
Psychological Questionnaires		
State Train Anxiety Inventory: State Anxiety, Trait Anxiety		
Arm Dystonia Disability Score		
NEO-FFI		

Motor Performance Tests		
Sub-Test	Measure	Right / Left / Bi-manual
Aiming	1) error number 2) error duration [ms] 3) total duration [s]	R, L, BR, BL
Steadiness	1) error number 2) duration [s]	R, L, BR, BL
Line Tracking	1) error number 2) error duration [ms]	R, L
Inserting of Long Pins	total duration [s]	R, L, BR, BL
Inserting of Short Pins	total duration [s]	R, L, BR, BL
Tapping	1) number of taps during first half of a 32 s recording 2) number of taps during second half 3) total number of taps	R, L, BR, BL

Writing Task		
Overall Writing Time	[s]	
Frequency of the Written Trace	[s^{-1}]	
Mean Frequency of Up- and Downstrokes	[s^{-1}]	
Mean Axial Pressure on Pen	[N]	
Writing Speed	[mm/s]	
Length of Pen on Paper	[mm]	
Doodling Circles		

Table 2 Overview of clinical data of examined WC patients *(Continued)*

Minimum Axial Pressure on Pen	[N]	
Difference of Minimum Axial Pressure while Doodling and Mean Axial Pressure during Writing Task	[N]	
Grip Force Tasks		
Maximum Grip Force (dystonic hand)	[N]	
Maximum kinematic acceleration (dystonic hand)	[N]	
Differential Load Force (dystonic hand)	[N]	
Differential Grip Force (dystonic hand)	[N]	
Mean Grip Force (dystonic hand)	[N]	
Difference of mean Grip Force and Slip Force (dystonic hand)	[N]	
Max Grip Force (non-dystonic hand)	[N]	
Maximum kinematic acceleration (non-dystonic hand)	[N]	
Differential Load Force (non-dystonic hand)	[N]	
Differential Grip Force (non-dystonic hand)	[N]	
Mean Grip Force (non-dystonic hand)	[N]	
Difference of mean Grip Force and Slip Force (non-dystonic hand)	[N]	
Grip force cyclic up-down Task (dystonic hand): min, max, mean and median	[N]	
Grip force cyclic up-down Task (non-dystonic hand): min, max, mean and median	[N]	

time and number of errors was recorded. This sub-test was only performed with the dominant hand.

The sub-test "Aiming" required the subjects to combine a fast vertical movement with a slower horizontal displacement of the limb by tapping successively on 20 adjacent metal circles with a metal rod as quickly as possible (circle diameter: 0.35 cm, midpoint-to-midpoint distance: 1.1 cm). Sliding the rod across the circles, as well as not touching a circle at all, was counted as an error. The number of errors and the required time were recorded.

For the "Tapping" sub-test, patients and controls tapped on a 50 mm × 50 mm metal surface with one of the metal rods as quickly as possible for 32 s. In this test, the number of taps was recorded separately for the first and second 16 s to account for possible fatigue effects, hypothesized to be higher in WC patients.

In the "Insertion" I and II sub-tests, subjects were asked to insert 25 pins, 50 mm and 10 mm long, respectively, into 25 target holes as quickly as possible. Longer pins were placed at a distance of 30 cm away

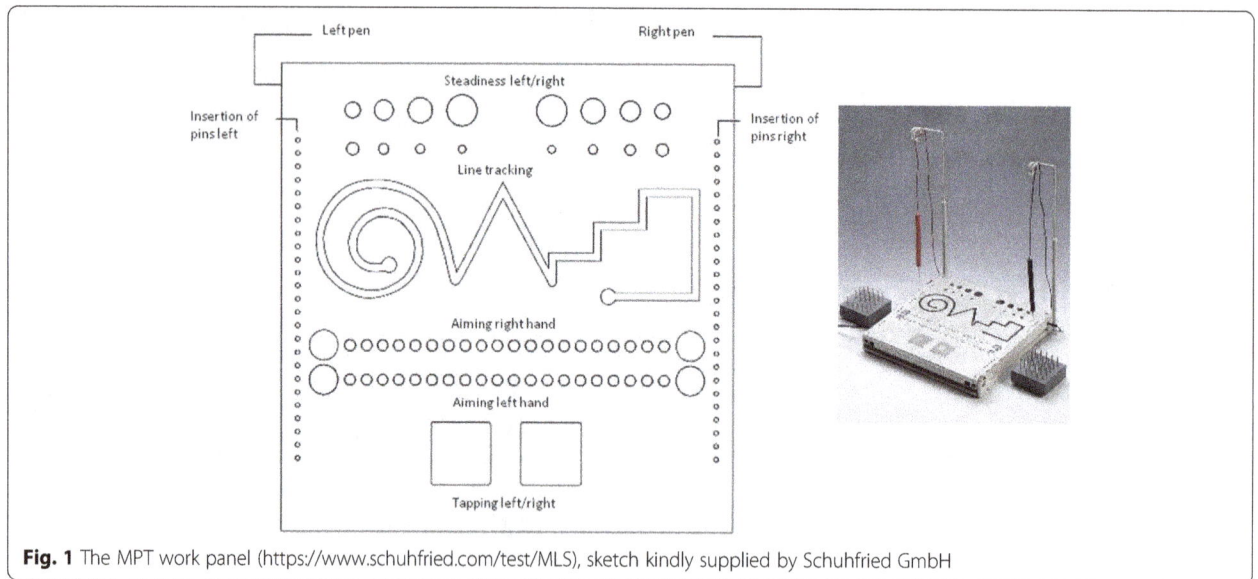

Fig. 1 The MPT work panel (https://www.schuhfried.com/test/MLS), sketch kindly supplied by Schuhfried GmbH

from the work panel, shorter pins 10 cm away. The required time was measured.

Writing tasks

Subjects wrote with a pressure-sensitive inking pen (WACOM Intuos3 pen, WACOM Europe, Krefeld, Germany) on a piece of ruled paper fixed on a digitizing tablet (WACOM Intuos3 A4 oversize with Grip Pen; WACOM Europe, Krefeld, Germany). Using this, we conducted a kinematic analysis of the writing to quantify the performed pressure, writing-speed and fluency. Registration and analysis of the data were done with CSWin Software (MedCom corp., Munich, Germany, version 2007). Resuming the writing tasks of Zeuner et al. [28], subjects performed 2 sub-tests. In the handwriting task, subjects wrote the sentence "Die Wellen schlagen hoch" ("The waves are surging high") ten times in their normal handwriting. We used this sentence because of its facilitating sequences of letters which enable a quick and smooth writing style [28]. The test had to be performed within three minutes, which increased motivation and psychological pressure in patients and controls, in order to detect latent writing impairment. Data were analyzed exclusively from the word "Wellen" of the three first and three last sentences. We registered overall writing time [ms], number of pencil lifts, mean of axial pressure [N], mean frequency [s^{-1}] of up- and downstrokes (vertical writing frequency), mean velocity [mm/s] and mean distance [cm] of the writing on the paper. The "Drawing Task" required subjects to draw as many superimposed circles with a diameter of about 2 cm as possible in 3 s, exerting as little vertical pressure on the pen tip as possible. We assumed that this task sensitively detects subtle changes in speed, smoothness and variability of successive movements [28], as circle drawing depends on the ability to accurately

reproduce a typical movement pattern over time. In this sub-test, only the axial pressure was recorded. To assess the subjects' ability of adaptation, the latter parameter was subtracted from the mean axial pressure obtained in the handwriting task.

Grip force tasks

In these tasks, a metal block with integrated force and acceleration sensors and a total weight of 306.5 g (see Fig. 2: The Grip Force object. W × H × D: 65 × 65 × 50 mm) was used. Similar objects have been used in several studies by Hermsdörfer et al. [29]. We

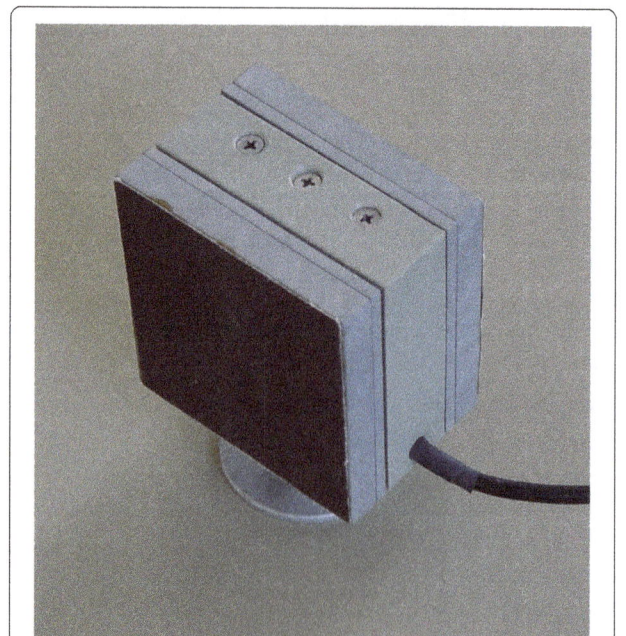

Fig. 2 The Grip Force object

recorded grip force (0 – 80 N, accuracy ±0.1 N) and acceleration (50 m/s^2, accuracy ±0.2 m/s^2). After a/d-conversion (National Instruments USB-6009, sampling width: 14 bits, sampling rate: 100 Hz), the analysis of the signals was carried out with GF-Win software (Christian Marquardt, Munich, Germany).

In all tasks, subjects were instructed to only use thumb, index and middle finger (i.e. a tripod grip) to hold the object. Both sub-tests were carried out consecutively, first with the affected and then with the unaffected hand in patients, and with the respective matched hands in the control group.

Lifting task

Subjects sat on a chair in front of a small object, holding the upper arm parallel to the trunk and the forearm unsupported to the front. When an acoustic cue sounded, the object was lifted approximately 4 cm above the table, held there for 5 s and then placed back on the desk [29]. Patients and controls repeated this task 30 times (15 trials per hand) with intervals of 2 s between trials. Patients began with their dystonic hand, the matched controls with their respective hand.

Slipping task

We applied a procedure to evaluate the minimal grip force needed to hold the object, originally introduced by Johansson and Westling [30]. Subjects were instructed to hold the object and reduce the grip force as slowly as possible until the object slipped from their fingers. This was repeated twice, resulting in a total of three slip force trials. Again, patients began with their dystonic hand.

During the lifting and slipping tasks, we measured various data, which were collected for all 30 trials. We recorded GFMax [N] (maximal force after the object had been lifted up), AccMax [m/s^2] (kinematic acceleration during lifting phase of the object), and MeanGF [N] (during the static phase). In addition to this, we calculated the ratio GFMax/LFMax (sensitive measurement for the efficiency of grip force in relation to the lifting-induced load) and TLift-off [ms] (time until object was lifted off). For the slipping task, we registered the mean slip force (GFSlip [N]) for all three trials and also calculated the difference of MeanGF and GFSlip to obtain a sensitive value for the subject's ability to adapt to the weight while grasping and lifting an object.

Cyclic movement task

Patients were instructed to lift the object and to move it up and down for a period of 15 s with an amplitude of approximately 30 cm and a tempo corresponding to 65BPM as paced by a metronome, beginning with their dystonic hand. Matched controls started with their respective hand. Every five trials hands were switched. To analyze the performance of this task, minimum, maximum, mean and median grip forces of the first 9000 ms of all trials of the cyclic up-down movements were taken into account.

Statistics

Psychological questionnaire data were compared between groups using Wilcoxon's signed rank test. To identify differences in motor performance between WC patients and healthy controls, the applied motor test battery scores of dystonic hands and the corresponding hands of the matched controls were compared. For investigating task-specificity of WC, variables were grouped test battery-wise and subjected to a random forest ensemble supervised learning algorithm [31]. Random forests are large collections or ensembles of many classification trees (10,000 in this study). A single classification tree partitions a data set recursively by locally assessing, at each node, which predictor or variable distinguishes best between patients and controls. The resulting two daughter nodes then exhibit a maximally reduced impurity with respect to the response variable. An error rate is obtained by randomly assigning observations to learning and testing subsets, respectively, followed by cross-validation after learning has taken place. This randomized pre-partitioning renders the results of single trees unreliable, as no two successive runs on the same data set will yield the same result. This shortcoming is resolved by adding randomness by growing many such trees (thus a random forest) on subsampled subsets of the data (average subsample size: 0.632 * n, with n the number of total observations [32]. In each tree and at each node, the best splitting variable from a random subset of all predictors is found. The forest's majority vote is then used to classify the observations as either patient or control. A conditional permutation importance measure is also provided, allowing an estimation of the relative influence of all predictors on the response variable [33]. For classification, the function "cforest" from the R package "party" was used [34].

This method provides tables listing the number of cases in which the algorithm correctly and incorrectly classified patients and controls. These confusion matrices were subjected to Pearson's Chi^2-test.

The advantage of using this data-driven classification rather than classical hypothesis-driven methods, like logistic regression, is its ability to determine complex interactions even in small n large p problems with more predictors than observations, where methods from the General Linear Model framework would fail.

To assess the degree of the "focal" character of WC, forests on Motor Performance and grip force data were examined separately for the left and right hand.

To determine which dependent variables contributed most to differentiation between patients and controls, the entire set of dependent variables (with a few exceptions) was used to grow a forest. To avoid trivial results, we excluded all WT and ADDS data before training. This resulted in a data set with 96 variables. As the hand movement in the line tracking task in the MPT battery vaguely resembles writing movements – though from right to left instead from left to right – we additionally excluded those data before running the classification algorithm a second time on then 88 dependent variables.

The level of significance for all tests was set to $\alpha = 0.05$. All statistical computations were done in R, version 3.0.1 [34].

Results
Task-specificity
Thirty-four randomly selected variables from the MPT data were used at each node to find a split. Nine of the 14 patients (64%) and 10 of 14 controls (71%) were correctly classified by the random forest ($\chi^2 = 2.297$, df = 1, $p > 0.05$). The WT data (8 variables used) yielded a correct classification rate of 100% and 86% for patients and controls, respectively ($\chi^2 = 17.65$, df = 1, $p < 0.05$). The variable importance measure showed the total duration of writing and the vertical writing frequency of the pen to be the most important variables used to split the data set successfully into patients and controls (see Fig. 3:Variable Importance of Writing Tasks.). Grip force data (16 variables) returned rates of 43% and 57% ($\chi^2 = 0$, df = 1, $p > 0.05$).

Focal nature of Dystonia
Correct classification rates on the basis of MPT subtests performed with the right hand scored 71% and 57%

in patients and controls, respectively ($\chi^2 = 1.312$, df = 1, $p > 0.05$). Those performed with the left reached 43% and 57% ($\chi^2 = 0$, df = 1, $p > 0.05$). Data in sub-tests performed bi-manually were analyzed independently for both hands. The correct classification rate for the bimanual right hand data amounted to 64% and 57% ($\chi^2 = 1.292$, df = 1, $p > 0.05$), while those for bi-manual left hand data reached 57% and 50% ($\chi^2 = 0.1436$, df = 1, $p > 0.05$). Right hand grip force data amounted to 36% and 43% ($\chi^2 = 1.292$, df = 1, $p > 0.05$), those from the left hand reached 64% and 57% ($\chi^2 = 1.292$, df = 1, $p > 0.05$).

Psychological questionnaires
The State Anxiety and the Trait Anxiety Inventory (STA-I) scores differed between both groups: Median difference [95% CI] -5.0 [-10.0, -1.5], $V = 13.5$, $p = 0.016$, and -6.5 [-11.5, -1], $V = 15$, $p = 0.02$, respectively. WC patients had more state and trait anxiety as compared to healthy subjects.

Our data did not provide evidence that groups differed in the Big-Five (Neuroticism: -5 [-11, 0.9], $V = 25$, $p = 0.09$; Extraversion: 3.5 [-2.5, 10.0], $V = 72.5$, $p = 0.22$; Openness: 1.5 [-7.0, 9], $V = 56$, $p = 0.85$; Agreeableness: 1.0 [-4.0, 3.5], $V = 27$, $p = 0.62$; Conscientiousness: -0.5 [-4.9, 3.5], $V = 41$, $p = 0.78$.

Data exploration
To explore the features separating patients and controls, a random forest was grown over the entire data set, including biographical data and the STAI questionnaire, amounting to 96 dependent variables. From these 96, 72 randomly selected variables were used at each node to

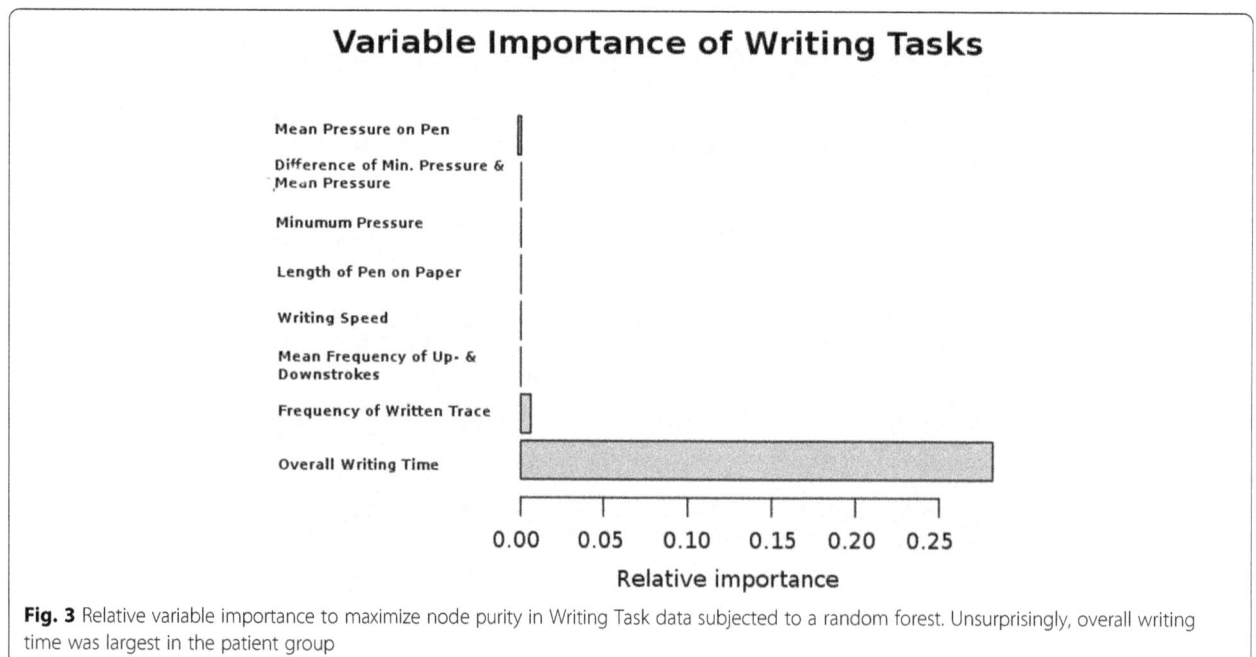

Fig. 3 Relative variable importance to maximize node purity in Writing Task data subjected to a random forest. Unsurprisingly, overall writing time was largest in the patient group

choose the best split point from. The resulting classification rates were 100% and 86% for patients and controls, respectively (χ^2 = 17.65, df = 1, p < 0.05). Not very surprisingly given the results in the Task-Specificity section, the total duration of writing and the vertical writing frequency of the pen significantly contributed to the splitting of the data set. Their predictive power was so pervasive that the classification rates and the result of the χ^2 test were identical to those in the above section. After the exclusion of WT data (66 randomly chosen variables from a total of 88), rates went down to 57% and 71% (χ^2 = 1.312, df = 1, p > 0.05).

Discussion

Task-specificity

Apart from the writing task, our extensive fine motor testing battery failed to detect any differences between WC and healthy controls. Although WC has previously been frequently described as focal and task-specific dystonia, other researchers found signs of reduced range of finger motion, or spread to secondary motor disturbances [9, 13]. It has been discussed whether, among these secondary motor disturbances, primarily movements similar to the major affected task could be affected [17]. This would confirm the notion that WC is more movement- than task-specific and would therefore have implications for therapies, e. g. retraining [35]. Here, we do not have any evidence that tasks closely related to writing, such as the drawing task or the steadiness task in the Vienna testing battery, displayed any differences. Furthermore, increased grip force, which is a hallmark of WC, was not present in the grip force and slipping tests. In the WT, only total duration of writing and vertical writing frequency of the pen explained most of the variance separating patients and controls, showing that patients had more difficulties performing the WT. We therefore explain the lack of further variables suitable to classify patients and controls in the MPT by the absence of spread of motor symptoms in our population of WC patients. This implies that our sample patients exhibit a task-specific and focal WC, thus supporting the results of Schneider et al. [19] With respect to grip-force, Nowak et al. claimed that increased grip-force levels are learned and context specific phenomena [36], and most probably subject to the sensory trick phenomena when tested in a short-time paradigm [37].

Even though we recruited a cohort with stable patients, many factors may have contributed to a possible heterogeneity of our patient group. Eight of 14 patients were amateur musicians and, though none were diagnosed with MD, difficulties in musician's performance had been reported by 5 patients. It should be mentioned that in Germany, about 18% of the population play a musical instrument, and even more in the WC population (mainly school-teachers, lawyers and doctors). We cannot exclude that musical performance as an environmental factor may have contributed to the triggering of WC [37, 38]. However, these amateurs did not practice more than 3 h a week and fine motor workload was probably much more increased by computer typing and handling smart phones. Moreover, since 12 of 14 patients in our study were diagnosed with WC more than 4 years ago, adaptation of the writing style over time may have occurred. Furthermore, as eight of 14 patients were treated with combination of at least 2 different therapeutic options, less motor impairment within our patient group in comparison to other severely affected cohorts must be considered.

Ideally, future studies should examine untreated WC patients with a shorter history of FD. Pen grip force should be additionally assessed, although we expect that this will be increased, as writing time was slowed in our study.

Psychological profile

Given that psychological symptoms have been demonstrated to be present in MD [20], it is widely discussed whether or not non-motor symptoms are also common in WC [21], demanding reconsideration of etiological factors and additional therapeutic approaches, for example behavioral training. In this context, it is noteworthy that our data suggest that at least state and trait anxiety seem to be elevated in WC patients as compared to healthy matched controls, whereas the NEO-FFI subscales did not provide evidence that the patients differ from the controls.

Classification of patients and controls using personality factors and anxiety traits was unsuccessful, thus failing to provide support for a possible connection between psychological and motor symptoms. This is in contrast to results of Ioannou et al., who could show that a majority of MD patients suffer from psychological symptoms, which might even trigger dystonic symptoms [20]. Such a clear connection between MD and certain personality traits [39] may be partially due to the impact of professional pressures in musicians, which is obviously less pronounced in WC patients. Moreover, the role of overuse and prolonged practice as triggering factors in WC seem to only play a minor role [21]. These results could, if confirmed with a new data set, support the notion that there are etiological differences within subtypes of FD, as the latter have been already discussed [13, 40].

However, as Enders et al. showed psychiatric comorbidities of FD [41], it is important to not disregard psychodynamic developments, psychoreactive aspects (especially the patients' experience of FD), as well as influences of the disorder concerning everyday activities and life quality [42, 43]. This can be achieved in future studies by using psychological and psychiatric case reports, and should be accomplished by obtaining thoroughly detailed anamnesis.

Conclusion

Only total duration of writing and vertical writing frequency of the pen correctly separated patients and controls, corroborating that patients had more difficulties performing the WT, indicating task-specificity within our patient group. We suggest that similar research should be performed on larger samples of simple WC patients in early stages of impairment without reported clinical secondary motor disturbances to verify our findings, using logistic regression techniques.

Our manuscript does not contain any individual persons data.

Abbreviations

ADDS: Arm Dystonia Disability Scale; GF: Grip Force; GFT: Grip Force Task; MD: Musician's Dystonia; MPT: Motor Performance Test; NeoFFI: Neo Five-Factor Inventory; STAI: State-Trait Anxiety Inventory; WC: Writer's cramp; WT: Writing Task

Acknowledgements

We are grateful to Aurélie Hofmann for setting up the motor test batteries and helping in calculating intermediate data, and to Caroline Seer, Anne-Kathrin Brehl and Marlehn Lübbert for data entry. We wish to thank Dr. Volker Baur for his enormous support in collection of clinical data, and calculation of statistics. We furthermore sincerely wish to thank Britta Westner for worthwhile and fruitful discussions on random forests, and Anthony Williams for language editing.

Funding

This research was funded by the University of Music Drama and Media Hannover (HMTM). The HMTM provided funding for purchasing the measurement devices and for a student assistant (AA) to conduct the measurements.

Authors' contributions

AA conceived the design of the study, recruited healthy subjects, carried out measurements and drafted the manuscript. MG conceived the design if the study, carried out the statistical analysis and drafted the manuscript. JH conceived the design of the study, developed the measurement devices and carried out the measurements, contributed to the statistical analysis and contributed to drafting the manuscript. EA conceived the design of the study, examined the patients neurologically, participated in data collection and data evaluation and drafted the manuscript. All authors read and approved the manuscript.

Authors' information

Ali Amouzandeh is a medical doctor currently specializing in movement disorders.
Dr. Michael Grossbach is a researcher and applied statistician.
Prof. Dr. Joachim Hermsdörfer is a sports scientist and motor control specialist with extensive expertise in movement disorders.
Prof. Dr. Eckart Altenmüller is a neurologist, specialized in movement disorders.

Competing interests

The authors declare that they have no competing interests.

Author details

[1]Institute of Music Physiology and Musicians' Medicine (IMMM), University of Music, Drama and Media, Emmichplatz 1, 30175 Hannover, Germany.
[2]Institute of Human Movement Science, Department of Sport and Health Sciences, Technical University of Munich, Munich, Germany.

References

1. Hallett M. Pathophysiology of writer's cramp. Hum Mov Sci. 2006;25:454–63.
2. Albanese A. Phenomenology and classification of dystonia: a consensus update. Mov Disord. 2013;28:863–73.
3. Torres-Russotto D. Focal Dystonias of the hand and upper extremity. J Hand Surg Am. 2008;33:1657–8.
4. Marsden CD, Sheehy MP. Writer's cramp. Trends Neurosci. 1990;13:148–53.
5. Steeves TD, Day L, Dykeman J, Jette N, Pringsheim T. The prevalence of primary dystonia: a systematic review and meta-analysis. Mov Disord. 2012;27:1789–96.
6. Nutt JG, Muenter MD, Aronson A, Kurland LT, Melton LJ. Epidemiology of focal and generalized dystonia in Rochester. Minnesota Mov Disord. 1988;3:188–94.
7. Pirio Richardson S, Altenmüller E, Alter K, Alterman RL, Chen R, Frucht S, et al. Research priorities in limb and task-specific Dystonias. Front Neurol. 2017;8:170. doi.org/10.3389/fneur.2017.00170
8. Gallea C, Horovitz SG, Najee-Ullah AM, Hallett M. Impairment of a parieto-premotor network specialized for handwriting in writer's cramp. Hum Brain Mapp. 2016;37:4363–75.
9. Sheehy MP, Marsden CD. Writers' cramp-a focal dystonia. Brain. 1982;105:461–80.
10. Shamim EA, Chu J, Scheider LH, Savitt J, Jinnah HA, Hallett M. Extreme task specificity in writer's cramp. Mov Disord. 2011;26:2107–9.
11. Jabusch HC, Altenmüller E. Focal dystonia in musicians: from phenomenology to therapy. Adv Cogn Psychol. 2006;2:207–20.
12. Song IU, Kim JS, Kim HT, Lee KS. Task-specific focal hand dystonia with usage of a spoon. Parkinsonism Relat Disord. 2008;14:72–4.
13. Stahl CM, Frucht SJ. Focal task specific dystonia: a review and update. J Neurol. 2016;30 doi:10.1007/s00415-016-8373-z.
14. Srivanitchapoom P, Shamim EA, Diomi P, Hattori T, Pandey S, Vorbach S, et al. Differences in active range of motion measurements in the upper extremity of patients with writer's cramp compared with healthy controls. J Hand Ther. 2016;29:489–95.
15. Wilson FR, Wagner C, Hömberg V. Biomechanical abnormalities in musicians with occupational cramp/focal dystonia. J Hand Ther. 1993;6:298–307.
16. Leijnse JN, Hallet M. Etiological musculo-skeletal factor in focal dystonia in a musician's hand: a case study of the right hand of a guitarist. Mov Disord. 2007;22:1803–8.
17. Rosset-Llobet J, Candia V, Fàbregas S, Ray W, Pascual-Leone A. Secondary motor disturbances in 101 patients with musician's dystonia. J Neurol Neurosurg Psychiatry. 2007;78(9):949-953.
18. Hofmann A, Grossbach M, Baur V, Hermsdörfer J, Altenmüller E. Musician's dystonia is highly task specific: no strong evidence for everyday fine motor deficits in patients. Med Probl Perform Art. 2015;30:38–46.
19. Schneider AS, Fürholzer W, Marquardt C, Hermsdörfer J. Task specific grip force control in writer's cramp. Clin Neurophysiol. 2013;125:786–97.
20. Ioannou CI, Altenmüller E. Psychological characteristics in musician's dystonia: a new diagnostic classification. Neuropsychologia. 2014;61:80–8.
21. Ioannou CI, Furuya S, Altenmüller E. The impact of stress on motor performance in skilled musicians suffering from focal dystonia: physiological and psychological characteristics. Neuropsychologia. 2016;85:226–36.
22. Oldfield RC. The assessment and analysis of handedness: the Edinburgh inventory. Neuropsychologia. 1971;9:97–113.
23. Truong D, Dressler D, Hallett M. Manual of Botulinum toxin therapy. Cambridge: Cambridge University Press; 2009. p. 195–204.
24. Costa PT, McCrae RR. Normal personality assessment in clinical practice: the NEO personality inventory. Psychol Assess. 1992;4:5–13.
25. Fahn S. Assessment of the primary dystonias. In: Munsat TL, editor. Quantification of neurologic deficit. London: Butterworths; 1989. p. 241–70.
26. Spielberger CD. State-trait anxiety inventory. Corsini encyclopedia of psychology, 2010.
27. Laux L, Glanzmann P, Schaffner, Spielberger CD. State-trait-Angstinventar. Göttingen: Hogrefe Verlag; 1995.
28. Zeuner KE, Peller M, Knutzen A, Holler I, Münchau A, Hallett M, et al. How to assess motor impairment in Writer's cramp. Mov Disord. 2007;22:1102–9.

29. Nowak DA, Hermsdörfer J. Grip force behavior during object manipulation in neurological disorders: toward an objective evaluation of manual performance deficits. Mov Disord. 2005;20:11–25.

30. Johansson RS, Westling G. Roles of glabrous skin receptors and sensorimotor memory in automatic control of precision grip when lifting rougher or more slippery objects. Expl Brain Res. 1984;56:550–64.

31. Breiman L. Random Forests Machine Learning. 2001;45:5–32.

32. Strobl, C. Statistical Issues in Machine Learning. Towards Reliable Split Selection and Variable Importance Measures. PhD thesis; Institut für Statistik der Fakultät für Mathematik, Informatik und Statistik der Ludwig-Maximilians-Universität München, 2008.

33. Hothorn T, Hornik K, Zeileis A. Unbiased recursive partitioning: a conditional inference framework. J Comput Graph Stat. 2006;15:651–74.

34. R Core Team (2012). R: a language and environment for statistical computing. R Foundation for Statistical Computing. Vienna, Austria. ISBN 3-900051-07-0, URL http://www.R-project.org/.

35. Zeuner KE, Molloy FM. Abnormal reorganization in focal hand dystonia-sensory and motor training programs to retrain cortical function. Neuro Rehabilitation. 2008;23:43–53.

36. Nowak DA, Rosenkranz K, Topka H, Rothwell J. Disturbances of grip force behaviour in focal hand dystonia: evidence for a generalised impairment of sensory-motor integration? J Neurol Neurosurg Psychiatry. 2005;76:953–9.

37. Cheng FP, Großbach M, Altenmüller E. Altered sensory feedbacks in pianist's dystonia: the altered auditory feedback paradigm and the glove effect. Front Hum Neurosci. 2013;17:7:868. doi:10.3389/fnhum.2013.00868.

38. Baur V, Jabusch HC, Altenmüller E. Behavioral factors influence the phenotype of musician's dystonia. Mov Disord. 2011;26:1780–1.

39. Jabusch HC, Müller SV, Altenmüller E. Anxiety in musicians with focal dystonia and those with chronic pain. Mov Disord. 2004;19:1169–75.

40. Rosenkranz K, Williamon A, Butler K, Cordivari C, Lees AJ, Rothwell JC. Pathophysiological differences between musician's dystonia and writer's cramp. Brain. 2005;128:918–31.

41. Enders L, Spector JT, Altenmüller E, Schmidt A, Klein C, Jabusch H-C. Musician's dystonia and comorbid anxiety: two sides of one coin? Mov Disord. 2011;26:539–42.

42. Windgassen K, Ludolph A. Psychiatric aspects of Writer's cramp. Eur Arch Psychiatry Clin Neurosci. 1991;241:170–6.

43. Schmidt A, Jabusch HC, Altenmüller E, Kasten M, Klein C. Challenges of making music: what causes musician's dystonia? JAMA Neurol. 2013;70:1456–9.

22

Embouchure dystonia: a video guide to diagnosis and evaluation

Steven J Frucht

Abstract

Background: Embouchure dystonia is an unusual focal task-specific dystonia affecting the muscles that control the flow of air into the mouthpiece of a brass or woodwind instrument. The complexity of the embouchure and the relative rarity of the condition pose barriers for recognition and management of the disorder.

Methods: Case review and video survey.

Results: This paper presents four video compilations that illustrate the rich phenomenology of embouchure dystonia, in order to enhance recognition and diagnosis.

Conclusion: The phenomenology of embouchure dystonia is discussed.

Keywords: Embouchure, Dystonia, Musician

Background

Embouchure dystonia (ED) is a focal task-specific cranial dystonia affecting the muscles of the lower face, tongue, jaw and pharynx used to control the flow of air into the mouthpiece of a brass or woodwind instrument. In three prior papers, we summarized the clinical phenomenology and natural history of ED [1–3]. ED may affect brass instrumentalists (trumpet, French horn, trombone, tuba) and woodwind players (piccolo, flute, oboe, clarinet, saxophone, bassoon). It typically presents as a painless deterioration in playing, progressing over months to years, and usually ends professional performance. Patients may be categorized by their predominant phenotype: task-specific tremor; lip-pulling; lip-lock; jaw; tongue; and task-specific Meige [2]. Playing difficulty is often limited to one register (pitch range) or to one specific technique, for example articulations (separated notes) or legato (connected notes). About 10 % of ED patients have coincident writer's cramp, suggesting a possible genetic predisposition to developing focal dystonia. Patients with ED involving the jaw or tongue frequently experience spread of dystonia to other oral tasks such as speaking or eating, and these dystonic features may persist even if they discontinue playing. ED may stem from a central disorder of cortical and subcortical sensorimotor networks that control the lower face, jaw, tongue and pharynx [4]. More recent work using a novel technique for rapid image acquisition demonstrated complex abnormalities in the activation of these muscles in ED patients relative to unaffected professional musicians [5].

The diagnosis of ED remains challenging even for experienced neurologists, and few neurologists are familiar with the mechanics of the embouchure. In this paper, we present a series of video compilations of ED patients to illustrate its rich phenomenology and to facilitate diagnosis (Fig. 1).

Methods/Consent to publish

Of 109 patients with ED evaluated by the author over a fifteen-year period, 65 available videos were reviewed and categorized. The Mount Sinai Medical Center Institutional Review Board approved the study. All patients shown in videos signed consent allowing publication of their videos in scientific format.

Results

Thirty-five patient videos were selected and edited into four composite video segments. The first segment (Additional file 1) illustrates practical features for evaluating patients, and the later three (Additional files 2–4) illustrate unique phenomenologic features of ED.

Correspondence: Steven.frucht@mssm.edu
5 East 98th Street, New York, NY 10029, USA

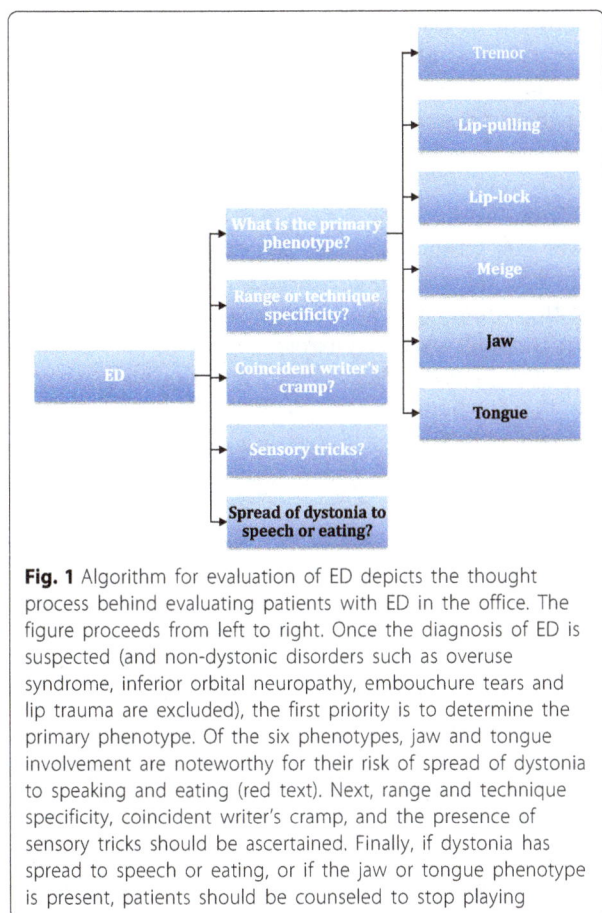

Fig. 1 Algorithm for evaluation of ED depicts the thought process behind evaluating patients with ED in the office. The figure proceeds from left to right. Once the diagnosis of ED is suspected (and non-dystonic disorders such as overuse syndrome, inferior orbital neuropathy, embouchure tears and lip trauma are excluded), the first priority is to determine the primary phenotype. Of the six phenotypes, jaw and tongue involvement are noteworthy for their risk of spread of dystonia to speaking and eating (red text). Next, range and technique specificity, coincident writer's cramp, and the presence of sensory tricks should be ascertained. Finally, if dystonia has spread to speech or eating, or if the jaw or tongue phenotype is present, patients should be counseled to stop playing

Additional file 1 presents three useful techniques that aid in the evaluation of patients with ED (Additional file 1: Techniques for the evaluation of the embouchure). In addition to carefully observing patients while they play, three approaches are useful when evaluating brass instrumentalists: free buzzing, using an O-ring, and playing using only the mouthpiece of the instrument. "Buzzing" refers to the exercise of vibrating the lips while forming the embouchure. Many brass players warm up before playing by "free buzzing" without a mouthpiece or instrument. Observing a patient's free buzz can be very informative since the lips are readily visible. The first patient (Free buzz 1) developed task-specific involuntary movements of the upper lip during playing French horn. When he free buzzes, irregular 2–3 Hz anterior protrusions of the upper lip are evident, consistent with lip-pulling dystonia. The next patient, a trombonist, developed loss of control of his embouchure. On free buzzing (Free buzz 2), the upper lip consistently pulls to the right. The next patient, also a trombonist, developed symptoms of ED with prominent tremor. On asking him to free buzz (Free buzz 3), a rapid tremor of the upper lip is visible and audible.

The next three patients illustrate the value of using an O-ring to evaluate brass players with ED. The O-ring is a practice device used by many brass players. It allows the performer to visualize their lips when they buzz: the lips are ordinarily hidden by the mouthpiece during instrumental performance. The first patient (O-ring 1), a trombonist with mild ED interfering with his ability to articulate notes, demonstrates the use of an O-ring. His lips vibrate normally, but there is a slight delay in vibration on starting notes. Legato or connected playing poses no difficulty. The next patient (O-ring 2) developed the tremor variant of ED on tuba. When he buzzes using the O-ring, a rapid tremor of the upper and lower lips is visible and audible. The third patient (O-ring 3) developed the lip-lock pattern of ED, in which his lips come together forcefully when he tries to initiate attacks. He is able to sustain legato playing with the O-ring without difficulty, however when he articulates individual separated notes a delay in initiation of sound is evident.

The final video segment of Additional file 1 ('Techniques for the evaluation of the embouchure') illustrates three patients using just their mouthpiece to play. The first patient (Mouthpiece 1) demonstrates a fast tremor of the upper and lower lips when he blows on his French horn mouthpiece. The next patient (Mouthpiece 2, identical to Free buzz 2), demonstrates a similar pattern using his trombone mouthpiece. The final patient (Mouthpiece 3, identical to Free Buzz 3), demonstrates a similar tremor with sustained notes in the middle register.

By definition, ED is a task-specific form of focal dystonia. Careful evaluation reveals that in many patients with ED, task-specificity is even further refined. In Additional file 2, we explore four aspects of "refined" task-specificity: register-specificity (dystonia occurring in only one pitch range on the instrument); technique-specificity (dystonia triggered selectively by sustained notes or by separated notes); speed (dystonia triggered by specific tempos); and instrument (dystonia triggered by playing one instrument but not by playing others) (Additional file 2: 'Task-specificity in ED').

The first video segment of Additional file 2 ('Task-specificity in ED') demonstrates four French hornists with register-specific ED. The first patient, (Task-specific 1 (TS 1)), develops a fine tremor as he plays a descending scale, affecting notes located within the interval of a perfect fifth. The second patient, TS 2, demonstrates a similar tremor in the same register, with minimal tremor when she plays in the higher registers. The next patient (TS 3) also demonstrates prominent tremor limited to the middle register. The last patient (TS 4) demonstrates inability to sustain airflow and sound only in the highest registers of the horn, a task that she previously accomplished with ease.

The next patient (TS 5) demonstrates technique-specificity in ED. Articulating (i.e., starting notes with a clear beginning) is difficult, producing an unwanted blur to the start of each note. Playing the same notes by slurring (legato playing) presents no problem. The next patient, a tuba player (TS 6, identical to O-ring 3), demonstrates an exquisite speed-dependent trigger for ED. Affected with lip-lock dystonia, his lips come together with excessive force when he articulates notes, producing a delay in the sound. He demonstrates exquisite velocity-dependence of dystonia with normal performance at faster speed, and triggering and worsening of dystonia as his speed slows. The final patient (TS 7) demonstrates exquisite instrument-dependence for ED. Previously able to play flute and saxophone with great fluency, he developed ED of the jaw type, selectively affecting his ability to form the embouchure of the saxophone. Flute playing remains unaffected.

Additional file 3 demonstrates seven ED patients who also possess prominent sensory tricks (Additional file 3: ED—geste maneuvers). Sensory gestes are relatively uncommon in ED, but their effect can be quite dramatic. In some instances, patients were unaware of the trick and the improvement was only discovered during the office evaluation. The first patient (Pt 1) is a trumpeter affected with task-specific Meige, a form of ED where cranial movements are specifically triggered only by playing the trumpet. Touching a particular area at the corner of the right side of his mouth markedly lessens his dystonia. External touch by the examiner to the same location is ineffective, illustrating an exquisite dependence of his dystonia on internal sensory input. The next two patients, both flautists, are affected with ED of the lip-pulling phenotype, with protrusion and forward pursing of the upper lips. In Pt 2, applying mild pressure to the upper lip with the examiner's fingers or with tongue depressors improves the dystonia, with audible improvement in the quality and volume of sound. Patient 3 displays a similar phenotype, with improvement in the control of airflow when gentle pressure is applied by the examiner to his upper lip.

The next three trombonists (Pts 4–6) developed ED that selectively impaired their ability to produce articulations. All three patients demonstrate improvement with application of a geste. In Pt 4, lip-pulling ED protrudes and pulls his lips apart, blurring his attacks. A gentle touch to the corners of his lips immediately improves his playing, and the improvement even lasts for several seconds after the fingers are removed. Patient 5, afflicted with lip-lock ED, discovered on his own that applying gentle pressure to the corner of the left side of his mouth markedly improves his ability to articulate notes. Similar to Pt 4, this improvement lasts for several seconds after the finger is withdrawn. Pt 6 developed ED affecting the jaw, with inability to maintain a seal on his mouthpiece. Touching the lower jaw, either by the patient or the examiner, improves the dystonia. The final patient, Pt 7, developed ED affecting the jaw related to playing the flute (Additional file 3). Gentle pressure to the lower jaw by the examiner substantially improves the dystonia. She also obtains partial benefit from imagining the sensory geste, a feature seen in some patients with torticollis and blepharospasm [6].

Additional file 4 demonstrates five unusual phenomena in ED (Additional file 4: ED—miscellaneous phenomenology). The first patient (Ph 1, identical to Pt 7 in Additional file 3) developed coincident writer's cramp twenty years prior to evaluation at our center. Dystonic flexion of the thumb and index finger are improved by holding the pen between her second and third fingers. Mirror dystonia demonstrated as flexion of the right thumb is also evident when she writes with the left hand. The next two patients (Ph 2 and 3), both flautists, developed ED affecting the tongue which first affected their ability to perform rapid tongue articulations on the flute (so called "double and triple tonguing"). By the time of their evaluations, dystonia had spread to involve speech and both had ceased playing. Tongue protrusion and mild movements of the upper and lower lips are triggered by speaking in Patient 2 (Ph 2). She discovered a sensory geste that improved her speech, confirmed in the office by having her hold a plastic syringe between her teeth, either on the left or right side. The next patient (Ph 3) demonstrates moderate dysarthria due to excess tongue tension. A notable improvement in his speech occurs when he employs a sensory trick, holding a plastic pipette between his teeth. He responded very well to treatment with trihexyphenidyl 6 mg daily. The next patient (Ph 4) developed involuntary jaw closure when paying saxophone, which spread over time to occur at rest. On exam, dystonic movements involve the lips, jaw and tongue at rest, but are paradoxically absent when she speaks or reads aloud. The last patient (Ph 5) illustrates the perils of using botulinum toxin to treat ED. Injected with 1.25 units of Botox to the right zygomaticus group, she developed significant right facial weakness which failed to improve her playing and even worsened her ability to compensate for the dystonia.

Conclusion

In this paper, we have presented four video compilations illustrating the rich phenomenology of ED. We close with a practical algorithm for evaluating patients with embouchure dysfunction in the office.

The first question facing the clinician is to distinguish ED from other embouchure disorders such as overuse syndrome, inferior orbital neuropathy, Satchmo syndrome and mechanical trauma to the lip (these have been extensively reviewed [3]). Once the clinician determines that a patient has ED, the primary phenotype should be defined, and range and technique-specificity should be assessed. The presence of coincident dystonia or sensory tricks should also be sought. Spread of dystonia to speech or eating, or the presence of ED affecting the jaw or tongue should lead to a firm recommendation to cease playing. For other patients, therapeutic approaches may be considered including pedagogic retraining, instrument modification and oral medications such as trihexyphenidyl or propranolol. These approaches are rarely satisfactory, and better treatments are sorely needed for this challenging disorder.

Abbreviations
ED: Embouchure dystonia.

Acknowledgement
The author wishes to acknowledge the tireless efforts of Glen Estrin in helping patients affected by embouchure dystonia throughout the world over the last fifteen years.

Author's contribution
The author contributed to all aspects of the manuscript, including data collection, video editing, drafting of the manuscript and revision.

Competing interests
The author declares that he has no competing interests.

References
1. Frucht SJ, Fahn S, Greene PE, et al. The natural history of embouchure dystonia. Mov Disord. 2001;16:899–906.
2. Frucht SJ. Embouchure dystonia—portrait of a task-specific cranial dystonia. Mov Disord. 2009;24:1752–62.
3. Termsarasab P, Frucht SJ. Evaluation of embouchure dysfunction: experience of 139 patients at a single center. Laryngoscope 2015. doi:10.1002/lary.25723
4. Haslinger B, Altenmuller E, Castrop F, Zimmer C, Dresel C. Sensoriomotor overactivity as a pathophysiologic trait of embouchure dystonia. Neurology. 2010;74:1790–7.
5. Itlis PW, Frahm J, Voit D, Joseph A, Schoonderwaldt E, Altenmuller E. Divergent oral cavity motor strategies between elite and dystonic horn players. J Clin Mov Dis. 2015;2:15. doi:10.1186/s40734-015-0027-2.
6. Greene PE, Bressman S. Exteroceptive and interoceptive stimuli in dystonia. Mov Disord. 1998;13:549–51.

23

Atrophy of the putamen at time of clinical motor onset in Huntington's disease: a 6-year follow-up study

Emma M. Coppen[1]* , Jeroen van der Grond[2] and Raymund A. C. Roos[1]

Abstract

Background: Striatal atrophy is detectable many years before the predicted onset of motor symptoms in premanifest Huntington's disease (HD). However, the extent of these neurodegenerative changes at the actual time of conversion from premanifest to a motor manifest disease stage is not known. With this study, we aimed to assess differences in degree and rate of atrophy between converters, i.e. premanifest individuals who develop clinically manifest HD over the course of the study, and non-converters.

Methods: Structural T1-weighted Magnetic Resonance Imaging (MRI) scans were used to measure volumes of seven subcortical structures. Images were acquired yearly over a maximum follow-up period of 6 years (mean 4.8 ± 1.8 years) in 57 participants (healthy controls $n = 28$, premanifest HD gene carriers $n = 29$). Of the premanifest HD gene carriers, 20 individuals clinically developed manifest HD over the course of the study, i.e. converters, whereas 9 individuals did not show any clinical signs. Differences between controls, converters and non-converters in volumetric decline over time were assessed using a one-way ANCOVA with age, gender and intracranial volume as covariates. All data were adjusted for multiple comparisons using Bonferonni correction.

Results: The putamen showed a significant difference in volume at the time of conversion in the converters group compared to the non-converters group (adjusted $p = 0.04$). Although, volumes of all other subcortical structures were smaller at time of conversion compared to non-converters and controls, these differences were not statistically significant. Over time, rate of volumetric decline in all subcortical structures in converters did not significantly differ from non-converters.

Conclusions: Putamen volume is smaller at the time of manifestation of motor symptoms compared with premanifest HD that not showed any clinical disease progression during the course of this 6-year follow-up study.

Keywords: Huntington's disease, Structural MRI, Converters, Motor onset, Putamen, Longitudinal study

Background

Huntington's disease (HD), an autosomal-dominant inherited neurodegenerative disease, causes widespread atrophy throughout the cerebral cortex and the striatum [1, 2]. The disease is clinically characterized by a manifest stage in which motor disturbances, cognitive decline and psychiatric symptoms progress gradually [3].

After the detection of the cytosine-adenine-guanine (CAG) repeat expansion causing a mutation of the Huntingtin gene on chromosome four [4], special interest emerged to identify and investigate premanifest HD gene carriers; individuals with a CAG repeat expansion without motor symptoms, but who gradually will develop manifest HD.

It is currently well known that atrophy of the striatum is the hallmark sign of HD, and is already detectable in the premanifest disease stage, many years before the onset of motor symptoms [5–8]. In addition to the striatum, other subcortical grey matter structures and cortical brain areas also show early signs of atrophy in premanifest HD gene carriers, but are less pronounced [7, 9, 10].

* Correspondence: e.m.coppen@lumc.nl
[1]Department of Neurology (J3-R-162), Leiden University Medical Center, PO Box 9600, 2300 RC Leiden, The Netherlands
Full list of author information is available at the end of the article

In this respect, subcortical volumetric measures have shown to be clinically useful in the prediction of time to onset at which individuals convert from premanifest HD to motor manifest HD [5, 6, 11]. Furthermore, it has been suggested that in addition to volume differences between various disease stages, the rate of decline in striatal volume may be an important factor in disease progression [6, 7].

Although cortical and subcortical atrophy are considered early markers of the disease, it is not known whether the absolute reduction in striatal volume is indicative for clinical conversion from a premanifest disease stage without motor symptoms into clinically manifest HD. Moreover, it is not unlikely that the rate of decline in volume, rather that atrophy itself, is involved in the process of initiating conversion. Such data, obtained at the actual time of conversion, rather than comparing premanifest HD gene carriers with manifest HD gene carriers, may elucidate the underlying process that could initiate clinical motor conversion. Currently, subcortical volume changes that are present at the time of conversion into motor manifest HD have not yet been fully investigated.

The aim of the present study was to characterize differences in striatal and extrastriatal grey matter atrophy at the time of conversion, between premanifest HD gene carriers that progress into the manifest stage of the disease and premanifest individuals that do not show any clinical signs. Furthermore, we assessed the rate of atrophy by examining the degree of volume loss over time. Therefore, we have investigated premanifest HD gene carriers on a yearly basis that were followed over a period of 6 years. Providing insight into the brain changes that occur as premanifest HD gene carriers become clinically affected by the disease might guide the timing of future therapeutic intervention.

Methods

Participants

A total of 57 participants (28 healthy controls and 29 premanifest HD gene carriers) were included in this longitudinal retrospective cohort study. Participants included in our study had at least one follow-up visit and were seen annually from 2008 till 2014, with a maximum of seven visits.

Premanifest HD gene carriers included in our study had a genetically confirmed expanded CAG repeat of 40 or more and a disease burden score of more than 250, based on CAG length and age, to ensure a premanifest HD group close to disease onset [12]. The estimated predicted years to disease onset were calculated using a survival analysis formula based on the participants' age at baseline and CAG repeat length

[13]. At baseline, all premanifest HD gene carriers showed no clinical motor symptoms indicating manifest HD. This was defined as a total motor score (TMS) of 5 or less on the Unified Huntington's Disease Rating Scale (UHDRS). The UHDRS-TMS is widely used for assessment of motor disturbances, ranging from 0 to 124, with higher scores indicating more increased motor impairment [14]. Certified movement disorder experts administered this scale and also assigned a score from 0 to 4 on the UHDRS Diagnostic Confidence Level (DCL), indicating the rater's level of confidence that motor abnormalities reflect the presence of HD. The HD motor diagnosis is defined as a score of 4 on the DCL, meaning that the rater has ≥99% confidence that the participant shows motor abnormalities that are unequivocal signs of HD [7, 14]. In our study, 20 premanifest participants received a motor diagnosis with a rating of 4 on the UHDRS-DCL sometime during the course of the study, further referred to as 'converters'. Partners and gene-negative relatives were recruited as healthy controls.

The local Medical Ethical Committee approved this study and written informed consent was obtained from all participants.

MRI acquisition

From 2008 to 2014, all participants underwent structural magnetic resonance imaging (MRI) scanning each year with a maximum of 7 time points. Imaging was performed on a 3 Tesla MRI scanner (Philips Achieva, Best, the Netherlands) using a standard 8-channel whole-head coil. Three-dimensional T1-weighted images were acquired with the following parameters: TR = 7.7 ms, TE = 3.5 ms, flip angle = 8 °, FOV 24 cm, matrix size 224 × 224 cm and 164 sagittal slices to cover the entire brain with a slice thickness of 1.0 mm with no gap between slices, resulting in a voxel size of 1,07 mm × 1,07 mm × 1,0 mm.

MRI post processing

All T1-weighted images were analyzed using software provided by FMRIB's software library (FSL, version 5.0.8, Oxford, United Kingdom) [15].

Volumes of subcortical structures were measured for each time point using FMRIB's Integrated Registration and Segmentation Tool (FIRST) [16]. Non-brain tissue was removed for all images using a semi-automated brain extraction tool implemented in FSL [17]. Subcortical regions include the accumbens, amygdala, caudate nucleus, hippocampus, pallidum, putamen and thalamus. T1-weighted images were registered to the MNI (Montreal Neurological Institute) 152-standard space image, using linear registration with 12 degrees of freedom [18].

Subsequently, segmentation of the subcortical regions was carried out using mesh models that are constructed from a large library of manually segmented images. Finally, a boundary correction was applied to prevent overlap with adjacent structures. Then, absolute volumes per structure were calculated. Visual inspection was performed during the registration and segmentation steps on randomly chosen images.

Whole brain intracranial volume, normalized for individual head size, was estimated with SIENAX [19]. Brain and skull images were extracted from the single whole-head input data. The brain images were then affine-registered to a MNI 152-space standard image [18], using the skull image to determine the registration scaling. Next, tissue-type segmentation with partial volume estimation was carried out in order to calculate the total volume of normalized brain tissue. Visual inspection of motion artifacts, registration and segmentation was performed for each brain-extracted image.

Statistics

Statistical analyses were performed using the Statistical Package for Social Sciences (SPSS for Mac, version 23, SPSS Inc.). Demographic group differences at baseline were analyzed using the χ2 test for gender and independent-samples t-test for age, CAG repeat length, disease burden score, and UHDRS-TMS. Group differences in absolute subcortical volumes were analyzed using a one-way analysis of covariance (ANCOVA) with age, gender and normalized intracranial volume (ICV) as covariates.

To assess the individual change over time, a linear regression analysis was performed for each subcortical structure in each participant to calculate the linear regression slope. To account for an individuals' total brain volume, we calculated for each individual and subcortical structure the ratio between subcortical volume and ICV by dividing the volume of the subcortical structure with the total ICV at each visit. With this volume/ICV ratio, we constructed a linear fitted coefficient that indicates the estimated change (increase or decrease) in volume per participant for every additional year adjusted for total brain volume. Then, this regression coefficient was used as a dependent variable in a one-way ANCOVA with age and gender as covariates.

The significance level was set at $p < 0.05$. Bonferonni correction for post-hoc analyses was performed to correct for multiple comparisons.

Results
Demographic characteristics

Demographic and clinical group characteristics at baseline are shown in Table 1. The mean follow-up period was 4.8 years (SD 1.8 years, range 0.9–6.6 years). Longitudinal data was collected for two or more years in 55 of the 57 participants. For the two remaining participants, the follow-up period was 1 year. Of all participants, 36 (63%) completed a follow-up period of 6 years.

There were no significant differences in gender and total motor score at baseline between controls and the whole group of premanifest HD gene carriers. Controls were significantly older compared to the premanifest HD group ($t(55) = 2.48$, $p = 0.016$).

The premanifest HD group was subsequently divided into converters ($n = 20$ with DCL = 4) and non-converters ($n = 9$ with DCL < 4). After baseline, converters had a median time of progression into manifest HD of 4.0 years (SD 1.5 years). Compared to non-converters, converters had a significantly higher mean disease burden score ($t(27) = -2.73$, $p = 0.011$) at baseline.

Subcortical volume at time of conversion

Mean volumes of seven subcortical structures (accumbens nucleus, amygdala, caudate nucleus, hippocampus, pallidum, putamen and thalamus) were calculated for converters at the time of conversion (Table 2), whereas absolute volume changes are shown in Fig. 1.

Table 1 Demographic and clinical baseline characteristics

	Premanifest HD			Controls
	Non-converters	Converters	Combined	
Number of participants	9	20	29	28
Gender (male/female)	3/6	9/11	12/17	13/15
Age (years)	41.6 (6.5)	44.2 (8.7)	43.3 (8.0)	48.6 (7.9) [†]
CAG repeat length	42.4 (1.8)	43.8 (2.6)	43.4 (2.4)	–
Disease burden score	286 (56.9)	352 (61.3)[*]	332 (66.6)	–
UHDRS - TMS	1.9 (1.8)	2.7 (1.3)	2.4 (1.5)	2.6 (2.4)

Data is given in mean (standard deviation). Premanifest HD gene carriers were divided into non-converters with a Diagnostic Confidence Level (DCL) below 4 and converters who progressed to manifest HD rated as a DCL of 4. CAG: cytosine-adenine-guanine. UHDRS-TMS: Unified Huntington's Disease Rating Scale – Total Motor Score. Disease burden score = age x (CAG length – 35.5) by Penney et al. [12]
[*] Significantly different between converters and non-converters at $p < 0.05$
[†] Significantly different between controls and premanifest HD combined group at $p < 0.05$

Table 2 Subcortical volumes

| | Controls | Premanifest HD gene carriers | | p – value non-converters vs. converters[a] |
		Non-converters	Converters	
Accumbens	0.92 (0.21)	0.86 (0.15)	0.72 (0.18)[*]	0.566
Pallidum	3.39 (0.44)	3.15 (0.50)	2.78 (0.54)[*]	0.149
Amygdala	2.19 (0.36)	2.31 (0.49)	2.01 (0.51)	0.157
Putamen	9.31 (1.30)	8.32 (1.34)[*]	7.24 (1.05)[*]	*0.040*
Caudate nucleus	6.67 (0.88)	5.65 (0.78)[*]	5.15 (0.73)[*]	0.367
Thalamus	14.79 (1.32)	14.76 (1.40)	13.87 (1.51)	0.402
Hippocampus	7.75 (0.80)	7.85 (0.97)	7.15 (0.86)	0.178

Uncorrected mean (standard deviation) subcortical volumes in ml are displayed. For converters, volumes at time of conversion are measured. For non-converters and controls, mean volumes across visits were calculated. Results of a one-way analysis of covariance (ANCOVA) for group differences with age, gender and intracranial volume as covariates. Significant difference between converters and non-converters is displayed in *Italic*.
[a]Post-hoc analyses were adjusted for multiple comparisons using a Bonferonni correction
[*]Significant difference compared to controls, $p < 0.05$

Converters showed a lower mean volume at time of conversion for all subcortical structures compared with the mean volume across visits in controls and non-converters. After correction for age, gender and intracranial volume, and adjustment for multiple comparisons, the accumbens nucleus (F(2,51) = 4.02, p = 0.020, η_p^2 = 0.14), pallidum (F(2,51) = 5.46, p = 0.007, η_p^2 = 0.18), putamen F(2,51) = 15.96, p < 0.001, η_p^2 = 0.39), and caudate nucleus (F(2,51) = 16.84, p < 0.001, η_p^2 = 0.40) were all smaller in converters compared with controls.

Volumes of the caudate nucleus and putamen in non-converters were also smaller compared to controls (p = 0.020 and p = 0.044 respectively). Converters only had a significantly smaller putamen volume at time of conversion compared with non-converters (p = 0.040).

Subcortical volume change over time

The caudate nucleus (F(2,50) = 4.37, p = 0.018, η_p^2 = 0.15) demonstrated a significantly steeper decrease in volume in both converters and non-converters compared with controls (Table 3, Fig. 1). The pallidum showed a higher decline in volume over time in converters compared to controls (F(2,50) = 4.61, p = 0.015, η_p^2 = 0.16). No significant differences in atrophy rate for any subcortical structure were found between converters and non-converters.

Discussion

Our results showed that putamen volume is reduced in individuals that converted to the manifest disease stage compared to individuals that did not show any clinical disease progression during the study period of 6 years. Although atrophy rate over time of the pallidum and caudate nucleus was higher in converters compared with controls, no differences in atrophy

rate were found between converters and non-converters for any of the subcortical structures.

The putamen is essential for regulation of movements and for learning and performance of motor skills. As the clinical diagnosis of HD is based on the presence of unequivocal motor signs, our results suggest that the putamen undergoes degeneration, when premanifest individuals approach clinical motor onset.

To our knowledge, one other study specifically focused on longitudinal brain changes in premanifest HD that converted into a manifest disease stage [11]. Their results showed that putamen volume could be used to improve the prediction of disease onset in addition to CAG repeat length and age [11]. We provide evidence of atrophy of the putamen at the actual time of clinical motor onset, instead of using predicted data. Nevertheless, our findings that premanifest individuals have a smaller volume of the putamen at the time of clinical motor onset confirm this suggestion of using putamen volume as a predictor for disease onset. The large multi-center observational Track-HD study also focused on identifying predictors of disease progression in early HD and premanifest HD gene carriers [7]. Here, baseline and longitudinal caudate nucleus, putamen and grey matter volumes showed a strong predictive value for the risk of future clinical diagnosis in a premanifest individual [7]. In our study, we found no difference in the rate of subcortical volume loss over time between converters and non-converters. An explanation for this finding could be that other factors, such as environmental, biochemical and genetic aspects, might play a more substantial role in clinical motor onset than striatal volume loss. Another explanation might be that the number of non-converters in our study was too minimal to detect such specific differences.

Compared with controls, the whole premanifest HD group did show a more rapid decline in volume loss over

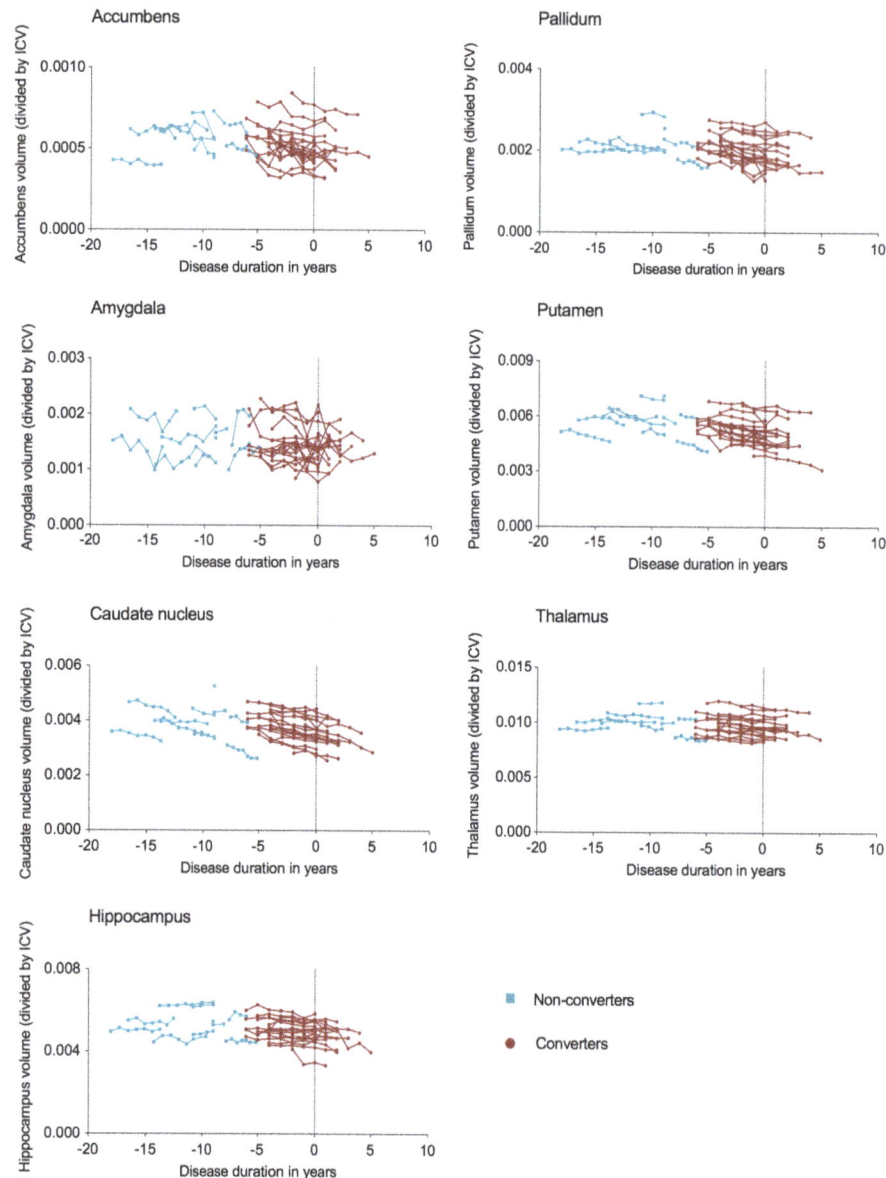

Fig. 1 Subcortical volume change over time. Individual volumes over time in premanifest HD for all seven subcortical structures. Disease duration (years) was calculated for converters with time of conversion based on the Diagnostic Confidence Level (DCL) of 4. For non-converters, estimated time to disease onset was calculated using the survival analysis formula of Langbehn et al. [13]. ICV: Intra-Cranial Volume

time for the pallidum and caudate nucleus. This finding is consistent with previous longitudinal studies [10, 20]. However, other longitudinal studies also showed that in premanifest HD gene carriers, the volume of the caudate nucleus declines more rapidly over time than the putamen volume [6, 21], which is contradictory to our findings. Specifically, the results of our study suggest that the *degree* of decline in subcortical volume might not be a reliable marker for clinical motor onset in premanifest HD, as we did not find any differences in rate of decline between converters and non-converters over time.

Our findings are strengthened by the fact that we used data of the actual time of clinical motor onset in the converter group rather than predicted data. Also, many studies that have been performed to date are cross-sectional and compare brain atrophy between different disease stages, such as premanifest and early manifest HD, to measure disease progression.

Striatal atrophy is one of the most recognized neurodegenerative signs in HD, and is associated with chorea severity. [22, 23] In our study, we have therefore focused on the progression of subcortical changes in premanifest HD. In manifest HD gene carriers, oculomotor

Table 3 Mean subcortical volume change in ml per year

	Controls	Premanifest HD gene carriers	
		Non-converters	Converters
Accumbens	- 0.018 (0.027)	- 0.035 (0.046)	- 0.020 (0.014)
Pallidum	0.006 (0.041)	- 0.054 (0.056)	- 0.049 (0.043)[*]
Amygdala	- 0.0012 (0.107)	0.031 (0.109)	- 0.020 (0.063)
Putamen	- 0.022 (0.082)	- 0.165 (0.128)	- 0.123 (0.066)
Caudate nucleus	- 0.023 (0.048)	- 0.086 (0.079)[*]	- 0.125 (0.052)[*]
Thalamus	- 0.067 (0.099)	- 0.015 (0.090)	- 0.106 (0.070)
Hippocampus	- 0.010 (0.123)	0.029 (0.041)	- 0.066 (0.084)

Mean individual linear regression coefficients (standard deviation) indicate the change (increase or decrease) in volume for each subcortical structure for every additional year. In the statistical regression analyses, the ratio between subcortical volume and total intracranial volume at each measurement was used to account for an individuals' brain volume. A one-way analysis of covariance (ANCOVA) for group differences was performed with age and gender as covariates. Post-hoc analyses were adjusted for multiple comparisons using a Bonferonni correction
[*]Significantly different compared to controls, $p < 0.05$

dysfunction, however, was related to volume changes in the occipital cortex. [23] It could therefore be of great interest to examine longitudinal cortical changes in relation to clinical symptoms in larger clinical trials. To assess clinical disease progression in premanifest HD, we defined clinical motor onset as the time that certified raters had a confidence of ≥99% that the participant showed motor abnormalities that are unequivocal signs of HD (measured with a DCL score of 4). Participants were rated each year at their annual follow-up visit, which included the MRI scan. We acknowledge that this might be a conservative classification of clinical motor onset, as other studies also defined a decline in functional capacity or increase in total motor score as disease progression [20, 24]. Still, the DCL score showed to be stable over time and was used previously to monitor disease progression [7, 11, 25]. Therefore, it would be interesting to assess volumetric changes over time in premanifest non-converters with DCL scores between 1 and 3 (e.g. non specific motor abnormalities or motor signs that are likely signs of HD), but our cohort consisted of a relatively small number of non-converters. In addition, this small number of non-converters might explain the non-significant findings in our longitudinal analyses. Future studies with larger samples sizes are necessary to confirm and extend the findings of our study. Then, there is also a possibility to assess if specific brain regions, independent of certain classifications into groups, can predict progression of motor symptoms. In this way, large longitudinal studies with longer follow-up periods can provide a better understanding of disease progression in HD as this might guide the timing of future therapeutic intervention.

Conclusion

In summary, we provide new insights in the difference in putamen volume between HD patients at the time of clinical motor onset and premanifest individuals that do not show any clinical progression. Our longitudinal study in premanifest HD demonstrates that the degree of atrophy in putamen volume, rather than rate of decline in volume, is involved in the process of conversion into clinically motor manifest HD.

This implies that putamen volume might be a suitable neuroimaging outcome measure for clinical trials as a marker for disease onset.

Abbreviations
ANCOVA: Analysis of Covariance; CAG: Cytosine-adenine-guanine; DCL: Diagnostic Confidence Level; FIRST: FMRIB's Integrated Registration and Segmentation Tool; FSL: FMRIB's Software Library; HD: Huntington's disease; ICV: Intracranial Volume; MNI: Montreal Neurological Institute; MRI: Magnetic Resonance Imaging; SPSS: Statistical Package for Social Sciences; TMS: Total Motor Score; UHDRS: Unified Huntington's Disease Rating Scale

Acknowledgements
The authors would like to thank all patients and their relatives who participated in this study, and the study-investigators for collecting all the data. Also, we would like to thank M. Jacobs, MSc for assisting with the statistical analyses and advising on the content of this article.

Funding
None.

Authors' contributions
EC was involved in the design and conceptualization of the study, analysis and interpretation of the data, and drafting the manuscript. JG was involved in the design and conceptualization of the study, interpretation of the data and drafting and revising the manuscript. RR was involved in the interpretation of the data and revising the manuscript. All authors read and approved the final manuscript.

Competing interests
Emma M. Coppen and Jeroen van der Grond report no competing interest. Raymund A.C. Roos receives grants from TEVA Pharmaceuticals, Cure Huntington's Disease Initiative (CHDI), Gossweiler Foundation, and is member of the advisory board of UniQure.

Author details
[1]Department of Neurology (J3-R-162), Leiden University Medical Center, PO Box 9600, 2300 RC Leiden, The Netherlands. [2]Department of Radiology, Leiden University Medical Center, Leiden, The Netherlands.

References

1. Tabrizi SJ, Langbehn DR, Leavitt BR, Roos RAC, Durr A, Craufurd D, et al. Biological and clinical manifestations of Huntington's disease in the longitudinal TRACK-HD study: cross-sectional analysis of baseline data. Lancet Neurol. 2009;8(9):791–801.

2. Vonsattel JP, Myers RH, Stevens TJ, Ferrante RJ, Bird ED, Richardson EP. Neuropathological classification of Huntington's disease. J Neuropathol Exp Neurol. 1985;44(6):559–77.

3. Roos RAC. Huntington's disease: a clinical review. Orphanet J Rare Dis. 2010; 5(1):40.

4. The Huntington's Disease Collaborative Research Group. A novel gene containing a trinucleotide repeat that is expanded and unstable on Huntington's disease chromosomes. Cell. 1993;72(6):971–83.

5. Aylward EH, Liu D, Nopoulos PC, Ross CA, Pierson RK, Mills JA, et al. Striatal volume contributes to the prediction of onset of Huntington disease in incident cases. Biol Psychiatry. 2012;71(9):822–8.

6. Hobbs NZ, Barnes J, Frost C, Henley SMD, Wild EJ, Macdonald K, et al. Onset and progression of pathologic atrophy in Huntington disease: a longitudinal MR imaging study. Am J Neuroradiol. 2010;31:1036–41.

7. Tabrizi SJ, Scahill RI, Owen G, Durr A, Leavitt BR, Roos RAC, et al. Predictors of phenotypic progression and disease onset in premanifest and early-stage Huntington's disease in the TRACK-HD study: analysis of 36-month observational data. Lancet Neurol. 2013;12(7):637–49.

8. Jurgens CK, Van De Wiel L, Van Es ACGM, Grimbergen YM, Witjes-Ané MNW, Van Der Grond J, et al. Basal ganglia volume and clinical correlates in "preclinical" Huntington's disease. J Neurol. 2008;255(11):1785–91.

9. van den Bogaard SJA, Dumas EM, Acharya TP, Johnson H, Langbehn DR, Scahill RI, et al. Early atrophy of pallidum and accumbens nucleus in Huntington's disease. J Neurol. 2011;258(3):412–20.

10. Kipps CM, Duggins AJ, Mahant N, Gomes L, Ashburner J, McCusker EA. Progression of structural neuropathology in preclinical Huntington's disease: a tensor based morphometry study. J Neurol Neurosurg Psychiatry. 2005; 76(5):650–5.

11. Paulsen JS, Long JD, Ross CA, Harrington DL, Erwin CJ, Williams JK, et al. Prediction of manifest huntington's disease with clinical and imaging measures: a prospective observational study. Lancet Neurol. 2014;13(12): 1193–201.

12. Penney J, Vonsattel JP, MacDonald M, Gusella JF, Myers RH. CAG repeat number governs the development rate of pathology in Huntington's disease. Ann Neurol. 1997;41(5):689–92.

13. Langbehn DR, Brinkman RR, Falush D, Paulsen JS, Hayden MR. A new model for prediction of the age of onset and penetrance for Huntington's disease based on CAG length. Clin Genet. 2004;65(4):267–77.

14. Huntington Study Group. Unified Huntington's disease rating scale: reliability and consistency. Mov Disord. 1996;11(2):136–42.

15. Smith SM, Jenkinson M, Woolrich MW, Beckmann CF, Behrens TEJ, Johansen-Berg H, et al. Advances in functional and structural MR image analysis and implementation as FSL. NeuroImage. 2004 Jan;23:S208–19.

16. Patenaude B, Smith SM, Kennedy DN, Jenkinson M. A Bayesian model of shape and appearance for subcortical brain segmentation. NeuroImage. 2011;56(3):907–22.

17. Smith SM. Fast robust automated brain extraction. Hum Brain Mapp. 2002; 17(3):143–55.

18. Jenkinson M, Bannister P, Brady M, Smith S. Improved optimization for the robust and accurate linear registration and motion correction of brain images. NeuroImage. 2002;17(2):825–41.

19. Smith SM, Zhang Y, Jenkinson M, Chen J, Matthews PM, Federico A, et al. Accurate, robust, and automated longitudinal and cross-sectional brain change analysis. NeuroImage. 2002;17(1):479–89.

20. Hobbs NZ, Henley SMD, Ridgway GR, Wild EJ, Barker RA, Scahill RI, et al. The progression of regional atrophy in premanifest and early Huntington's disease: a longitudinal voxel-based morphometry study. J Neurol Neurosurg Psychiatry. 2010;81(7):756–63.

21. Aylward EH, Nopoulos PC, Ross CA, Langbehn DR, Pierson RK, Mills JA, et al. Longitudinal change in regional brain volumes in prodromal Huntington disease. J Neurol Neurosurg Psychiatry. 2011;82(4):405–10.

22. Biglan KM, Ross CA, Langbehn DR, Aylward EH, Stout JC, Queller S, et al. Motor abnormalities in premanifest persons with Huntington's disease: the PREDICT-HD study. Mov Disord. 2009;24(12):1763–72.

23. Coppen EM, Jacobs M, van den Berg-huysmans AA, van der Grond J, Roos RAC. Grey matter volume loss is associated with specific clinical motor signs in Huntington's disease. Park Relat Disord. 2018;46:56–61.

24. Tabrizi SJ, Reilmann R, Roos RA, Durr A, Leavitt B, Owen G, et al. Potential endpoints for clinical trials in premanifest and early Huntington's disease in the TRACK-HD study: analysis of 24 month observational data. Lancet Neurol. 2012;11(1):42–53.

25. Rupp J, Blekher T, Jackson J, Beristain X, Marshall J, Hui S, et al. Progression in prediagnostic Huntington disease. J Neurol Neurosurg Psychiatry. 2010; 81(4):379–84.

24

Italian validation of the Belastungsfragebogen Parkinson kurzversion (BELA-P-k): a disease-specific questionnaire for evaluation of the subjective perception of quality of life in parkinson's disease

Paola Ortelli[1*], Roberto Maestri[2], Marianna Zarucchi[1], Veronica Cian[1], Elisa Urso[1], Francesca Giacomello[1], Davide Ferrazzoli[1] and Giuseppe Frazzitta[1]

Abstract

Background: Quality of life (QoL) is the sense of well-being perceived by people. The improvement of parkinsonian patient's QoL is a crucial goal for clinicians involved in rehabilitative care. In order to provide an appropriate endpoint for the assessment of the effectiveness of rehabilitation treatments on QoL of patients with Parkinson's Disease (PD), in this study we have first translated and then validated the Belastungsfragebogen Parkinson kurzversion (BELA-P-k). This tool allows evaluating separately two crucial aspects: i) the loss of personal autonomy in activities of daily life and ii) the psychological and psychosocial impact of the disease.

Methods: The BELA-P-k was translated from Dutch into Italian. Subsequently 202 PD patients filled out the questionnaire. Patients were also evaluated by using the Parkinson Disease Questionnaire –39 (PDQ39), the Unified Parkinson's Disease Rating Scale (UPDRS), the Mini Mental State Examination (MMSE) and the Frontal Assessment Battery (FAB).

Results: The internal consistency for total of two different scores *Bothered by* (Bb) and *Need for Help* (NfH) was excellent ($p = 0.91$) for both categories. The correlation between Bb and NfH categories was significant and strong, very-strong, ranging from 0.78 to 0.88 (all $p < 0.0001$). Finally, the value of Spearman r for the relationship between Bb and NfH items and PDQ 39 values were significant ($p \leq 0.003$).

Conclusions: In conclusion, we validated the BELA-P-k and demonstrated that it is an appropriate and potentially useful tool for assessing QoL in the management of PD.

Keywords: Quality of life, Wellbeing, Rehabilitation treatment

* Correspondence: ortellipaola73@gmail.com
[1]Department of Parkinson's disease, Movement Disorders and Brain Injury Rehabilitation, "Moriggia-Pelascini" Hospital, Via Pelascini, 3, Gravedona ed Uniti, 22015 Como, Italy
Full list of author information is available at the end of the article

Background

Parkinson's disease (PD) is a chronic and neurodegenerative disorder characterized by motor and non-motor symptoms. An impaired ability to acquire and express automatic actions, rigidity, resting tremor, bradykinesia, hypokinesia and postural instability are the cardinal motor symptoms of the disease. However, other non-motor cognitive, emotional and motivational symptoms, such as dysexecutive syndrome, mood dysregulation disorders, anxiety and behavioural alterations affect PD patients [1, 2].

The interaction between these motor and non-motor symptoms is responsible for a negative impact on patients' daily life. Indeed, a chronic condition such as PD affects the motor abilities, the cognitive domains and the social functioning, which are features that equally contribute to determine the subjects' quality of life (QoL) [3–5].

QoL is the sense of well-being perceived by people and it depends not only on the presence or absence of a disease, but also on personal, social and environmental factors [6, 7]. An improvement in patients QoL is generally considered a crucial goal for the clinicians.

As a matter of fact, there is not a cure for PD: dopamine replacement therapy (DRT) represents the gold standard for the medical treatment of PD, but its long-term use side effects (such as dyskinesia, motor fluctuations, dopamine dysregulation syndrome) and its inefficacy on the axial disturbances do not provide patients with a curative treatment. Surgical therapies for PD are now largely widespread, but at the moment, several critical issues regarding its use remain open [8]. Recently, rehabilitation has been highlighted as a feasible, effective and complementary treatment for the management of PD. In this course, several studies have suggested the need for a multidisciplinary and intensive rehabilitative approach in order to achieve better results in PD patients [9–13].

In order to evaluate the effectiveness of a specific rehabilitation treatment for PD, a valid and appropriate assessment of QoL is crucial.

There is a great number of available tools for the assessment of QoL. By using some of them, QoL has been assessed in the general population [14, 15]. Other tools have been specifically designed to assess QoL in specific conditions, such as PD [16, 17]: the most widely adopted tool for the evaluation of QoL in parkinsonian subjects in clinical and research context is the Parkinson Disease Questionnaire –39, PDQ39 [18].

The most important advantage of this questionnaire is the possibility to investigate specific sub-dominions of QoL and specific problems for each sub-dominion. The most important limit is the failure to distinguish two different aspects: the impact of loss of personal autonomy in daily life and the psychological and psychosocial impact of specific disease symptoms. The questionnaire *Belastungsfragebogen Parkinson kurzversion* (BELA-P-k)

was developed by the Max- Planck Institute in Munich, as part of a standardized psychological diagnostic routine test for PD patients [19]. This dutch version validates separately the questionnaire, that has the advantage of to evaluate the above-mentioned both aspects [20].

Similar to the PDQ39, the BELA-P-k allows the evaluation of different aspects of the disease, but also the impact of loss of the personal autonomy in daily life and the psychological and psychosocial impact of specific disease symptoms. Thus, we believe that BELA-P-k could be an appropriate tool for evaluating the impact of rehabilitation treatment in QoL of parkinsonian patients.

The present study aims at translating the Bela-P-k for the Italian population and at testing both its internal consistency reliability and its validity.

Methods

Two hundred and two PD patients hospitalized at the Department of Parkinson's disease and Brain Injury Rehabilitation of the "Moriggia-Pelascini" Hospital (Gravedona ed Uniti, Italy) were enrolled for the study. The Parkinsonian patients were diagnosed according to the UK Brain Bank criteria [21] and were evaluated by a neurologist with expertise in movement disorders field.

The exclusion criteria were: i) Mini Mental State examination (MMSE) [22] < 24, ii) any focal brain lesion detected in brain imaging studies (CT or MRI) performed in the previous 12 months, iii) other chronic diseases with a known impact in QoL.

The study design and protocol were approved by the local Ethics Committee (*Comitato Etico Interaziendale delle Province di Lecco, Como e Sondrio - Italy)* and were in accordance with the World Medical Association's code of Ethics (Declaration of Helsinki, 1967). The clinicians explained the study protocol. A written informed consent that was obtained by the patients before their participation in the study. This trial was retrospectively registered with ClinicalTrials.gov, NCT03073044.

Study instruments and data collection

The patients' evaluation was performed at admission to the hospital: it included a neurological and neuropsychological examination in order to define the disease stage in accordance with the Hoehn & Yahr (H & Y) classification and assess the following measures: the Unified Parkinson's Disease Rating Scale (UPDRS), the MMSE and the Frontal Assessment Battery (FAB) [23] the PDQ39 and the Bela-P-k. All patients were assessed in the morning, medication "on"-state, 1 h after they had taken the first dopaminergic drug dose.

The BELA-P-k questionnaire was translated from Deutch into Italian, by using the *translation and back-translation* method and following the guidelines for cross-cultural adaptation of QoL measures defined by Guyatt [24] and by Guillemin and colleagues [25].

The validation was determined by comparing the outcome with the PDQ-39.

The BELA-P-k consists of 19 items grouped into 4 subscales:

1. Achievement capability/physical symptoms (Questions 1–5)
2. Fear/emotional symptoms (Questions 6–9)
3. Social functioning (Questions 10–14)
4. Partner-bonding/family (Questions 15–19).

Each question aims at investigating three specific aspects. First of all, the presence of a certain problem, which is evaluated by a a dichotomous value, that is "yes" or "no". For every highlighted problem, patient has to describe i) the perceived discomfort related to the problem ("Bothered by" -Bb- and ii) the possible loss of personal autonomy due to that problem ("Need for Help" -NfH-). Both of these aspects are scored on a 5-point Likert scale and permit to obtain two sub-total scores by summing every single question scores.

Statistics

Clinical data are reported as mean ± SD, while Bela-P-k results are expressed both as mean ± SD and median (lower quartile, upper quartile). Numbers (frequency) are reported for categorical variables. The internal consistency reliability of the Italian version of the Bela-P-k questionnaire was assessed by means of Cronbach's alpha coefficient. Both the global Bb and the global NfH sub-scale scores of all items (physical symptoms, emotional functioning, social functioning and partner-bonding/family) were tested.

Convergent and discriminant validity were assessed by Multitrait Scaling Analysis [26]. Item convergence was supported if the correlation, corrected for overlap with the trait, that it is hypothesized to represent, was ≥0.4. Item discrimination was supported if the correlation between the item and the trait, that it is hypothesized to represent, was the highest. The discriminant validity was also assessed by the method of known group comparison, testing for differences between mean values for patients grouped according to H & Y stages. This analysis was carried out by a one-way analysis of variance applied to the global Bb and global NfH scores and to all items.

Finally, the relationship between Bela-P-k and the PDQ39 was assessed by Spearman rank correlation coefficient.

The chosen level of statistical significance was 0.05. When appropriate, a false discovery rate was controlled at 5% employing the Benjamini-Hochberg method. All

analyses were carried out by using the SAS/STAT statistical package, release 9.2.

Results

Table 1 reports the demographic and clinical characteristics of patients. The 57% of patients were in Hoehn and Yahr stage, 3, 37% in stage 2 and 6% in stage 4.

Descriptive statistics and internal consistency results are reported in Table 2 for all Bb and NfH scores. The Spearman r for the relationship between Bb and NfH scores is also given.

The internal consistency was acceptable (>0.70) for all items of Bb and NfH category scores. A tendency towards values in NfH higher than in Bb was observed with regards to all items. The internal consistency for total Bb and NfH was 0.91 for both categories. The correlation between Bb and NfH categories was significant and strong very-strong, ranging from 0.78 to 0.88 (all $p < 0.0001$).

Table 3 shows the percentage of patients who judged each question as relevant. The most endorsed question was Q1: 80% of patients who thought the problem was relevant to them, with percentages very similar in males and females and with a greater frequency as HY increases, but without reaching statistical significance (Table 4). On the contrary, the least endorsed question was Q18 (28%), with significantly higher occurrences in males (36 vs 19%, adjusted $p = 0.027$). Significant differences between gender were observed also for Q9, Q13, Q16 and Q19 (adjusted $p = 0.004$, $p = 0.045$, $p = 0.004$, $p < 0.0001$, respectively) and between HY stages for Q5 and Q14 (adjusted $p = 0.006$ and $p = 0.036$, respectively).

Item convergence and discrimination were supported for all items of both Bb and NfH category scores (corrected correlation with the trait hypothesized to represent ranging from 0.46 to 0.78 for Bb category scores and from 0.46 to 0.82 for NfH category scores).

Table 1 Demographical and clinical data of patients

Variable	N	
Gender (M)	202	105 (52%)
Age (yrs)	202	65.8 ± 9.0
Hoehn and Yahr	185	2.7 ± 0.6
Education (yrs)	202	11.3 ± 4.2
MMSE[a] [22]	201	28.3 ± 1.6
FAB[b] [23]	201	14.5 ± 2.6
Total UPDRS	135	39.7 ± 13.1
UPDRS III	135	19.3 ± 6.2
UPDRS II	135	14.2 ± 5.7
UPDRS IV	135	4.2 ± 3.7

The MMSE and FAB scores have been corrected for normative data from Italian population. See reference [a][22] for the validation of Italian version of MMSE and reference [b][23] for the validation of Italian version of FAB

Table 2 Descriptive statistics, internal consistency for Bb (Bothered by) and NfH (Need for Help) score and relationship between the both scores

Variable	N	Bb Mean ± SD	Bb Median (Q1, Q3)	Bb int cons	NfH Mean ± SD	NfH Median (Q1, Q3)	NfH Int cons	Spearman r
Total	198	22.1 ± 16.5	19.0 (10.0,31.0)	0.91	19.7 ± 16.0	15.0 (7.0,28.0)	0.91	0.84
Physical Symptoms	201	6.6 ± 4.8	6.00 (3.00,9.25)	0.72	6.0 ± 4.9	5.00 (2.00,9.00)	0.75	0.78
Emotional Symptoms	201	6.0 ± 4.4	5.00 (2.00,9.00)	0.74	5.1 ± 4.3	4.00 (2.00,8.00)	0.76	0.80
Social Support	201	5.0 ± 5.2	4.00 (1.00,8.00)	0.79	4.6 ± 5.0	3.00 (0.50,7.00)	0.80	0.88
Partner Bonding/Family	198	4.5 ± 4.8	3.00 (1.00,7.00)	0.71	4.1 ± 4.7	2.00 (0.00,6.00)	0.73	0.88

The Italian version of Bela-P-k scores showed discrimination between patients with different disease severity according to the H & Y stage, only for the Achievement capability/physical symptoms with a borderline significance ($p = 0.056$) for Bb category and a clear significance ($p = 0.022$) for NfH category.

Table 5 reports the value of Spearman r for the relationship between Bb and NfH items and PDQ 39 values (total score and 3 sub-scores: mobility; well being and social support). All associations were significant ($p \leq 0.003$).

Discussion

A multidisciplinary rehabilitation treatment helps the patients to reduce both the functional impact and the discomfort due to the disease symptoms in everyday living activities and allows patients to acquire strategies to face with their motor difficulties [2, 12, 25, 27].

QoL is a crucial endpoint in the evaluation of the effectiveness of any therapeutic approach, since it explores the personal well-being perceived by patients.

Even if the PDQ39 is a specific and widely used tool for the assessment of QoL in parkinsonian patients, this instrument does not allow to distinguish between the impact of loss of personal autonomy in activities of daily life and the psychological and psychosocial impact of specific disease symptoms.

This is an important distinction in the rehabilitation field, since it permits to evaluate both the functional impact of the symptoms on everyday living and the perceived discomfort.

In this context, we have translated and validated the Bela-P-k. This questionnaire, which requires a short period of administration, permits to obtain two different scores: "Bothered by" (Bb) and "Need for Help" (NfH).

Table 3 Percentage of "relevant judgment" to each question for patients

Variable	presence (%)	M presence (%)	F presence (%)	HY 2 presence (%)	HY 3 presence (%)	HY 4 presence (%)
PS1q	162 (80%)	86 (82%)	76 (78%)	51 (75%)	86 (81%)	10 (91%)
PS2q	131 (65%)	64 (61%)	67 (69%)	40 (59%)	72 (68%)	7 (64%)
PS3q	107 (53%)	55 (52%)	52 (54%)	30 (44%)	58 (55%)	10 (91%)
PS4q	112 (55%)	60 (57%)	52 (54%)	39 (57%)	56 (53%)	8 (73%)
PS5q	107 (53%)	53 (50%)	54 (56%)	22 (32%)	65 (61%)	8 (73%)
ES6q	128 (63%)	69 (66%)	59 (61%)	43 (63%)	69 (65%)	6 (55%)
ES7q	106 (52%)	60 (57%)	46 (47%)	38 (56%)	54 (51%)	5 (45%)
ES8q	147 (73%)	73 (70%)	74 (76%)	53 (78%)	76 (72%)	9 (82%)
ES9q	117 (58%)	52 (50%)	65 (67%)	42 (62%)	59 (56%)	7 (64%)
SF10q	113 (56%)	66 (63%)	47 (48%)	38 (56%)	57 (54%)	7 (64%)
SF11q	90 (45%)	52 (50%)	38 (39%)	30 (44%)	45 (42%)	6 (55%)
SF12q	70 (35%)	39 (37%)	31 (32%)	22 (32%)	37 (35%)	6 (55%)
SF13q	98 (49%)	63 (60%)	35 (36%)	30 (44%)	48 (45%)	8 (73%)
SF14q	79 (39%)	44 (42%)	35 (36%)	15 (22%)	50 (47%)	4 (36%)
PB-F15q	103 (51%)	61 (58%)	42 (44%)	31 (46%)	56 (53%)	8 (73%)
PB-F16q	64 (32%)	45 (43%)	19 (20%)	12 (18%)	39 (37%)	5 (45%)
PB-F17q	74 (37%)	32 (30%)	42 (44%)	24 (35%)	40 (38%)	4 (36%)
PB-F18q	56 (28%)	38 (36%)	18 (19%)	23 (34%)	27 (26%)	4 (36%)
PB-F19q	85 (43%)	68 (65%)	17 (18%)	28 (41%)	44 (42%)	6 (55%)

PS Physical Symptoms, *ES* Emotional symptoms, *SF* Social Functioning, *PB-F* Partner-Bonding\Family, *q* question

Table 4 Discriminant validity to Bb (Bothered by) and NfH (Need for Help) scores for patients grouped according to H%Y stages

Variable	HY 2	HY 3	HY 4	p val ANOVA
Total_Bb	21.0 ± 17.0	22.3 ± 16.1	29.1 ± 18.9	0.33
Physical Symptoms_Bb	5.8 ± 4.7	6.7 ± 4.7	9.4 ± 4.8	0.056
Emotional Symptoms_Bb	6.1 ± 4.3	5.9 ± 4.5	6.7 ± 4.9	0.84
Social Functioning_Bb	4.6 ± 5.3	5.2 ± 5.2	6.5 ± 5.5	0.55
Partner Bonding\Family_Bb	4.3 ± 4.8	4.6 ± 4.8	6.5 ± 5.6	0.38
Total_NfH	18.3 ± 17.4	19.7 ± 15.0	28.1 ± 18.1	0.18
Physical Symptoms_NfH	5.2 ± 5.0	6.0 ± 4.7	9.5 ± 4.5	0.022
Emotional Symptoms_NfH	5.1 ± 4.2	5.0 ± 4.2	6.9 ± 5.4	0.38
Social Functioning_NfH	4.1 ± 5.3	4.6 ± 4.7	5.8 ± 5.8	0.56
Partner Bonding\Family_NfH	3.9 ± 4.9	4.1 ± 4.6	5.9 ± 5.4	0.42

In accordance with previous studies [20], our data indicate that the internal consistency of Bela-P-k is excellent for both total scores of Bb and NfH and is also acceptable for the both scores in each singular question. The correlation between Bb and NfH scores was strong, but it never corresponded to 1.0. For this reason we confirm the advantage in assessing both issues separately.

Table 5 Relationship between Bela-p-K and PDQ39

	PDQ_39	PDQ Mobility	PDQ Emotional Well-being	PDQ Social Support
Total_Bb	0.63	0.49	0.59	0.51
Physical Symptoms_Bb	0.62	0.55	0.47	0.39
Emotional Symptoms_Bb	0.56	0.40	0.66	0.44
Social Functioning_Bb	0.52	0.38	0.50	0.45
Partner Bonding\Family_Bb	0.43	0.31	0.38	0.48
Total_NfH	0.54	0.46	0.48	0.33
Physical Symptoms_NfH	0.58	0.56	0.40	0.27
Emotional Symptoms_NfH	0.49	0.38	0.56	0.30
Social Functioning_NfH	0.46	0.36	0.44	0.33
Partner Bonding\Family_NfH	0.35	0.26	0.31	0.36

Bb Bothered by, *NfH* Need for Help

There was a positive correlation between the QoL assessment obtained by Bela-P-k and PDQ39: this confirms that Bela-P-k is a good tool for clinicians.

In parkinsonian patients, the interindividual differences are often quite striking. In order to evaluate which symptoms are most common, we analysed the frequencies of relevance for each item. The most frequent issue reported by patients is the loss of efficiency in daily living: 80% of parkinsonian people complain about this, with a greater incidence in the advanced stage of the disease, as highlighted in precedent studies [28, 29]. People in the more advanced stages reported more frequently problems in requiring caregiver's assistance in daily living activities and the need of delegating their duties to others.

We found no gender differences in QoL. However, between the males and females some differences were detected: while a greater fear for the future was found in women, males show a greater loss of identity, a greater influence of the family in their daily lives and sexual difficulties.

We suggest that these differences are due to the different tendency between female and male: the first tends to develop affective symptoms while the males tend to develop behavioural symptoms [30].

Conclusions

In conclusion, we found that the BELA-P-k is a suitable, valid and easily administrable test. This questionnaire provides the clinicians with an instrument that make possible to distinguish between the specific life's aspects (Achievement skills, emotional status, social functioning and integration and quality of relationship with partner and relatives) and the components that worsen the Qol (the loss of personal autonomy in daily life and the perceived discomfort of each symptom). Given these features, BELA-P-k could represent a good outcome in a rehabilitative care context, allowing the clinicians to tailor specific rehabilitation treatments.

Abbreviations
Bb: Bothered by; BELA-p-K: Belastungsfragebogen Parkinson kurzversion; CT: Computed tomography; DRT: Dopamine replacement therapy; FAB: Frontal Assessment Battery; MMSE: Mini Mental State Examination; MRI: Magnetic resonance imaging; NfH: Need for help; PD: Parkinson's Disease; PDQ-39: Parkinson Disease Questionnaire −39; QoL: Quality of life; UPDRS: Unified Parkinson's Disease Rating Scale

Acknowledgements
Not applicable.

Funding
This study has no sponsors or funding support.

Authors' contributions

PO wrote the text, conceived and designed the experiments, provided substantial contributions to discussion of the content and edited the manuscript before submission. RM wrote the text, conceived and designed the experiments analysed the data and did the statistical analysis. MZ researched data for the article. VC researched data for the article. EU researched data for the article. FG researched data for the article. DF wrote the text, conceived and designed the experiments, provided substantial contributions to discussion of the content and edited the manuscript before submission. GF wrote the text, conceived and designed the experiments, provided substantial contributions to discussion of the content. All authors read and approved the final manuscript.

Competing interests

The authors declare that they have no competing interests.

Author details

[1]Department of Parkinson's disease, Movement Disorders and Brain Injury Rehabilitation, "Moriggia-Pelascini" Hospital, Via Pelascini, 3, Gravedona ed Uniti, 22015 Como, Italy. [2]Department of Biomedical Engineering, Istituti Clinici Scientifici Maugeri Spa Società Benefit, IRCCS, Via per Montescano 31, Montescano, 27040 Pavia, Italy.

References

1. Tysnes OB, Storstein A. Epidemiology of Parkinson's disease. J Neural Transm (Vienna). 2017. doi:10.1007/s00702-017-1686-y.
2. Frazzitta G, Maestri R, Bertotti G, Riboldazzi G, Boveri N, Perini M, et al. Intensive rehabilitation treatment in early Parkinson's disease: a randomized pilot study with a 2-year follow-up. Neurorehabil Neural Repair. 2015;29:123–31.
3. Gomez-Esteban JC, Zarranz JJ, Lezcano E, Tijero B, Luna A, Velasco F, et al. Influence of motor symptoms upon the quality of life of patients with Parkinson's disease. Eur Neurol. 2007;57:161–5.
4. Global Parkinson's Disease Survey Steering Committee. Factors impacting on quality of life in Parkinson's disease: results from an international survey. Mov Disord. 2002;17:60–7.
5. Soh SE, McGinley JL, Watts JJ, Iansek R, et al. Determinants of health-related quality of life in people with Parkinson's disease: a path analysis. Qual Life Res. 2013;22:1543–53.
6. Schrag A, Jahanshahi M, Quinn N. What contributes to quality of life in patients with Parkinson's disease? J Neurol Neurosurg Psychiatry. 2000;69:308–12.
7. Schrag A, Jahanshahi M, Quinn N. How does Parkinson's disease affect quality of life? A comparison with quality of life in the general population. Mov Disord. 2000;15:1112–8.
8. Smith Y, Wichmann T, Factor SA, DeLong MR. Parkinson's disease therapeutics: new developments and challenges since the introduction of Levodopa. Neuropsychopharmacology. 2012;37:213–46. Published online 28 Sept 2011. doi:10.1038/npp.2011.212
9. Tomlinson CL, Patel S, Meek C, Clarke CE, Stowe R, Shah L, et al. Physiotherapy versus placebo or no intervention in Parkinson's disease. Cochrane Database Syst Rev. 2012;11:CD002817. doi:10.1002/14651858. CD002817. pub2. Review. Update in: Cochrane Database Syst Rev. 2012;(8): CD002817. PubMed PMID: 22786482
10. Bloem BR, de Vries NM, Ebersbach G. Nonpharmacological treatments for patients with Parkinson's disease. Mov Disord. 2015;30:1504–20. doi:10.1002/mds.26363.
11. Goodwin VA, Richards SH, Taylor RS, Taylor AH, Campbell JL. The effectiveness of exercise interventions for people with Parkinson's disease: a systematic review and meta-analysis. Mov Disord. 2008;23:631–40. doi:10.1002/mds.21922.
12. Frazzitta G, Bertotti G, Riboldazzi G, Turla M, Uccellini D, Boveri N, et al. Effectiveness of intensive inpatient rehabilitation treatment on disease progression in parkinsonian patients: a randomized controlled trial with 1-year follow-up. Neurorehabil Neural Repair. 2012;26:144–50. doi:10.1177/1545968311416990.
13. Ekker MS, Janssen S, Nonnekes J, Bloem BR, de Vries NM. Neurorehabilitation for Parkinson's disease: future perspectives for behavioural adaptation. Parkinsonism Relat Disord. 2016;22(Suppl 1):S73–7. doi:10.1016/j.parkreldis.2015.08.031.
14. Wood-Dauphinee S. Assessing quality of life in clinical research: from where have we come and where are we going? J Clin Epidemiol. 1999;52:355–63.
15. McKenna SP, Doward LC. The needs-based approach to quality of life assessment. Value Health. 2004;7:S1–3.
16. Soh S-E, McGinley JL, Morris ME. Measuring quality of life in Parkinson's disease: selection of an appropriate health-related quality of life instrument. Physiotherapy. 2011;97:83–9.
17. Ellgring H, Seiler S, Perleth B, Frings W, Gasser T, Oertel W. Psychosocial aspects of Parkinson's disease. Neurology. 1993;43(Suppl):41–4.
18. Peto V, Jenkinson C, Fitzpatrick R, Greenhall R. The development and validation of a short measure of functioning and well being for individuals with Parkinson's disease. Qual Life Res. 1995;4:241–8.
19. Ringendahl H, Werheid K, Leplow B, Ellgring H, Annecke R, Emmans D. Vorschlage fur eine standardisierte psychologische Diagnostik bei Parkinsonpatienten. Nervenarzt. 2000;71:946–54.
20. Spliethoff-Kamminga NG, Zwinderman AH, Springer MP, Roos RA. Psychosocial problems in Parkinson's disease: evaluation of a disease-specific questionnaire. Mov Disord. 2003;18:503–9.
21. National Collaborating Centre for Mental Health (UK). Dementia: a NICE-SCIE guideline on supporting people with dementia and their carers in health and social care. Leicester: British Psychological Society; 2007.
22. Measso G, Cavarzeran F, Zappalà G, Lebowitz BD, Crock TH, Pirozzolo FJ, et al. The mini-mental state examination: normative study of an italian random sample. Neuropsychol. 1993;9:77–85. doi:10.1080/87565649109540545.
23. Appollonio I, Leone M, Isella V, Piamarta F, Consoli T, Villa ML, et al. The frontal assessment battery (FAB): normative values in an Italian population sample. Neurol Sci. 2005;26:108–16. doi:10.1007/s10072-005-0443-4.
24. Guyatt GH. The philosophy of health related QoL translation. Qual Life Res. 1993;2:461–5.
25. Guilleman F, Bombardier C, Beaton D. Cross-cultural adaptation of health related QoL measures: literature review and proposed guidelines. J Clin Epidemiol. 1993;46:1417–32.
26. Hays RD, Hayashi T. Beyond internal consistency reliability: rationale and user's guide for Multitrait scaling analysis program on the microcomputer. Behav Res Methods Instrum Comput. 1990;22:167–75.
27. Rafferty MR, Schmidt PN, Luo ST, Li K, Marras C, Davis TL, Guttman M, Cubillos F, Simuni T; all NPF-QII Investigators. Regular Exercise, Quality of Life, and Mobility in Parkinson's Disease: A Longitudinal Analysis of National Parkinson Foundation Quality Improvement Initiative Data. J Parkinsons Dis. 2017;7(1):193–202. doi:10.3233/JPD-160912.
28. De Boer AGEM, Wijker W, Speelman JD, de Haes JCJM. Quality of life in patients with Parkinson's disease: development of a questionnaire. J Neurol Neurosurg Psychiatry. 1996;61:70–4.
29. Zhu K, van Hilten JJ, Marinus J. Onset and evolution of anxiety in Parkinson's disease. Eur J Neurol. 2016;29. doi:10.1111/ene.13217.
30. Heller J, Dogan I, Schulz JB, Reetz K. Evidence for gender differences in cognition, emotion and quality of life in Parkinson's disease? Aging Dis. 2014;5:63–75. Published online 22 Oct 2013. doi:10.14366/AD.2014.050063

25

Crossing barriers: a multidisciplinary approach to children and adults with young-onset movement disorders

Martje E. van Egmond[1,2*†] (iD), Hendriekje Eggink[1†], Anouk Kuiper[1], Deborah A. Sival[3], Corien C. Verschuuren-Bemelmans[4], Marina A. J. Tijssen[1] and Tom J. de Koning[1,3,4]

Abstract

Background: Diagnosis of less common young-onset movement disorders is often challenging, requiring a broad spectrum of skills of clinicians regarding phenotyping, normal and abnormal development and the wide range of possible acquired and genetic etiologies. This complexity often leads to considerable diagnostic delays, paralleled by uncertainty for patients and their families. Therefore, we hypothesized that these patients might benefit from a multidisciplinary approach. We report on the first 100 young-onset movement disorders patients who visited our multidisciplinary outpatient clinic.

Methods: Clinical data were obtained from the medical records of patients with disease-onset before age 18 years. We investigated whether the multidisciplinary team, consisting of a movement disorder specialist, pediatric neurologist, pediatrician for inborn errors of metabolism and clinical geneticist, revised the movement disorder classification, etiological diagnosis, and/or treatment.

Results: The 100 referred patients (56 males) had a mean age of 12.5 ± 6.3 years and mean disease duration of 9.2 ± 6.3 years. Movement disorder classification was revised in 58/100 patients. Particularly dystonia and myoclonus were recognized frequently and supported by neurophysiological testing in 24/29 patients. Etiological diagnoses were made in 24/71 (34%) formerly undiagnosed patients, predominantly in the genetic domain. Treatment strategy was adjusted in 60 patients, of whom 43 (72%) reported a subjective positive effect.

Conclusions: This exploratory study demonstrates that a dedicated tertiary multidisciplinary approach to complex young-onset movement disorders may facilitate phenotyping and improve recognition of rare disorders, with a high diagnostic yield and minimal diagnostic delay. Future studies are needed to investigate the cost-benefit ratio of a multidisciplinary approach in comparison to regular subspecialty care.

Keywords: Multidisciplinary, Young-onset movement disorders, Diagnosis, Dystonia, Myoclonus, Clinical phenotyping

Background

Young-onset movement disorders (YMDs) is a relatively new field in neurology, comprising clinical neurological syndromes presenting with involuntary movements manifesting before the age of 18. As with movement disorders (MDs) in adults, YMDs are subdivided into hyperkinetic movements (dystonia, myoclonus, chorea, ballism, tremor and tics), hypokinetic (parkinsonism) movements, and ataxia [1–5]. Recognition of common YMDs, such as tics and stereotypies, is usually straightforward for most clinicians. However, diagnosis of less common and more complex YMDs, such as disorders presenting primarily with myoclonus or dystonia, is often difficult, both for pediatric and adult neurologists [1, 6, 7].

The recognition and classification of YMDs present some unique challenges. Firstly, YMDs are often embedded in a complex clinical phenotype. For example, the occurrence of mixed MDs (more than one MD present)

---

* Correspondence: m.e.van.egmond@umcg.nl
†Equal contributors
[1]Department of Neurology, University of Groningen, University Medical Center Groningen, Groningen, the Netherlands
[2]Department of Neurology, Ommelander Ziekenhuis Groningen, Delfzijl and Winschoten, PO Box 30.001, 9700, RB, Groningen, the Netherlands
Full list of author information is available at the end of the article

or co-existence of a variety of symptoms such as psycho-motor retardation or behavioral abnormalities are commonly seen [5, 8, 9]. Secondly, in young children the developing nervous system may produce a variety of motor patterns that would be labeled as pathologic in older children and adults, but are simply a manifestation of brain immaturity in younger patients [1]. For instance, chorea is a normal feature in healthy infants and toddlers, and (subtle) signs of overflow dystonia and ataxia are found in healthy children up till the age of 12 years or even older [10, 11]. Finally, YMDs can be caused by a broad spectrum of both acquired and genetic disorders, including infections, auto-antibody and auto-immune disorders, as well as rare metabolic disorders and other inherited defects [7, 12–14].

The complexity of the diagnosis and management of YMDs is becoming increasing clear, which has resulted in a growing number of specialized pediatric neurologists. Despite this development, the diagnostic process in complex YMDs often remains challenging, a burden for patients and their families, and costly for our health care system as patients often remain undiagnosed for many years [1, 6, 7, 14, 15]. This has been reflected in a recent study in a tertiary referral center that showed a mean delay of diagnosis of $11.1 \pm 12,5$ years in a cohort of 260 patients with non-tic YMDs [7].

In other heterogeneous or rare diseases in children such as epilepsy or neuromuscular disorders, a beneficial effect of a multidisciplinary approach has been reported. [16–20] We hypothesized that such an approach might be a possibility to tackle the complexity of children and young adults with MDs. A multidisciplinary team may enable to overcome the three difficulties experienced in this patient group: a complex clinical phenotype (movement disorder specialist), the variety of motor patterns produced by the developing brain (pediatric neurologist), and a broad spectrum of both acquired and genetic disorders (pediatrician for inborn errors of metabolism and a clinical geneticist).

In this exploratory study, we report on the first 100 patients with YMDs who visited our multidisciplinary outpatient clinic. Our aim was to share our experience of a new multidisciplinary approach in terms of changes in MD classification, diagnostic yield and targeted treatment strategies.

Methods
Design and setting of the study
In this retrospective, single center, observational study we evaluated the first 100 patients who visited our multidisciplinary outpatient clinic for YMDs. It was situated in a tertiary referral center, the University Medical Center Groningen, in the Netherlands. The study was performed according to the ethical standards and regulations of our institute.

Patients
All patients had a confirmed or suspected MD with an onset before the age of 18 years and were referred for an expert opinion regarding MD classification, etiology or treatment of involuntary movements (Table 1).

Multidisciplinary outpatient clinic
The clinic was initiated in 2012 with a team consisting of an adult neurologist specialized in MDs (MT), a pediatric neurologist specialized in developmental neurology and YMDs especially ataxia (DS), a pediatrician specialized in metabolic diseases (TK) and a clinical neuro-geneticist (CV). In addition, clinical fellows in movement disorders and residents attend the clinic to gain skills and knowledge from the different medical specialties involved as part of their clinical training.

The pediatrician for inborn errors of metabolism received the referrals as the coordinating medical specialist, which were subsequently discussed within the team. Prior to the consultation, referral letters and medical reports containing previous diagnostic and treatment strategies were read carefully by the clinical fellow, who sent a summary to all team members.

During the consultation, patients were seen by all team members at once. In a separate meeting, the team members reviewed the video images, discussed the movement disorder classification and the results of the additional investigations, and developed joint diagnostic and therapeutic recommendations. In all cases the team members reached consensus. The main diagnostic steps were laboratory investigations, (neuro-)imaging, clinical neurophysiology or genetic testing. The key therapeutic options comprised pharmacological treatment, botulinum toxin injections, paramedical interventions (e.g. physiotherapy, occupational therapy, speech therapy), ketogenic diet, and deep brain stimulation.

The primary purpose of the multidisciplinary team was not to take over the clinical care provided by the referring medical specialist, but preferably to see a patient once and provide an all-in-one expert opinion. The presence of the clinical geneticist enabled direct genetic counseling in case genetic testing was considered. Results of additional investigations and genetic diagnostics were shared with the patient or caregivers by one of the team members via a follow-up consult or, if preferred by the family, by a telephone consultation. The team aimed to leave further management and follow-up to the referring specialist, but in case of unresolved issues patients were welcome to return to the multidisciplinary outpatient clinic.

Table 1 Baseline characteristics

Patient characteristics	
Sex (male/female)	56/44
Age (years)[a]	12.5 ± 6.3; 1–33
Age at symptom-onset (years)[a]	3.3 ± 4.6; 0–18
Duration of symptoms (years)[a]	9.2 ± 6.3; 1–32
Referral questions	
Movement disorder classification	50
Etiology	38
Treatment	42
MD classification	
Ataxia	9
Dystonia	32
Myoclonus	11
Other[b]	12
Unclassified	36
Etiological diagnosis	
Inherited etiologies	17
Monogenic	
ARX mutation	1
Ataxia telangiectasia	1
Coffin Lowry syndrome	1
Glutaric aciduria type 1	2
GLI2 mutation	1
GOSR2 mutation	1
GTPCH deficiency (DYT5)	1
Proprionacidemia	1
SCN1A mutation	2
THAP1 mutation (DYT6)	2
TITF1 mutation	1
Structural chromosomal abnormality	
Microdeletion 19p13.2p13.13 (*NFIX* and *CACNA1A* gene)	1
Partial deletion chromosome 7q (*SCGE* gene)	1
Uniparental disomia chromosome 7 (*SCGE* gene)	1
Acquired etiologies	12
Infectious	2
Perinatal asphyxia	9
Functional	2

[a]Age in years ± standard deviation; range
[b]Chorea, tics, tremor, parkinsonism and if no MD was present
Abbreviations: ARX, Aristaless related homeobox; *GOSR2*, Golgi SNAP receptor complex member 2; *GTPCH*, Guanosine Triphosphate Cyclohydrolase; *SCN1A*, sodium channel voltage gated type I alpha subunit; *TITF1*, Thyroid transcription factor-1; *NFIX*, nuclear factor I/X; *CACNA1A*, calcium channel voltage-dependent, P/Q type, alpha 1A subunit; *SCGE*, epsilon-sarcoglycan

Data collection

We evaluated the first 100 patients who visited our multidisciplinary clinic for YMDs between June 2012 and May 2014. Medical records were reviewed for patient characteristics and previous phenotypical classifications. The severity of the YMDs present was assessed by the team members using the global clinical impression scale of severity (GCI-S). This commonly used 7-point scale enables a clinician to rate the extent movement disorders with no movement disorder (1), slight (2), mild (3), moderate (4), marked (5), severe (6), and among the most severest (7) [21]. We compared the classification of the most prominent MD and etiological diagnosis before and after assessment by the multidisciplinary team. In addition, we studied the treatment strategies and whether the patients or their caregivers reported any positive effects of therapies 3–6 months after initiation. Since many patients were not under our primary care, and/or living at a distance from our center, we performed follow-up using a semi-structured interview during a telephone consultation. Patients and/or caregivers were asked (1) whether they experienced benefit with regard to motor symptoms, (2) since when they experienced this, (3) extent of improvement (none/slight/moderate/good), and (4) if any adverse effects were present.

Results
Patient characteristics
A total of 56 male and 44 female patients visited the multidisciplinary clinic (Table 1). Patients had a mean age of 12.5 years (SD 6.3) and a mean duration of symptoms of 9.2 years (SD 6.3). Referring specialists were predominantly pediatric neurologists, pediatricians and rehabilitation doctors with questions concerning the MD classification, etiology or treatment options. We had 36 patients referred with an unclassified MD, documented as dyskinesias, trembling, involuntary movements, or restlessness. A confirmed etiological diagnosis (17 inherited, 12 acquired) already explained the phenotype of 29 patients upon referral.

Movement disorder classification
Mean severity of the MDs present was 4.3 ± 1.7 on the global clinical impression scale (range 1–7), corresponding with a moderate to marked MD severity. The multidisciplinary team revised the initial classification in 58/100 patients (Table 2). These revisions reduced the number of patients with an unclassified MD from 36 down to 4. Compared to the referring clinicians, the team more frequently classified the patients' involuntary movements as dystonia (from 32 to 41) and myoclonus (from 11 to 31). The number of ataxic and tremor patients dropped (from 9 to 1 and 6 to 1, respectively),

Table 2 Overview of classification of most prominent MD before and after visiting the multidisciplinary outpatient clinic

		Observed MD classification by the multidisciplinary team					
		Dystonia	Myoclonus[a]	Ataxia	Other[b]	Unclassified	Total
Referral MD classification	Dystonia	26	1	0	4	1	32
	Myoclonus[a]	0	10	0	1	0	11
	Ataxia	0	8	0	1	0	9
	Other[b]	2	5	0	5	0	12
	Unclassified	13	7	1	12	3	36
	Total	41	31	1	23	4	100

[a]Isolated myoclonus, myoclonus ataxia and myoclonus dystonia
[b]Comprises chorea, tics, tremor, parkinsonism and if no MD was present

whereas the number of patients with chorea increased (from 4 to 6). The multidisciplinary team observed no MDs in eleven patients (e.g. the movements were related to agitation or caused by behavioral abnormalities). Simultaneous non-invasive surface electroencephalography/electromyography (EEG/EMG) was performed in 29 predominantly myoclonic patients and this confirmed or supported the MD classification observed by the team in 24/29 patients. In the remaining five cases, EEG/EMG was not conclusive due to an absence of symptoms during registration ($n = 3$) or the patient being unable to comply with the registration protocol ($n = 2$).

Associated neurological and non-neurological features
Only 26/100 patients presented with a (mixed) MD without associated features, whereas the majority of patients also had additional neurological symptoms ($n = 35$), non-neurological symptoms ($n = 9$) or both ($n = 30$). The most important additional features were intellectual disability, epilepsy, spasticity, skin abnormalities, deafness, dysmorphias, and skeletal and growth abnormalities.

Etiological diagnosis
At presentation, 29/100 patients had a confirmed genetic or acquired cause explaining their phenotype (Table 1). The multidisciplinary team established a diagnosis in 24 additional patients (Table 3), particularly in the genetic domain, where the number of diagnoses more than doubled from 17 to 37. Monogenetic etiologies were found using single-gene testing in nine cases, by targeted resequencing in three cases and using whole exome sequencing in five cases. Biochemical testing led to a diagnosis of non-ketotic hyperglycinemia in one case in which confirmation of the molecular defect is still pending.

Among the acquired causes, oral contraceptive-induced chorea was diagnosed in one patient and three patients turned out to have functional MDs. Despite an increase in confirmed etiological diagnoses from 29 to 53, we still had 35 patients categorized with a suspected

genetic diagnosis (defined as strong suspicion of a genetic cause based on a severe clinical phenotype, early onset, family history, and absence of any of the known acquired causes). In these cases, multiple genetic tests, including whole exome sequencing, have not yet

Table 3 Confirmed etiological diagnoses after assessment by the multidisciplinary team

Diagnosis	*N*
Inherited etiologies	20
Monogenic	
ACTB mutation	1
CTNNB1 mutation	1
GLRA1 mutation	1
GOSR2 mutation	6
HSD17B10 mutation	1
MECP2 mutation	1
OFD-1 mutation	1
OTC-deficiency	1
PRRT2 mutation	1
SPTBN2 mutation	1
TH mutation	1
TITF-1 mutation	1
Laboratory abnormalities	
Non-ketotic hyperglycinemia	1
Syndrome diagnosis	
Gilles de la Tourette	1
Linear naevus syndrome	1
Acquired etiologies	4
Drug-induced	1
Functional	3

Abbreviations: ACTB, beta-actin; *CTNNB1*, catenin (cadherin-associated protein) beta 1; *GLRA1*, glycine receptor alpha 1; *GOSR2*, Golgi SNAP receptor complex member 2; *HSD17B10*, 17beta-hydroxysteroid dehydrogenase type 10; *MECP2*, methyl CpG binding protein 2; *OFD-1*, oral-facial-digital syndrome 1; OTC, ornithine carbamoyltransferase; *PRRT2*, proline-rich transmembrane protein 2; *SPTBN2*, spectrin beta non-erythrocytic 2; TH, tyrosine hydroxylase; *TITF1*, thyroid transcription factor-1; HSD17B10 or 2-methyl-3-hydroxybytyryl-CoA dehydrogenase deficiency.

revealed a causative molecular defect. For 21 of these 35 patients we are awaiting elucidation of the causal mutation in a research setting, the other 14 patients (or their caregivers) decided not to participate in this research.

Treatment strategies

More than half of the 100 patients (61%) had not been given any specific treatment for their MD before visiting our clinic. The multidisciplinary team initiated or changed the treatment strategy in 60/100 of the patients. Table 4 gives an overview of changes in the treatment strategy, categorized by MD type. In 30/60 cases (50%), the new treatment strategy was based on the revised MD classification. In the other 30 patients the team initiated or adjusted the treatment strategy, despite an unchanged MD classification: for example symptomatic treatment with trihexyphenidyl in dystonic cerebral

Table 4 Overview of treatment strategies that were changed by the multidisciplinary team

Movement disorder	Treatment category	Treatment specifics	N	Positive effect (n)
Dystonia				
	Pharmacological			
		Clonazepam	1	1
		Gabapentin	3	3
		L-dopa	2	1
		Trihexyphenidyl	8	3
		Cessation of drug	1	1
	Botulinum toxin		5	5
	Deep brain stimulation		5	4
	Paramedical		2	2
	Total dystonia		27	20
Myoclonus				
	Pharmacological	Clonazepam	10	10
	Ketogenic diet		4	1
	Paramedical		4	2
	Total myoclonus		18	12
Other				
	Pharmacological			
		L-dopa	4	4
		Acetozolamide	1	1
		Cessation of drug	4	2
	Botulinum toxin		1	1
	Paramedical		3	2
	Total other		13	10
Difficult to classify			2	
	Pharmacological	L-dopa	2	1
Total			60	43

palsy. We advised six patients to stop their medication, which led to unchanged clinical symptoms in two patients and an improvement of symptoms in three others. An example of the latter was advice to stop taking oral contraceptives, which led to an almost complete disappearance of adolescent-onset chorea. In the group of 60 patients who had new or adjusted treatment, 72% of them or their caregivers reported a positive effect therapy after 3–6 months. Five patients were advised to stop their medication at the 3–6 months evaluation, because of limited benefit and or potential aggravation of other symptoms and side effects, such as effects on mood, behavior or constipation.

Discussion

To our knowledge, this is the first study describing the experience with a multidisciplinary team approach towards children and adults with YMDs. Based on the results it is likely that patients with YMDs benefit from a multidisciplinary team strategy with regard to MD classification, diagnostic yield and targeted treatment strategies.

The multifaceted nature of YMDs served as an impulse for setting up our multidisciplinary outpatient clinic, because the complexity of YMDs often leads to a time-consuming and burdensome diagnostic process [1, 6, 7]. This issue is reflected by a mean symptom duration of 74% of our patients' life spans, which is in line with the results of a previous study [7]. In 58% of the patients, the team revised the MD classification or defined another MD as the most prominent clinical symptom. We think this high percentage of revisions may be due to the combined expertise of a pediatric neurologist, trained to distinguish normal developmental from abnormal movements, and a movement disorder specialist, trained to establish the phenomenology of clinical MD syndromes [1, 8]. Although we are aware that there is no gold standard for clinical MD classification, additional investigations such as EEG/EMG for myoclonus confirmed the clinical diagnosis in 24/29 of our cases [22]. The presence of non-neurological features in 39% of our YMD cohort underscores the complexity of the clinical presentations in a significant part of this population, and the combined expertise of a pediatrician and a clinical geneticist to include all symptoms, facilitated the diagnostic process.

The team identified a etiological diagnosis in 24/71 (34%) previously undiagnosed patients, of which 17 were found to have monogenetic disorders. In contrast, in a study with 260 patients non-tic YMDs patients, who were referred to a neurologist specialized in YMDs between 2004 and 2013, a definitive genetic diagnosis was made in 17%. [7]. We realize that the genetic advances of the past decade are likely to have contributed to the higher yield in our sample, however we hypothesize that the team's broad and combined expertise has also been an important contributing factor. Furthermore, the diagnostic yield was obtained in a relatively short period of time, as a multidisciplinary team strategy facilitates immediate decision-making in comparison to the normal serial process involving multiple referrals, therefore minimizing the burden for the patients and their families.

After critical appraisal of phenotype and etiology, therapeutic strategies were considered and tailored to individual patient needs. The team gave specific advice on treatment for 60% of patients, with 72% ($n = 42$) of them or their caregivers reporting a subjective positive effect of the suggested treatment on follow-up. The effectiveness of treatment was only assessed through a semi-structured questionnaire and it was therefore not possible to draw more detailed conclusions on objective and/or long-term outcome measures of its effectiveness. Nevertheless, the large number of patients in which treatment was initiated at our clinic may reflect a potential under-treatment of YMDs, likely to significantly impact the patient's quality of life. The low number of patients that were already treated for their MD is remarkable, in particular when taking into account that the mean MD severity of these 60 cases was significant (5 on a scale of 7). Low treatment rates and potential under-treatment have also been reported in MDs in children with inborn errors of metabolism, [13] despite the fact that it has been shown that symptomatic treatment may significantly improve patients' daily functioning and quality of life [14, 23, 24].

The results of this exploratory study indicate that YMDs patients might benefit from a multidisciplinary team approach in terms of diagnosis and treatment in comparison to the referring specialists. However, interpretation of the results is limited by the lack of a control group of patients' receiving assessment by a pediatric movement disorder specialist, or in comparison to assessments by an alternative team consisting of two or three specialists. Inclusion of such a control group was not feasible in our center. Nevertheless, we think that this single-institution experience indicates that a dedicated multidisciplinary approach to YMDs disorders may facilitate phenotyping and improve recognition of rare disorders.

Notably, in this study, the age at presentation at our outpatient clinic ranged from 1 to 33 years, which is beyond the standard upper limit of 18 years for pediatric care. Distinguishing early-onset from later-onset MDs is useful for diagnostic purposes [3, 4]. However, we believe that the age of symptom-onset in these patients is a more important inclusion criterion than the age at time of referral, especially because long delays between symptom-onset and diagnosis have been reported. [7] Therefore, we propose to consider patients

with YMDs as a spectrum, irrespective of the age of referral, and to allow all complex YMD patients to benefit from the combined expertise of a multidisciplinary team, crossing barriers between pediatric and adult neurology.

Conclusion

In summary, our results suggest that a multidisciplinary approach might help tackle the complexity of diagnosis and managing complex YMDs. Our experience indicates that this approach may improve recognition of rare disorders, with a good diagnostic yield and a minimal diagnostic delay. Future studies are needed to investigate the cost-benefit ratio of a multidisciplinary approach in comparison to regular subspecialty care, preferably using a prospective study design with standardized clinical assessments to systematically evaluate treatment effects.

Abbreviations
EEG/EMG: Electroencephalography/electromyography; MD: Movement disorder; YMD: Young-onset movement disorder

Acknowledgements
The authors thank Jackie Senior (University Medical Center Groningen, Department of Genetics) for editing the manuscript, and Maria Fiorella Contarino (Department of Neurology, Leiden University Medical Centre, and Department of Neurology, Haga Teaching Hospital, The Hague, the Netherlands) for her valuable comments on the manuscript.

Funding
No funding was received for this study.

Authors' contributions
HE and MvE attended the outpatient clinic, collected and analyzed the data and wrote the first version of the manuscript (1A-C; 2A-C; and 3 A-B). AK attended the outpatient clinic as PhD student (1A-C; 3B). DS, CV, MT and TdK formed the multidisciplinary team for the outpatient clinic for young-onset movement disorders (1 A-C, 3B). All authors were involved in the conception and design of the work and interpretation of the data. All authors participated critically revised the manuscript and approved the final version. All authors agree to be accountable for all aspects of the work in ensuring that questions related to the accuracy or integrity of any part of the work are appropriately investigated and resolved.

Competing interests
The authors declare that they have no competing interests. Full financial disclosures of all authors: Dr. van Egmond received a travel grant from Medtronic; Prof Tijssen received research grants from Fonds Nuts-Ohra, Stichting Wetenschapsfonds Dystonievereniging, Prinses Beatrix Foundation, STW Technology society (NeuroSIPE), and Phelps Stichting voor Spastici. Unrestricted grants were received from Allergan Pharmaceuticals, Actelion, Ipsen Pharmaceuticals. An unrestricted grant was received from Medtronic for a dystonia nurse, and from DystonieNet for a teaching course. Dr. de Koning received a research grant from Metakids Foundation, Ride4Kids Foundation, and Metabolic Power Foundation (non-profit) and a research grant from Actelion (for profit). The other authors have indicated they have no financial relationships to disclose.

Author details

[1]Department of Neurology, University of Groningen, University Medical Center Groningen, Groningen, the Netherlands. [2]Department of Neurology, Ommelander Ziekenhuis Groningen, Delfzijl and Winschoten, PO Box 30.001, 9700, RB, Groningen, the Netherlands. [3]Department of Pediatrics, University of Groningen, University Medical Center Groningen, Groningen, the Netherlands. [4]Department of Genetics, University of Groningen, University Medical Center Groningen, Groningen, the Netherlands.

References

1. Singer HS, Mink JW, Gilbert DL, Jankovic J. Movement Disorders in Childhood. 2nd ed. Philadelphia: Saunders Elsevier; 2016.
2. Sanger TD, Chen D, Fehlings DL, et al. Definition and classification of hyperkinetic movements in childhood. Mov Disord. 2010;25:1538–49.
3. Fahn S. Classification of movement disorders. Mov Disord. 2011;26:947–57.
4. Albanese A, Bhatia K, Bressman SB, Delong MR, Fahn S, Fung V, et al. Phenomenology and classification of dystonia: a consensus update. Mov Disord. 2013;28:863–73.
5. Delgado MR, Albright AL. Movement disorders in children: definitions, classifications and grading systems. J Child Neurol. 2003;15(Suppl):1–8.
6. van Egmond ME, Kuiper A, Eggink H, Sinke RJ, Brouwer OF, Verschuuren-Bemelmans CC, et al. Dystonia in children and adolescents: a systematic review and a new diagnostic algorithm. J Neurol Neurosurg Psychiatry. 2015;86:774–81.
7. Bäumer T, Sajin V, Münchau A. Childhood-onset movement disorders: a clinical series of 606 cases. Mov Disord Clin Prac. 2017;4:437–40.
8. Abdo WF, van de Warrenburg BPC, Burn DJ, Quinn NP, Bloem BR. The clinical approach to movement disorders. Nat Rev. Neurol. 2010;6:29–37.
9. Sanger TD, Chen D, Fehlings DL, Hallett M, Lang AE, Mink JW, et al. Definition and classification of hyperkinetic movements in childhood. Mov Disord. 2010;25:1538–49.
10. Brandsma R, Spits AH, Kuiper MJ, Lunsing RJ, Burger H, Kremer HP, et al. Ataxia rating scales are age-dependent in healthy children. Dev Med Child Neurol. 2014;56:556–63.
11. Kuiper MJ, Vrijenhoek L, Brandsma R, Lunsing RJ, Burger H, Eggink H, et al. The Burke-Fahn-Marsden Dystonia Rating Scale is Age-Dependent in Healthy Children. Mov Disord Clin Pract. 2015;3:580–6.
12. Gascon GG, Ozand PT, Brismar J. Movement disorders in childhood organic acidurias. Clinical, neuroimaging, and biochemical correlations. Brain & Development. 1994;16(Suppl):94–103.
13. García-Cazorla A, Wolf NI, Serrano M, Pérez-Dueñas B, Pineda M, Campistol J, et al. Inborn errors of metabolism and motor disturbances in children. J Inherit Metab Dis. 2009;32:618–29.
14. Eggink H, Kuiper A, Peall KJ, Contarino MF, Bosch AM, Post B, et al. Rare inborn errors of metabolism with movement disorders: a case study to evaluate the impact upon quality of life and adaptive functioning. Orphanet J Rare Dis. 2014;9:177.
15. Bertram KL, Williams DR. Diagnosis of dystonic syndromes – a new eight-question approach. Nat Rev. Neurol. 2012;8:275–83.
16. Shapiro BS, Cohen DE, Covelman KW, Howe CJ, Scott SM. Experience of an interdisciplinary pediatric pain service. Pediatrics. 1991;88:1226–32.
17. Bent N, Tennant T, Swift T, Posnett J, Scuffham P, Chamberlain MA, et al. Team approach versus ad hoc health services for young people with physical disabilities: a retrospective cohort study. Lancet. 2002;360:1280–6.
18. Ladner TR, Mahdi J, Attia A, Froehler MT, Le TM, Lorinc AN, et al. A multispecialty pediatric neurovascular conference: a model for interdisciplinary management of complex disease. Pediatric Neurol. 2016;52:165–73.
19. Geerlings R, Aldenkamp AP, Gottmer-Welschen LM, et al. Long-term effects of a multidisciplinary transition intervention from paediatric to adult care in patients with epilepsy. Seizure. 2016;38:46–53.
20. Paganoni S, Nicholson K, Leigh F, et al. Developing multidisciplinary clinics for neuromuscular care and research. Muscle Nerve. 2017 Nov;56(5):848–58.
21. Busner J, Targum SD. The Clinical Global Impressions Scale: Applying a Research Tool in Clinical Practice. Psychiatry (Edgmont). 2007;4:28–37.
22. Zutt R, van Egmond ME, Elting JW, van Laar PJ, Brouwer OF, Sival DA, et al. A novel diagnostic approach to patients with myoclonus. Nat Rev. Neurol. 2015;12:687–97.
23. Egmond ME, Elting JWJ, Kuiper A, Zutt R, Heineman KR, Brouwer OF, et al. Myoclonus in childhood-onset neurogenetic disorders: The importance of early identification and treatment. Eur J Paediatr Neurol. 2015;19:726–9.
24. Liow NY, Gimeno H, Lumsden D, Marianczak J, Kaminska M, Tomlin S, et al. Gabapentin can significantly improve dystonia severity and quality of life in children. Eur J Paediatr Neurol. 2016;20:100–7.

26

Economics of botulinum toxin therapy: influence of the abobotulinumtoxinA package size on the costs of botulinum toxin therapy

Dirk Dressler* and Fereshte Adib Saberi

Abstract

Background: AbobotulinumtoxinA (Dysport®) was distributed for many years in vials containing 500MU (D500). Recently a new 300MU vial (D300) was additionally introduced (introduction). We wanted to explore whether more differentiated package sizes allow for more economic use of Dysport® in a large neurological botulinum toxin (BT) outpatient clinic.

Methods: The study followed a retrospective chart review design based on our digital BT therapy data bank. All patients receiving Dysport® exclusively in a constant dose during the observation period (introduction ± 7 months) were included. Economic calculations are based on Dysport® prices as officially advertised in Germany. Sharing of vials between patients was not allowed.

Results: Altogether 83 patients (51 with dystonia, 25 with spasticity, 3 with hemifacial spasm, 4 with other diagnoses) were included in this study. The total amount of BT used before and after introduction was 102525MU, the amount prescribed 138000MU and 116300MU (−21700MU, −15.7%), the costs €146103 and €125250 (−€ 20853, −14.3%). The price for D500 before and after introduction was €529.36, for D300 €339.71. The D500 price for 1MU before and after introduction is €1.0587, the D300 price for 1MU €1.1324 (+ €0.073, +7.0% against D500).

Conclusions: More flexible packaging reduces drug costs for BT therapy considerably. Introducing smaller packaging sizes is technically possible and should be encouraged. Extra costs for registration and logistics are moderate. Further cost reductions may be possible by introduction of even smaller packaging sizes. They can be calculated based on our model.

Keyword: AbobotulinumtoxinA, Package size, Economics, 300MU vial, 500MU vial, Botulinum toxin therapy, Dysport®

Background

Botulinum Toxin (BT) type A for therapeutic purposes is provided by several international manufacturers: Allergan (Dublin, Ireland) manufactures Botox® (onabotulinumtoxinA), Merz Pharmaceuticals (Frankfurt/M, Germany) Xeomin® (incobotulinumtoxinA) and Ipsen (Boulogne Bilancourt, France) Dysport® (abobotulinumtoxinA). BT type A drugs are sold as freeze-dried powders contained in vials [1]. Before application they need to be reconstituted with normal saline. BT content in the vials varies. The original content was 100MU for Botox® and Xeomin® and 500MU for Dysport® (D500).

* Correspondence: dressler.dirk@mh-hannover.de
Movement Disorders Section, Department of Neurology, Hannover Medical School, Carl-Neuberg-Str. 1, D-30625, Hannover, Germany

Over time package sizes were differentiated. Recently, an additional package size of 300MU was introduced for Dysport® (D300). We wanted to explore whether more differentiated package sizes allow for more economic use of Dysport® in a large neurologic BT outpatient clinic.

Methods

Setting

The study took place at the Movement Disorders Section of Hannover Medical School (HMS-MDS), Hannover, Germany. HMS-MDS is specialised in neurological BT therapy and attracts patients from the region and beyond. BT therapy is used in all neurological BT motor indications including dystonia, spasticity, infantile cerebral palsy, tremor and tics. It is also used in all hypersecretory indications of BT including hyperhidrosis, hypersalivation and hyperlacrimation. Other BT indications covered include chronic migraine as well as numerous special and experimental indications. BT therapy is used in registered indications as well as in in off-label indications. All three BT type A drugs are used. BT type B is used in special circumstances only. Annual BT consumption of HMS-MDS currently exceeds 12000 standard vials per year (1 standard vial = 1 vial Botox® 100MU = 1 vial Xeomin® 100MU = 1/3 vial Dysport® 500MU). Composition of patients treated is outlined in the results section and in Table 1.

Definitions

Introduction was the day when D300 became available and was used at HMS-MDS, i.e. January 1st 2014. Observation period was the time period from June 1st 2013 (introduction minus 7 months) to July 30th 2014 (introduction plus 7 months). Injection series is the set of BT injections given at one appointment. Interinjection interval is the time between two subsequent injection series.

BT therapy

D500 is reconstituted with 5.0 ml 0.9% NaCl/H_2O, D300 with 3.0 ml 0.9% NaCl/H_2O. BT therapy is applied following international guidelines and the algorithms developed at HMS-MDS during the past decades. Most applications are performed under anatomical guidance. Where necessary, electromyography and ultrasound [2] is used for this purpose.

Design

The design of the study followed a retrospective chart review design. All data evaluated were prospectively and continuously collected as part of our digital BT therapy data base. Data were retrieved using pre-programmed retrieval algorithms. During the observation period all patients of HMS-MDS fulfilling the inclusion criteria were included in this study. Inclusion criteria consisted of: (1) BT therapy with Dysport® exclusively during the observation period. (2) Constant Dysport® dose throughout the observation period. In eligible patients equal number of injection series before and after introduction were selected and used for further evaluation. Within the limits of the observation period either 1 or 2 injection series before and after introduction were selected.

Economics

Economic calculations are based on Dysport® prices as officially advertised in Germany. They are inclusive of German value added tax (VAT) at currently 19%.

Results

Patients

Table 1 gives an overview about the patients' demographic data and the composition of the patient base. Altogether 83 patients are included in this study. They reflect about 60% of all patients treated with Dysport® at HMS-MDS during the observation period. About 40% of all patients had to be excluded because of variable BT doses within the observation period and because of insufficient number of injection series. 51 patients (29 females, 22 males, age 60.3 ± 13.5 years) suffered from dystonia. 37 of them had cervical dystonia,

Table 1 Composition of the patient base included in this study

Diagnosis	Patients				Dose
	number [n]	female [n]	male [n]	age mean ± SD [years]	mean ± SD [MU]
Dystonia	51	29	22	60.3 ± 13.5	499.5 ± 371.4
Cervical Dystonia	37	23	14		610.4 ± 371.4
Blepharospasm	10	6	4		189.0 ± 156.5
Bruxism	4	0	4		250.0 ± 115.5
Spasticity	25	12	15	56.7 ± 14.6	1180.0 ± 574.4
Arm Spasticity	16	7	9		985.0 ± 569.3
Hemispasticity	6	2	4		1341.7 ± 399.3
Paraspasticity	3	1	2		1600.0 ± 624.5
Tetraspasticity	2	2	0		1625.0 ± 671.8
Hemifacial Spasm	3	2	1	65.4 ± 16.0	43.3 ± 22.5
Others	4	4	0	48.1 ± 20.8	600.0 ± 294.4
Hyperhidrosis	2	2	0		500.0 ± 70.7
Stump Pain	1	1	0		300
Focal Dystonia	1	1	0		1000

10 blepharospasm and 4 bruxism. 25 patients (12 females, 15 males, age 56.7 ± 14.6 years) suffered from spasticity. 16 of them had arm spasticity, 6 hemispasticity, 3 paraspasticity and 2 tetraspasticity. 3 patients were treated for hemifacial spasm (2 females, 1 male, age 65.4 ± 16.0 years). 4 patients (2 females, 2 males, age 48.1 ± 20.8 years) were treated for other diagnoses including hyperhidrosis (n = 2), stump pain (n = 1) and focal myokymia (n = 1).

Economics

All economics data are shown in Table 2. The total amount of BT used before and after introduction was 102525MU. The identical figure reflects the study design. Before introduction the total amount of BT prescribed was 138000MU, after introduction it was 116300MU. With the introduction the total amount of BT prescribed was reduced by 21700MU (–15.7%). Before introduction there were 276 D500 prescribed, afterwards 175 D500 and 96 D300. The costs of the BT therapy were €146103 before introduction and €125250 afterwards. With the introduction the costs of BT therapy was reduced by €20853 (–14.3%). The price of D500 is €529.36, of D300 €339.71. The D500 price for 1MU is €1.0587. This price was not changed with the introduction. The D300 price for 1MU is €1.1324. This reflects a surcharge against the D500 price for 1MU of €0.073 (7.0%).

Discussion

BT therapy has some unique features not found in other pharmacological therapies:

1) BT therapy is costly. D500, an average dose for neurological indications, costs €529.36 in Germany. Although daily treatment costs calculated on an average interinjection interval of 90 days are €5.88 only, economic use of BT drugs is mandatory. 2) BT therapy is performed in numerous indication groups throughout numerous medical specialties and in a therapeutic dose range seen in no other drug [3, 4]. Whilst lowest doses in spasmodic dysphonia may be below Dysport® 10MU, highest doses used in wide-spread dystonia or spasticity may be as high as Dysport® 2000MU. The same is true for other BT type A drugs. This makes adequate pricing very difficult. Whilst Dysport® treatment for one patient with spasmodic dysphonia may cost less than €10.00, Dysport® treatment for one patient with wide-spread dystonia or spasticity may cost over €2000.00. This spread would be economically unjustifiable as costs for development, registration, marketing and distribution are identical in both conditions and actual drug production costs are negligible. Applying pure economic considerations would discriminate all patients with BT low dose indications. Finding an average price reflecting this enormous spread, however, is difficult. 3) Another specific feature of BT drugs is their biologically active ingredient, the botulinum neurotoxin. As it is extremely toxic therapeutic doses have to be extremely low. For example, the BNT content per D500 is 12.5 ng only [1]. This excessive low amount makes BNT susceptible to various physical interactions. Reducing BNT per vial has therefore been a long-term manufacturing challenge. Additionally, providing long-term stability data for registration of new package sizes is costly. 4) BT drugs are distributed as freeze-dried powder requiring reconstitution with 0.9% NaCl/H_2O before use. After reconstitution the shelf life of all BT drugs is limited to avoid potential bacterial contaminations and general decay. In most countries spread of the reconstituted vial amongst several patients is prohibited for legal (mostly reimbursement) reasons and for general hygienic considerations. In Germany this drug use is specified by the Arzneimittelverschreibungsverordnung (AMVV). Within the framework of economic, marketing and manufacturing challenges we wanted to study the economic effects

Table 2 Economic parameters of botulinum toxin therapy with Dysport® before and after introduction of an additional Dysport®300MU vial

Item	Before D300 introduction	After D300 introduction	Difference
D300 price [€]	n/a	339.71	n/a
D300 price per MU [€]	n/a	1.1324	n/a
D500 price [€]	529.36	529.36	0
D500 price per MU [€]	1.0587	1.0587	0
D300 price per MU vs D500 price per MU [€]	n/a	n/a	0.073 (7.0%)
total BT used [MU]	102525	102525	0
total BT prescribed [MU]	138000	116300	−21700 (−15.7%)
D500 prescribed [n]	276	175	−101 (−36.7%)
D300 prescribed [n]	nil	96	96 (+100%)
costs [€]	146103	125250	−20853 (−14.3%)
cost reduction in D500 price per MU [€]	n/a	n/a	−22974 (−15.7%)

of the D300 introduction. For this, we controlled interfering treatment variabilities by applying rigorous inclusion criteria. Generalisation of our findings and relevance for other BT therapy centres is based on the typical constitution of the patient pool treated at HMS-MDS including a mix of patients covering all major neurological indications including dystonia, spasticity, hemifacial spasm and others. With the exemption of few patients shown under 'others' all Dysport® applications followed indications registered in Germany.

In summary, D300 introduction reduced the costs of Dysport® by 14.3%. It would have reduced them by 15.7%, if the D300 price per MU would not have been increased against the D500 price per MU by 7%. Considering the additional costs for registration of D300 and more complicated logistics a surcharge of 7% seems moderate and adequate.

Conclusions

More flexible packaging reduces drug costs for BT therapy considerably. Introduction of smaller packaging sizes is technically possible and should be encouraged. Extra costs for registration and more complicated logistics are moderate. Further cost reductions may be possible by introduction of even smaller packaging sizes. They can be calculated based on our model.

Abbreviations
€: Euro; BT: Botulinum toxin; D300: Dysport® 300MU vial; D500: Dysport® 500MU vial; HMS-MDS: Hannover Medical School Movement Disorders Section; MU: Mouse units; VAT: Value added tax

Acknowledgements
There are no acknowledgements.

Funding
There was no external funding.

Authors' contributions
DD and FAS designed the concept of the study, acquired the data and evaluated the data. All authors read and approved the final manuscript.

Competing interests
DD received honoraria for services provided to Allergan, Ipsen, M, Desitin, Syntaxin, Abbvie, Medtronic, St Jude, Boston Scientific, Almirall, Bayer, Sun, Teva, UCB, IAB-Interdisciplinary Working Group for Movement Disorders. He is shareholder of Allergan and holds patents on botulinum toxin and botulinum toxin therapy.
FAS is founder and owner of IAB - Interdisciplinary Working Group for Movement Disorders.

References

1. Dressler D. Pharmacology of botulinum toxin drugs. In: Mayer N, Brashear A, editors. Spasticity: etiology, evaluation, management, and the role of botulinum toxin. New York: We Move Press; 2009.
2. Walter U, Dressler D. Ultrasound guided botulinum toxin injections in neurology. Expert Rev Neurother. 2014;14:923–36.
3. Dressler D. Clinical applications of botulinum toxin. Curr Opin Microbiol. 2012;15:325–36.
4. Truong D, Dressler D, Hallett M, Zachary C. Manual of botulinum toxin therapy. 2nd ed. Cambridge: Cambridge University Press; 2013.

27

The effects of dopamine on digit span in Parkinson's disease

Clara Warden[1,2], Jaclyn Hwang[2], Anisa Marshall[2,3], Michelle Fenesy[2,4] and Kathleen L. Poston[2,5*]

Abstract

Background: Parkinson's disease patients are at an elevated risk of developing cognitive impairment. Although cognitive impairment is one of the strongest predictors of quality of life, dopaminergic anti-parkinsonian medications are designed to target motor symptoms. However, there is substantial evidence that dopamine also impacts cognition, in particular working memory. It is therefore critical for movement disorders physicians to understand the potential dopaminergic effects on working memory when prescribing these medications.

Verbal digit span tasks offer a potentially straightforward and quick assessment of baseline working memory. Moreover, Digit Span Backward was recently validated as a screening tool for mild cognitive impairment in Parkinson's disease when participants were medicated. Research indicates that the interaction between dopamine and working memory follows an Inverted-U shaped curve, but the effect of dopamine on Digit Span has not been well studied.

Our study seeks to: (1) determine the validity of verbal Digit Spans for detecting cognitive impairment in Parkinson's disease patients both ON and OFF medications; and (2) ascertain the effects of dopaminergic medications on verbal Digit Span.

Methods: We recruited 64 Parkinson's disease patients and 22 age-and education-matched controls. Parkinson's patients completed Digit Span Backward and Digit Span Forward ON and OFF medications, while healthy controls completed them once. All participants were categorized by cognitive diagnosis using level-II consensus criteria.

Results: Digit Span Backward successfully identified mild cognitive impairment in Parkinson's disease, both ON and OFF medications. Combining patients with and without cognitive impairment, we found that dopamine significantly improved performance on Digit Span Backward, but not Forward. In a secondary analysis, we found this dopaminergic improvement was restricted to the Low baseline working memory group; the High baseline working memory group was unaffected.

Conclusions: This study provides evidence for Digit Span Backward as a screening tool for working memory impairment in Parkinson's disease and for its utility in measuring baseline working memory. Moreover, it reveals a partial beneficial effect of dopamine on Digit Span in Parkinson's disease patients.

Keywords: Parkinson's disease, PD, Digit span backward, Digit span forward, Dopamine, Working memory, Cognitive impairment, Dementia

Background

Parkinson's disease (PD) patients are at an elevated risk of developing cognitive impairment and dementia [1, 2]. One common, early impairment is a working memory (WM) deficit [3]. WM is the ability to hold and manipulate information in short-term storage for task-relevant purposes; WM is crucial to many higher level cognitive processes such as learning, language comprehension, and reasoning [4, 5]. Although cognitive impairment is one of the strongest predictors of quality of life [6, 7], there are limited treatments targeting PD cognitive symptoms [8]. In the clinic, motor symptoms are treated with dopaminergic medications that alleviate the chronic dopamine depletion that defines PD; however, the effects of these medications on cognition are still poorly understood.

* Correspondence: klposton@stanford.edu
[2]Department of Neurology & Neurological Sciences, Stanford University, Stanford, CA, USA
[5]Department of Neurosurgery, Stanford University, Stanford, CA, USA
Full list of author information is available at the end of the article

In 1979, Brozoski et al first demonstrated that dopamine depletion from the striatum to the prefrontal cortex in monkeys led to severe impairment on a delayed response task [9]. In the intervening years, there has been growing evidence that dopamine and WM are closely linked [10–17]. Today, research indicates that WM impairment in PD is likely a down-stream effect of nigrostraital dopamine depletion [18]. However, it remains unclear if dopamine depletion is universally detrimental to WM and whether dopamine replacement leads to improvement for all individuals. In a recent review, Cools and D'Esposito argued that poor WM reflects an imbalance between the striatum and the prefrontal cortex, both of which are modulated by dopamine [10, 16, 17, 19–23]. They proposed a double Inverted-U model to describe the relationship between dopamine and WM. This model predicts that dopamine's effect on WM depends on both individual baseline WM and the specific task being tested [24]. The model holds strong implications for the effects of dopaminergic medications on cognition in PD patients in particular; individuals with intrinsic deficits might benefit from dopamine replacement while those with more superior baseline WM capabilities might suffer. For this reason, it is crucial for clinicians to be able to accurately determine baseline levels of WM in PD patients and predict the effects of dopaminergic medications on WM.

Verbal digit span tasks offer a potentially straightforward and quick assessment of baseline WM. Biundo et al recently validated Digit Span Backward as a diagnostic tool for determining cognitive impairment in PD [25]. However, this study did not consider the possible effects of dopamine since all individuals were tested ON dopaminergic medications. Owing to the strong evidence for a dopaminergic effect on WM, it is pertinent to investigate whether Digit Span remains a valid diagnostic tool OFF medications. Moreover, previous studies that examined the effect of dopamine and PD on Digit Span Backward and Digit Span Forward have reported conflicting findings [11, 26]. It is important to examine the effect of dopaminergic medications on both tasks in a large PD sample.

Our study seeks to: (1) determine the validity of verbal Digit Spans for detecting cognitive impairment in PD patients; and (2) ascertain the effects of dopaminergic medications on verbal Digit Span. In a secondary analysis, we explored the possibility of an Inverted-U effect of dopamine on verbal Digit Span. We tested 64 PD participants ON and OFF medications on Digit Span Forward and Backward.

Methods

Subjects

We recruited 64 participants with idiopathic Parkinson's disease from the Stanford Movement Disorders Clinic and the surrounding community (Table 1). Inclusion criteria were as follows: (1) Age between 45–90 years, (2) fluency in English, (3) right-handed, (4) diagnosis of PD by a board-certified neurologist with specialty training in movement disorders (KLP) based on UK Parkinson's Disease Society Brain Bank criteria [27], (5) at least two years of a PD diagnosis, (6) at least 20 % improvement in the Movement Disorders Society-United Parkinson's disease Rating Scale motor score (MDS-UPDRS-III) [28] when ON dopaminergic medications, and (7) no history of other significant neurological disease, serious psychiatric illness, substance abuse, or head trauma.

In addition, we recruited 22 age- and education-matched healthy controls (HC). Inclusion criteria were as follows: (1) Age between 45–90 years, (2) fluency in English, (3) right handed, (4) no history of significant neurological disease, serious psychiatric illness, substance abuse, or head trauma and (5) no history of cognitive impairment during phone screening.

All participants provided written informed consent to participate in the study following protocols approved by the Stanford Institutional Review Board.

Clinical evaluation

All PD and HC participants performed a neuropsychological battery that included at least two tests for each of the five cognitive domains (memory, language, executive function, visuospatial, working memory/attention), a Montreal Cognitive Assessment (MoCA), and the Clinical Dementia Rating (See Table 2). PD participants were categorized as PD without cognitive impairment (PD no-MCI), PD with mild cognitive impairment (PD-MCI), or PD with dementia (PDD) according to published criteria [27, 29]. PD-MCI was defined as exceeding 1.5 standard deviations below age- and education-matched normative values on two tests, either in the same domain or separate ones [27]. A designation of dementia was reserved for those individuals who received a score of greater than or equal to 1 on the CDR [29]; all dementia patients were independently categorized as impaired on multiple domains [30]. As recommended by current criteria [27], the comprehensive neuropsychological testing was performed ON medications to minimize motoric interference in testing.

In order to determine the effect of dopamine on Verbal Digit Span, PD participants performed the WAIS-IV Digit Span Backward and Digit Span Forward twice, once in the OFF and once in the ON state, counterbalanced, and with a least a two week interval period. The Digit Span OFF and ON was performed on the same day as the MDS-UPDRS-III OFF and ON, respectively, to control for potential motor fluctuations. The Neuropsychological battery was performed in the ON medication state, as recommended, and on a separate day [31]. Critically, we administered the oral version of

Table 1 Demographics for healthy control and Parkinson's disease participants

	HC	PD ALL	PD no-MCI	PD-MCI	PDD	p
N	22	64	28	22	14	
Male/Female	8/14	35/29	13/15	14/8	8/6	
Age (years)^	65.10 ± 6.89	68.36 ± 7.91	65.11 ± 7.21	69.14 ± 7.98	73.21 ± 6.68	* #
Education (years)^	16.81 ± 2.03	16.44 ± 2.42	16.48 ± 2.36	16.41 ± 2.56	16.71 ± 2.16	NS
Duration (years)^	n/a	5.92 ± 4.18	5.04 ± 3.47	6.64 ± 4.82	6.57 ± 4.38	NS
MDS-UPDRS III (OFF)^	n/a	37.47 ± 10.94	35.79 ± 10.53	34.00 ± 9.40	46.79 ± 9.37	# %
MDS-UPDRS III (ON)^	n/a	21.54 ± 11.11	19.81 ± 9.62	18.89 ± 10.32	29.85 ± 11.67	# %
LEDD^	n/a	695.4 ± 366.1	657.8 ± 382.7	831.8 ± 325.8	556.2 ± 344.1	NS
BDI^	3.64 ± 3.88	11.13 ± 8.34	9.26 ± 7.58	11.09 ± 7.08	13.92 ± 11.39	**
BAI^	2.68 ± 2.85	11.09 ± 8.80	11.43 ± 9.00	11.32 ± 8.34	10.04 ± 9.63	**

PD Parkinson's disease, *PDD* PD with Dementia, *PD-MCI* PD with mild cognitive impairment, *PD no-MCI* PD with no cognitive impairment, *HC* healthy controls, *MDS-UPDRS III* Movement Disorders Society-Unified Parkinson's disease Rating Scale, motor scale, *LEDD* levodopa equivalent daily dose, *BDI* Beck's Depression Inventory, *BAI* Beck's Anxiety Inventory
^ = mean ± standard deviation; * = $p < .05$ PDD vs HC; # = $p < .05$ PDD vs PD no-MCI; % = $p < .05$ PDD vs PD-MCI; ** = $p < 0.05$ HC vs All PD groups; NS = not significant

the Digit Span to minimize potential bias from bradykinesia or dyskinesias.

In PD participants, the OFF state was defined as ≥ 72 h off extended release dopamine agonists, selective MAO-B inhibitor, and long-acting levodopa, and ≥ 12 h off short acting dopamine agonists and levodopa. The ON state was defined as the patients taking their normal daily medications in the optimally medicated state, as determined by both the patient and the movement disorders neurologist. We took steps to minimize the influence of motor fluctuations on the tests performed ON medications. First, the researchers documented the patient's last dose of medications, and the next scheduled dose, to confirm the testing was during the optimal time in relation to scheduled medications. Second, it was documented that the patient remained in the ON state throughout the 30 min of the MDS-UPDRS-III and Digit Span. With regards to dopamine replacement therapy, 41 participants were taking levodopa and a dopamine agonist, 2 were taking levodopa and a MAO-B inhibitor, 18 were taking levodopa, a dopamine agonist, and a MAO-B inhibitor, 1 was taking a dopamine agonist and a MAO-B inhibitor, 1 was taking only an MAO-B inhibitor, and 1 was taking a combination of

Table 2 Neuropsychological battery

	HC	PD no-MCI	PD MCI	PDD	p-valueHC vs PD no-MCI
MoCA	27.52 ± 1.97	27.57 ± 2.01	23.50 ± 2.72	16.79 ± 1.97	0.93
DRS	140.19 ± 2.99	139.43 ± 2.81	135.45 ± 5.60	118.43 ± 16.01	0.37
CVLT LD Free	12.19 ± 2.71	11.07 ± 3.1	5.82 ± 2.75	3.29 ± 3.87	0.19
BVMT-R	10.1 ± 2.45	10.25 ± 1.92	5.64 ± 2.66	1.92 ± 2.47	0.80
JLO	26.24 ± 3.79	25.04 ± 3.39	21.14 ± 5.16	17.73 ± 5.85	0.25
HVOT	26.71 ± 1.91	25.88 ± 2.38	22.14 ± 4.28	17.69 ± 6.72	0.19
SDMT Oral	57.14 ± 9.46	56.46 ± 13.09	40.32 ± 11.98	17.75 ± 9.02	0.84
COWAT	46.43 ± 12.29	49 ± 12.96	33.77 ± 18.14	22.43 ± 10.06	0.49
WAIS-IV Digit total	17.43 ± 3.34	18.93 ± 3.89	15.82 ± 4.86	11.43 ± 2.24	0.16
Trails B	67.62 ± 23.44	68.39 ± 26.12	161.41 ± 91.46	280.5 ± 48.82	0.92
Stroop	-2.16 ± 14.76	-3.29 ± 7.57	-7.55 ± 9.55	-12.07 ± 5.63	0.73
BNT	29.14 ± 0.91	27.82 ± 3.94	24.64 ± 4.96	25.43 ± 2.93	0.14
DKEFs Verbal	20.9 ± 5.12	22.32 ± 6.34	17.09 ± 6.22	10 ± 5.39	0.41

Table depicts the mean ± standard deviation for the demographic information and neuropsychological test data, with p-values derived from independent-sample t-test between HC and PD no-MCI
PD Parkinson's disease, *HC* Healthy control, *MoCA* Montreal Cognitive Assessment, *CVLT LD Free* California Verbal Learning Test, Long Delay Free Recall, *BVMT-R* The Brief Visuospatial Memory Test-Revised, *JLO* Judgment of Line Orientation, *HVOT* Hooper Visual Organization Test, *SDMT Oral* Symbol Digit Modalities Test, oral, *COWAT* Controlled Oral Word Association Test, *WAIS-IV Digit total* Wechsler Adult Intelligence Scale, Digit combined total, *Trails B* Trail Making Test B, *Stroop* Golden version of Stroop test, Interference score, *BNT* Boston Naming Test, *DKEFs Verbal* Delis-Kaplan Executive Function System, Verbal score

levodopa, a dopamine agonist, a MAO-B inhibitor and a COMT inhibitor.

Statistical analysis

All statistical analysis were conducting using IBM SPSS Statistics version 22.0 [32].

Results

Demographics

HC participants were age-matched with the overall PD group and with the PD no-MCI and PD-MCI groups.) HC and PD no-MCI groups were significantly younger than the PDD group. There were no significant differences in education, duration of disease, levodopa equivalent doses (LEDD), depression, or anxiety across all PD groups (Table 1). In addition, there were no significant differences between the HC and PD no-MCI groups on any of the neuropsychological tests administered (Table 2). 59 participants completed the digit span ON and OFF dopaminergic medications, 1 completed it only OFF medications, and 4 completed it only ON medications. Only participants with both an ON and an OFF session were included in the analysis of medication effects. 34 participants were tested ON medications first while 25 were tested OFF medications first. Repeat measure ANOVAs with repeated factor Medications (ON, OFF) and between-subjects factors Session (ON first, OFF first) and Baseline WM (High, Low) did not reveal any session effects.

Between group analysis

Due to the non-normal distribution of the PDD group, Kruskal-Wallis tests with between-subjects factor Group (HC, PD no-MCI, PD-MCI, PDD) and post-hoc stepwise step-down procedures were used to analyze the differences in Digit Span Forward and Backward scores between clinical groups (Fig. 1). Four separate Kruskal-Wallis tests were conducted: Digit Span Forward with PD OFF, Digit Span Forward with PD ON, Digit Span Backward with PD OFF, and Digit Span Backward with PD ON. Moreover, we conducted a Kruskal-Wallis test with between-subject factor Group (HC, PD no-MCI, PD-MCI, PDD) for the abbreviated digit span on the MoCA.

Digit span forward, PD OFF

The effect of Group was significant ($p < .005$). Post-hoc analysis revealed that PDD performed significantly worse than PD no-MCI ($p < .05$). No other groups were significantly different (Fig. 1a).

Digit span forward, PD ON

The effect of Group was significant ($p < .001$). Post-hoc analysis revealed that PDD performed significantly worse

than PD no-MCI, PD-MCI, and HC ($p < .05$ in all cases). No other groups were significantly different (Fig. 1c).

Digit span backward, PD OFF

The effect of Group was significant ($p < .001$). Post-hoc analysis revealed that PDD performed significantly worse than HC, PD no-MCI, and PD-MCI ($p < .05$ in all cases). Moreover, the PD-MCI group performed significantly worse than PD no-MCI and HC (both $p < .05$). PD no-MCI was not significantly different from HC (Fig. 1b).

Digit span backward, PD ON

The effect of Group was significant ($p < .001$). Post-hoc analysis revealed that PDD performed significantly worse than HC, PD no-MCI, and PD-MCI ($p < .05$ in all cases). PD-MCI also performed significantly worse than PD no-MCI ($p < .05$). PD no-MCI and PD-MCI were not significantly different from HC (Fig. 1d).

MoCA digit span sub-score

The effect of Group was not significant. The majority of individuals, from all groups, achieved a perfect score of 2/2: 78.6 % of PDD, 90.9 % of PD-MCI, 89.3 % of PD no-MCI and 100 % of HC.

Effect of dopaminergic medication

In order to isolate the effect of dopaminergic medications on WM, as measured by Digit Spans, we compared performance within groups ON and OFF medications. For PD-MCI and PD no-MCI groups we conducted paired sample Student's T-tests between ON and OFF sessions. For the PDD group we conducted the Related-Samples Wilcoxon Signed Rank Test. There was no significant effect of dopaminergic medications in Digit Span Backward or Forward in PD no-MCI, PD-MCI, or PDD (Fig. 2a). However, when PD no-MCI and PD-MCI were combined, a significant effect of the medications was detected. In Digit Span Backward, PD participants performed significantly better ON compared to OFF dopaminergic medications ($p = .043$) (Fig. 2b).

Effect of baseline WM

Prior PD studies have shown that WM can have an Inverted-U response to dopamine, where patients with poor baseline (OFF dopamine) performance show improvement after dopamine replacement and those with good baseline performance show worsening [21, 22, 24, 33]. Therefore, we conducted a secondary analysis to explore a possible interaction between baseline WM and the effect of dopaminergic medications on Digit Span performance in our sample. We only included PD no-MCI and PD-MCI in this analysis due to the non-normal distribution of the PDD group and to eliminate the possible confounding factors of mixed pathology, elevated age, and severe impairment in

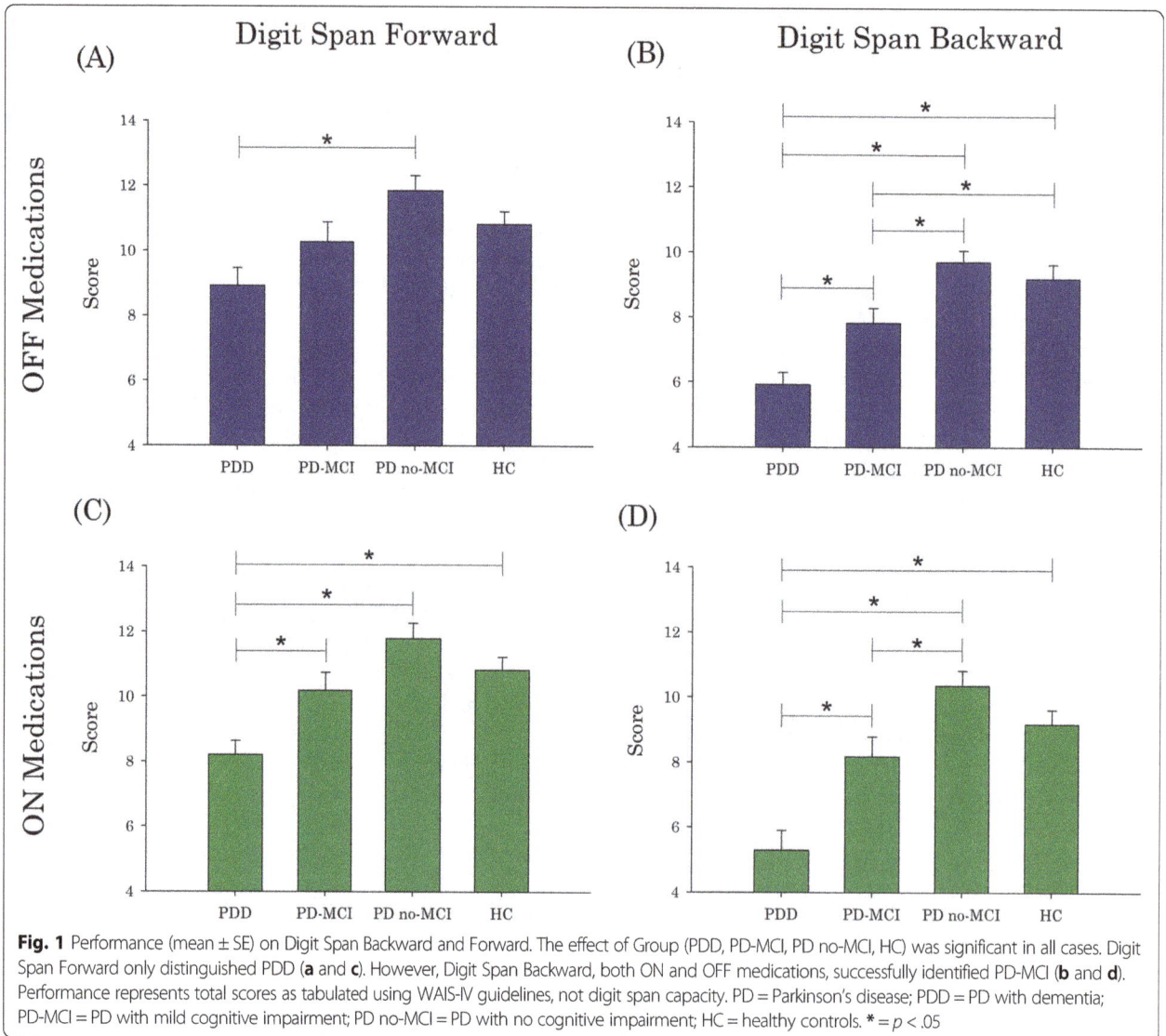

Fig. 1 Performance (mean ± SE) on Digit Span Backward and Forward. The effect of Group (PDD, PD-MCI, PD no-MCI, HC) was significant in all cases. Digit Span Forward only distinguished PDD (**a** and **c**). However, Digit Span Backward, both ON and OFF medications, successfully identified PD-MCI (**b** and **d**). Performance represents total scores as tabulated using WAIS-IV guidelines, not digit span capacity. PD = Parkinson's disease; PDD = PD with dementia; PD-MCI = PD with mild cognitive impairment; PD no-MCI = PD with no cognitive impairment; HC = healthy controls. * = $p < .05$

alternate cognitive domains that could impact performance (e.g. severe episodic memory or executive impairment that prohibits encoding). As the cross-sectional nature of our study prohibited evaluating premorbid WM performance, we followed the protocol of previous studies and used the median of the combined group Digit Span Backward OFF to determine the cut-off score differentiating High versus Low baseline WM in our cohort [33]. Digit Span Backward ≥ 9 categorized an individual as High WM while < 9 was categorized as Low WM. Of the PD-MCI group, 16 were determined to have Low baseline WM and 6 to have High baseline WM. Of the PD no-MCI group, 9 fell into the Low baseline WM group and 19 in the High baseline WM group. There were no significant differences between motor, depression, or anxiety scores between the High and Low groups (Table 3). We conducted separate analysis of Digit Span Forward and Backward, each using a mixed measures ANOVA with between-subjects factor Group

(High Baseline WM, Low Baseline WM) and within-subjects factor Medication (ON, OFF).

Digit span forward

There was a main effect of Group ($p < .001$), but no main effect of Medications. There was no interaction effect (Fig. 3a).

Digit span backward

There was a main effect of Group ($p < .001$), a main effect of Medication ($p = .042$), and no interaction effect; however post-hoc Student's T-tests revealed the Medication effect was only in the Low WM group ($p = .002$). Indeed, the Low WM group performed significantly better ON compared to OFF dopaminergic medications (Fig. 3b).

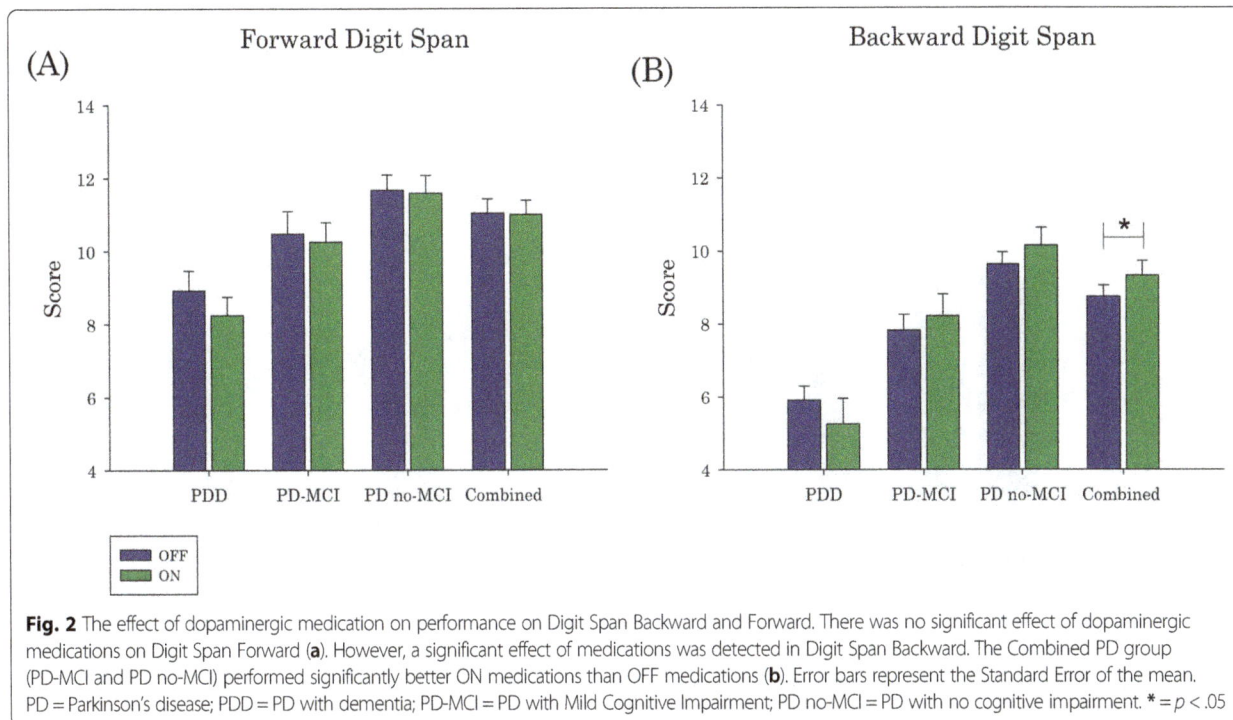

Fig. 2 The effect of dopaminergic medication on performance on Digit Span Backward and Forward. There was no significant effect of dopaminergic medications on Digit Span Forward (**a**). However, a significant effect of medications was detected in Digit Span Backward. The Combined PD group (PD-MCI and PD no-MCI) performed significantly better ON medications than OFF medications (**b**). Error bars represent the Standard Error of the mean. PD = Parkinson's disease; PDD = PD with dementia; PD-MCI = PD with Mild Cognitive Impairment; PD no-MCI = PD with no cognitive impairment. * = $p < .05$

Discussion

We investigated the utility of Digit Span Backward and Digit Span Forward as tools for identifying cognitive impairment in PD and the effects of dopaminergic medications on Digit Span in PD. We found that Digit Span Backward best distinguished cognitive classification (no-MCI, MCI and dementia) in our cohort. Moreover, exploratory analysis revealed a partial beneficial effect of dopaminergic medications on Digit Span Backward, with low WM individuals improving on dopamine and

high WM individuals demonstrating no benefit. Our research provides evidence for Digit Span Backward as a screening tool for WM impairment in PD and for its utility in measuring baseline WM.

Digit span backwards in PD

Our findings corroborate those of Biundo et al., who reported that Digit Span Backward was one of five cognitive assessments that reached diagnostic and screening validity for PD-MCI, while Digit Span Forward failed to do so [25]. While this study only tested participants ON dopaminergic medications, our study provides further evidence that Digit Span Backward successfully distinguishes between PD no-MCI, PD-MCI, and PDD regardless of whether performed ON or OFF medications. By contrast, we found Digit Span Forward was only abnormal in PDD.

Moreover, we found Digit Span Backward offers greater insight into WM impairment than the limited digit span conducted in the MoCA. Currently, the MoCA is among the most commonly used tools for screening PD cognitive impairment in the clinical setting [34]. However, our findings indicate the limited digit span in the MoCA is a very weak detector of WM impairment, especially among a population of highly educated individuals. This is in accordance with the finding that education is a strong predictor of verbal Digit Span, with higher educational attainment leading to greater span capacity [35]. Years of education in our cohort averaged 16 and the limited digit span on the MoCA failed to differentiate between any of

Table 3 High versus low baseline working memory

	Low Baseline Working Memory	High Baseline Working Memory	p
N	25	25	
PD no-MCI/PD-MCI	9/16	19/6	
Age (years)	65.36 ± 7.26	68.72 ± 8.07	NS
Education (years)	16.16 ± 2.90	16.56 ± 2.08	NS
Duration (years)	6.17 ± 5.02	5.20 ± 3.18	NS
MDS-UPDRS III (OFF)	33.32 ± 9.22	36.68 ± 9.89	NS
MDS-UPDRS III (ON)	19.83 ± 9.22	18.75 ± 10.76	NS
BDI	11.13 ± 6.84	9.80 ± 7.99	NS
BAI	11.72 ± 10.54	11.04 ± 6.38	NS

Table depicts the mean ± standard deviation for the demographics of the High and Low Baseline Working Memory groups

PD Parkinson's disease, *PD-MCI* PD with mild cognitive impairment, *PD no-MCI* PD with no cognitive impairment, *MDS-UPDRS III* Movement Disorders Society-Unified Parkinson's disease Rating Scale, motor scale, *BDI* Beck's Depression Inventory, *BAI* Beck's Anxiety Inventory, *NS* not significant between groups on t-test

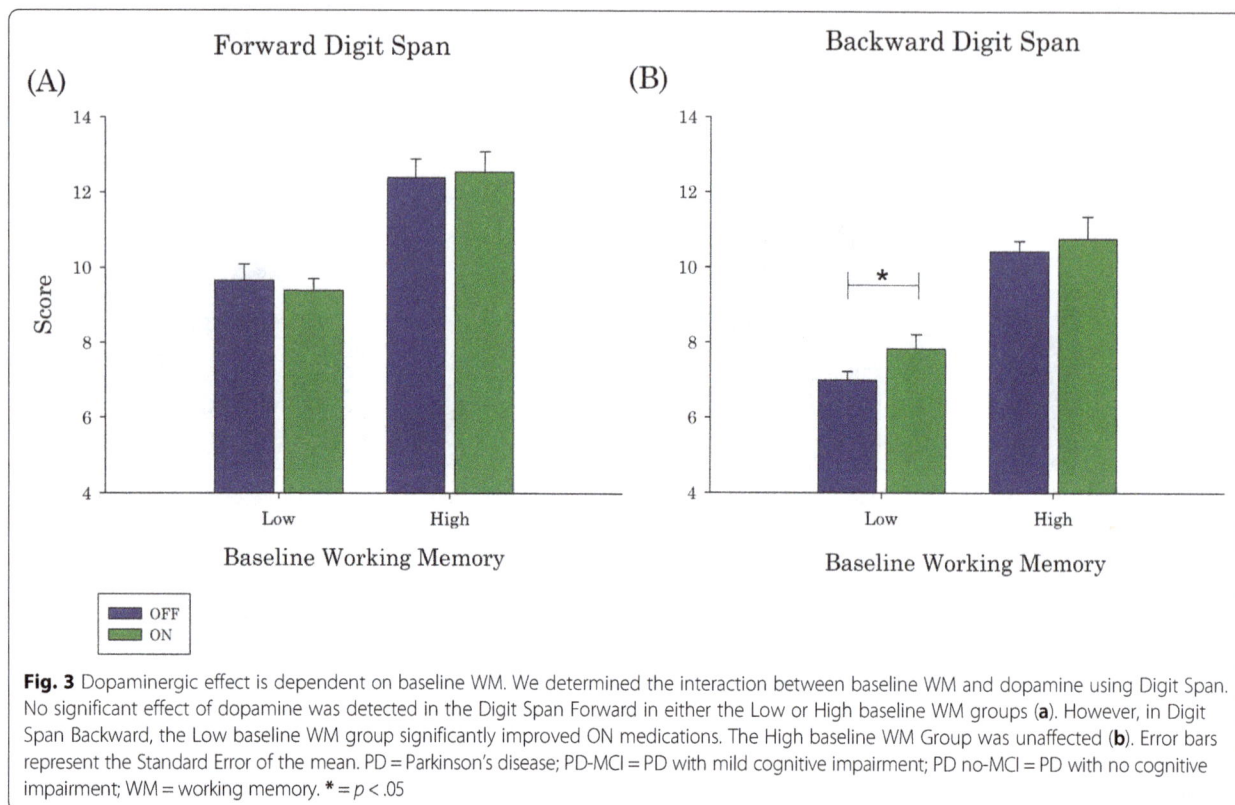

Fig. 3 Dopaminergic effect is dependent on baseline WM. We determined the interaction between baseline WM and dopamine using Digit Span. No significant effect of dopamine was detected in the Digit Span Forward in either the Low or High baseline WM groups (**a**). However, in Digit Span Backward, the Low baseline WM group significantly improved ON medications. The High baseline WM Group was unaffected (**b**). Error bars represent the Standard Error of the mean. PD = Parkinson's disease; PD-MCI = PD with mild cognitive impairment; PD no-MCI = PD with no cognitive impairment; WM = working memory. * = p < .05

the cognitive groups; even the vast majority of participants with dementia achieved a perfect score. Thus, we suggest Digit Span Backward could be a relatively simple compliment to the MoCA and could be used in clinic to screen highly educated PD patients who are suspected of a WM deficit.

Dopaminergic effect on digit span

Prior studies in PD have reported conflicting effects of dopaminergic medications on the verbal Digit Span, likely due to small sample sizes. Zokaei et al previously reported a significant dopaminergic improvement in WM in PD patients as detected by a WM precision task, but indicated this improvement was not detected in Digit Span Backward or Forward [26]. On the other hand, Cools et al found PD patients OFF medications performed worse than healthy controls on Digit Span Backward, but this impairment was rectified by dopaminergic medications [11]. Our study found a modest degree of dopaminergic improvement similar to that of Cools et al, but validates their finding in a much larger cohort. In addition, our study expands upon Cools et al by including a full neuropsychological assessment to confirm that the dopaminergic improvement is seen in both cognitively impaired and cognitively normal PD patients, depending on the baseline working memory.

An Inverted-U effect of dopaminergic medications has previously been described in other WM tasks, such as delay-response [36], and attentional set shifting [23, 33, 37]. We conducted a secondary analysis to determine a possible interaction between baseline WM and the effect of dopaminergic medications specifically on the Digit Span. In accordance with other studies exploring the Inverted-U model [21, 24], we only detected a dopaminergic improvement when groups were divided by baseline WM (Low versus High) and not by global cognitive classification (MCI versus no-MCI). This is likely because we our Low and High WM groups included a distribution of both PD no-MCI and PD-MCI individuals; 9 out of 28 PD no-MCI had low baseline WM and 16 out of 22 PD-MCI had low baseline WM. While it may seem counterintuitive that patients categorized as no-MCI have low WM, this is likely due to the threshold for determining PD no-MCI (1.5 SD below age- and education- normative values in at least two out of 10 tests), which allows patients to have one test more than 1.5 SD below normative values, or have sub-threshold poor performance on multiple tests. By contrast, PD patients who are globally categorized as cognitively impaired do not necessarily have poor WM, as they could have visuospatial or episodic memory impairments. Thus, our study highlights the limitations of using global cognitive categorization when examining a dopaminergic effect on a specific cognitive ability and the value of identifying validated tests for PD patients in individual cognitive domains. Due to the cross-sectional nature of our study, baseline WM was determined using performance on Digit Span Backward OFF medications. Although pre-morbid WM would have been a preferable baseline, using performance when OFF medications enabled us to isolate the effect of dopamine from that of the primary disease.

The Inverted-U hypothesis predicts that the effect of dopamine depends upon baseline WM and the nature of the cognitive task being performed. Specifically, tasks that require high levels of stabilization should benefit from high levels of dopamine in the prefrontal cortex relative to the striatum [10, 22, 24, 38]. Therefore, poor baseline WM suggests an imbalance of dopamine between the prefrontal cortex and striatum, and high baseline WM indicates an optimized balance [22, 24, 38]. In addition, this hypothesis suggests that low WM individuals should benefit from dopaminergic medications on straightforward WM tasks that require cognitive stabilization, such as Digit Span, while high WM individuals should be detrimentally affected. Our study was not optimized to fully explore this relationship because we could only divide our cohort into two groups (high and low WM) and a true Inverted-U effect would ideally show those who improve, those who do not change, and those who are detrimentally affected; however some of our findings can be explained within this framework. For instance, dopaminergic medications might have benefited the low WM individuals by shifting the dopamine balance between the prefrontal cortex and the striatum to a more optimal level [24, 38]. Our high WM individuals were unaffected by dopamine, possibly because dopaminergic medications did not alter the balance (i.e. they were already optimized). An alternative explanation is that, unlike other WM tasks, Digit Span Backward does not follow an Inverted-U dopaminergic response due to the simplicity of the task. Further studies optimized to explore this question, ideally with more difficult WM tasks, could clarify this distinction.

Practical applications for the digit span backward

As described above, we established Digit Span Backward as an accurate predictor of baseline WM. In concordance with Lewis et al, which revealed effects of dopaminergic medications on the manipulation but not maintenance stage of WM, the Inverted-U was only detected in Digit Span Backward and not Digit Span Forward [15]. Our findings indicate that Digit Span Backward can be used to differentiate between low and high WM individuals in clinical and research settings.

An important consequence of the detected dopaminergic effect on the Digit Span Backward is that the task is a more sensitive determinate of baseline WM when it is conducted OFF medications. As the medications improve performance in the Low WM group but do not

affect the High WM group, they effectively blur the line between high and low WM individuals such that in the ON medications state some low WM individuals could inadvertently be categorized as high WM. As such, we recommend the Digit Span Backward be conducted OFF medications if possible when being used to primarily identify low baseline WM individuals.

Methodology and limitations

Our study has several limitations. It should be noted that our PDD group was significantly older than our PD no-MCI and HC groups. The age difference, in addition to possible mixed-pathology, confounds our ability to determine whether the significantly impaired performance of the PDD group on Digit Span Forward was a direct effect of PDD or influenced by the effect of age. We were also unable to determine baseline WM for the PD patients prior to onset of disease. This limits our ability to determine whether impairments represent an individual's pre-morbid cognitive ability or are a result of PD. However, our findings remain significant for clinical purposes as they offer clinicians a tool to predict the effects of dopaminergic medications on WM. Moreover, it is difficult to generalize our findings to all PD patients since our cohort was not necessarily representative. Notably, our PD no-MCI and PD-MCI groups did not perform significantly differently than HC on any task, regardless of medication status. This could be due to motivation of PD patients to perform well [39–41], or because 6 out of 22 PD MCI participants had high baseline WM. Generalizability of our findings is also a concern; PD patients were primarily recruited from an academic tertiary care center, resulting in a highly educated cohort.

Finally, we recognize that Digit Span Backward does not test all aspects of WM and cognition. Notably, Cools et al previously reported that improvement in WM on Digit Span Backward was counterbalanced by increased distractibility in PD patients, indicating dopaminergic medications were beneficial to some aspects of cognition and detrimental to others [11]. Further studies should investigate the longitudinal validity of Digit Span Backward and the effects of dopaminergic medications on other cognitive functions, such as attentional control. Moreover, neuroimaging studies can lead to a deeper understanding of whether the dopaminergic effect we detected represents a stabilization of the balance between the prefrontal cortex and the striatum [24].

Conclusions

Our research supports the use of Digit Span Backward to screen for mild cognitive impairment, particularly among highly educated PD patients, and to detect baseline WM.

It also suggests a partial beneficial effect of dopaminergic medications on verbal Digit Span Backward in PD.

Abbreviations

ANOVA: analysis of variance; BNT: Boston naming test; BVMT-R: the brief visuospatial memory test-revised; COMT: Catechol-O-methyl transferase; COWAT: controlled oral word association test; CVLT LD Free: California verbal learning test long delay free recall; DKEFs Verbal: Delis-Kaplan executive function system, verbal score; HC: healthy controls; HVOT: Hooper visual organization test; JLO: judgment of line orientation; MAO-B: Monoamine oxidase B; MoCA: Montreal cognitive assessment; PD: Parkinson's disease; PD no-MCI: Parkinson's disease without cognitive impairment; PDD: Parkinson's disease with dementia; PD-MCI: Parkinson's disease with mild cognitive impairment; SDMT Oral: symbol digit modalities test, oral; Stroop: golden version of Stroop test, Interference score; Trails B: trail making test B; WAIS-IV Digit total: Wechsler adult intelligence scale, digit combined total; WM: working memory.

Competing interests

KLP has been a consultant for Acadia Pharmaceuticals and has received research support from Sangamo Biosciences Inc. and AstraZeneca. No other authors have competing interests to declare.

Authors' contributions

CW contributed to study design, data analysis, creation and editing of figures, manuscript preparation, editing, and critical revision. JW contributed to, data analysis, creation of figures, and critical revision of the manuscript. AM and MF contributed to participant recruitment, data acquisition, data analysis, and critical revision of the manuscript. KLP contributed to study design, participant recruitment, data acquisition, data analysis, manuscript preparation and critical revision. All authors contributed in accordance with authorship criteria, read and approved the final draft.

Acknowledgments

We thank David Everling and Sophie YorkWilliams for their assistance with administering the Digit Spans OFF medications. We also thank Nahri Ahn and Kali Xu for their assistance in documenting and recording the data. This research was supported by grants from the NIH/NIA (AG047366), NIH/NIAAA (AA023165), NIH/NINDS (NS075097, NS091461, NS086085, and NS071675), and Michael J. Fox Foundation for Parkinson's disease Research.

Author details

[1]Department of Psychology, Stanford University, Stanford, CA, USA. [2]Department of Neurology & Neurological Sciences, Stanford University, Stanford, CA, USA. [3]Department of Neuroimaging, King's College London, London, UK. [4]Department of Psychology, University of California, Los Angeles, CA, USA. [5]Department of Neurosurgery, Stanford University, Stanford, CA, USA.

References

1. Hely MA, Morris JG, Reid WG, Trafficante R. Sydney multicenter study of Parkinson's disease: non-L-dopa-responsive problems dominate at 15 years. Mov Disord. 2005;20(2):190–9. doi:10.1002/mds.20324.

2. Hely MA, Reid WG, Adena MA, Halliday GM, Morris JG. The Sydney multicenter study of Parkinson's disease: the inevitability of dementia at 20 years. Mov Disord. 2008;23(6):837–44. doi:10.1002/mds.21956.

3. Goldman JG, Williams-Gray C, Barker RA, Duda JE, Galvin JE. The spectrum of cognitive impairment in Lewy body diseases. Mov Disord. 29(5):608-21. doi:10.1002/mds.25866.

4. Baddeley A. Working memory: looking back and looking forward. Nat Rev Neurosci. 2003;4(10):829–39. doi:10.1038/nrn1201.

5. Baddeley A. Working memory and language: an overview. J Commun Disord. 2003;36(3):189–208.

6. Schrag A, Jahanshahi M, Quinn N. What contributes to quality of life in patients with Parkinson's disease? J Neurol Neurosurg Psychiatry. 2000;69(3):308–12.

7. Aarsland D, Litvan I, Salmon D, Galasko D, Wentzel-Larsen T, Larsen JP. Performance on the dementia rating scale in Parkinson's disease with dementia and dementia with Lewy bodies: comparison with progressive supranuclear palsy and Alzheimer's disease. J Neurol Neurosurg Psychiatry. 2003;74(9):1215–20.

8. Thanvi BR, Munshi SK, Vijaykumar N, Lo TC. Neuropsychiatric non-motor aspects of Parkinson's disease. Postgrad Med J. 2003;79(936):561–5.

9. Brozoski TJ, Brown RM, Rosvold HE, Goldman PS. Cognitive deficit caused by regional depletion of dopamine in prefrontal cortex of rhesus monkey. Science. 1979;205(4409):929–32.

10. Cools R, Barker RA, Sahakian BJ, Robbins TW. Enhanced or impaired cognitive function in Parkinson's disease as a function of dopaminergic medication and task demands. Cereb Cortex. 2001;11(12):1136–43.

11. Cools R, Miyakawa A, Sheridan M, D'Esposito M. Enhanced frontal function in Parkinson's disease. Brain. 2010;133(Pt 1):225–33. doi:10.1093/brain/awp301.

12. Lange KW, Robbins TW, Marsden CD, James M, Owen AM, Paul GM. L-dopa withdrawal in Parkinson's disease selectively impairs cognitive performance in tests sensitive to frontal lobe dysfunction. Psychopharmacology (Berl). 1992;107(2-3):394–404.

13. Owen AM, Iddon JL, Hodges JR, Summers BA, Robbins TW. Spatial and non-spatial working memory at different stages of Parkinson's disease. Neuropsychologia. 1997;35(4):519–32.

14. Owen AM, James M, Leigh PN, Summers BA, Marsden CD, Quinn NP, et al. Fronto-striatal cognitive deficits at different stages of Parkinson's disease. Brain. 1992;115(Pt 6):1727–51.

15. Lewis SJ, Slabosz A, Robbins TW, Barker RA, Owen AM. Dopaminergic basis for deficits in working memory but not attentional set-shifting in Parkinson's disease. Neuropsychologia. 2005;43(6):823–32. doi:10.1016/j.neuropsychologia. 2004.10.001.

16. Sawaguchi T, Goldman-Rakic PS. D1 dopamine receptors in prefrontal cortex: involvement in working memory. Science. 1991;251(4996):947–50.

17. Williams GV, Goldman-Rakic PS. Modulation of memory fields by dopamine D1 receptors in prefrontal cortex. Nature. 1995;376(6541):572–5. doi:10.1038/376572a0.

18. Halliday GM, Leverenz JB, Schneider JS, Adler CH. The neurobiological basis of cognitive impairment in Parkinson's disease. Mov Disord. 29(5):634-50. doi:10.1002/mds.25857.

19. Frank MJ. Dynamic dopamine modulation in the basal ganglia: a neurocomputational account of cognitive deficits in medicated and nonmedicated Parkinsonism. J Cogn Neurosci. 2005;17(1):51–72. doi:10.1162/0898929052880093.

20. Chudasama Y, Robbins TW. Functions of frontostriatal systems in cognition: comparative neuropsychopharmacological studies in rats, monkeys and humans. Biol Psychol. 2006;73(1):19–38. doi:10.1016/j. biopsycho.2006.01.005.

21. Vijayraghavan S, Wang M, Birnbaum SG, Williams GV, Arnsten AF. Inverted-U dopamine D1 receptor actions on prefrontal neurons engaged in working memory. Nat Neurosci. 2007;10(3):376–84. doi:10.1038/nn1846.

22. Cools R, Gibbs SE, Miyakawa A, Jagust W, D'Esposito M. Working memory capacity predicts dopamine synthesis capacity in the human striatum. J Neurosci. 2008;28(5):1208–12. doi:10.1523/JNEUROSCI.4475-07.2008.

23. Kimberg DY, D'Esposito M, Farah MJ. Effects of bromocriptine on human subjects depend on working memory capacity. Neuroreport. 1997;8(16):3581–5.

24. Cools R, D'Esposito M. Inverted-U-shaped dopamine actions on human working memory and cognitive control. Biol Psychiatry. 2011;69(12):e113–25. doi:10.1016/j.biopsych.2011.03.028.

25. Biundo R, Weis L, Pilleri M, Facchini S, Formento-Dojot P, Vallelunga A et al. Diagnostic and screening power of neuropsychological testing in detecting mild cognitive impairment in Parkinson's disease. J Neural Transm.120(4): 627-33. doi:10.1007/s00702-013-1004-2.

26. Zokaei N, Burnett Heyes S, Gorgoraptis N, Budhdeo S, Husain M. Working memory recall precision is a more sensitive index than span. J Neuropsychol. doi:10.1111/jnp.12052.

27. Litvan I, Bhatia KP, Burn DJ, Goetz CG, Lang AE, McKeith I. et al. SIC Task Force appraisal of clinical diagnostic criteria for parkinsonian disorders. Mov Disord. 2003;18(5):467–486.

28. Goetz CG, Tilley BC, Shaftman SR, Stebbins GT, Fahn S, Martinez-Martin P, et al. Movement Disorder Society-sponsored revision of the Unified Parkinson's Disease Rating Scale (MDS-UPDRS): Scale presentation and clinimetric testing results. Mov Disord. 2008;23(15):2129–70. doi:10.1002/mds.22340.

29. Morris JC. The Clinical Dementia Rating (CDR): current version and scoring rules. Neurology. 1993;43(11):2412–4.

30. Emre M, Aarsland D, Brown R, Burn DJ, Duyckaerts C, Mizuno Y, et al. Clinical diagnostic criteria for dementia associated with Parkinson's disease. Mov Disord. 2007;22(12):1689–707. doi:10.1002/mds.21507. quiz 837.

31. Litvan I, Goldman JG, Troster AI, Schmand BA, Weintraub D, Petersen RC, et al. Diagnostic criteria for mild cognitive impairment in Parkinson's disease: movement disorder society task force guidelines. Mov Disord. 2012;27(3):349–56. doi:10.1002/mds.24893.

32. IBM SPSS Statistics for Windows, Version 22.0. Armonk, NY: IBM Corp.; Released 2013.

33. Costa A, Peppe A, Mazzu I, Longarzo M, Caltagirone C, Carlesimo GA. Dopamine treatment and cognitive functioning in individuals with Parkinson's disease: the "cognitive flexibility" hypothesis seems to work. Behav Neurol. 2014;2014:260896. doi:10.1155/2014/260896.

34. Hoops S, Nazem S, Siderowf AD, Duda JE, Xie SX, Stern MB, et al. Validity of the MoCA and MMSE in the detection of MCI and dementia in Parkinson disease. Neurology. 2009;73(21):1738–45. doi:10.1212/WNL.0b013e3181c34b47.

35. Orsini A, Grossi D, Capitani E, Laiacona M, Papagno C, Vallar G. Verbal and spatial immediate memory span: normative data from 1355 adults and 1112 children. Ital J Neurol Sci. 1987;8(6):539–48.

36. Gibbs SE, D'Esposito M. Individual capacity differences predict working memory performance and prefrontal activity following dopamine receptor stimulation. Cogn Affect Behav Neurosci. 2005;5(2):212–21.

37. Frank MJ, O'Reilly RC. A mechanistic account of striatal dopamine function in human cognition: psychopharmacological studies with cabergoline and haloperidol. Behav Neurosci. 2006;120(3):497–517. doi:10.1037/0735-7044.120.3.497.

38. Moustafa AA, Sherman SJ, Frank MJ. A dopaminergic basis for working memory, learning and attentional shifting in Parkinsonism. Neuropsychologia. 2008;46(13):3144–56. doi:10.1016/j.neuropsychologia.2008.07.011.

39. Avlar B, Kahn JB, Jensen G, Kandel ER, Simpson EH, Balsam PD. Improving temporal cognition by enhancing motivation. Behav Neurosci. 2015;129(5):576–88. doi:10.1037/bne0000083.

40. Bahlmann J, Aarts E, D'Esposito M. Influence of motivation on control hierarchy in the human frontal cortex. J Neurosci. 35(7):3207-17. doi:10.1523/JNEUROSCI.2389-14.2015.

41. Szatkowska I, Bogorodzki P, Wolak T, Marchewka A, Szeszkowski W. The effect of motivation on working memory: an fMRI and SEM study. Neurobiol Learn Mem. 2008;90(2):475–8. doi:10.1016/j.nlm.2008.06.001.

28

Inpatient care for stiff person syndrome in the United States: a nationwide readmission study

James A. G. Crispo[1,2*], Dylan P. Thibault[1,2,3], Yannick Fortin[4] and Allison W. Willis[1,2,3,5]

Abstract

Background: Stiff person syndrome (SPS) is a progressive neurological disorder characterized by axial muscle rigidity and involuntary spasms. Autoimmune and neoplastic diseases are associated with SPS. Our study objectives were to describe inpatient care for SPS in the United States and characterize 30-day readmissions.

Methods: We queried the 2014 Nationwide Readmission Database for hospitalizations where a diagnosis of SPS was recorded. For readmission analyses, we excluded encounters with missing length of stay, hospitalization deaths, and out-of-state and December discharges. National estimates of index hospitalizations and 30-day readmissions were computed using survey weighting methods. Unconditional logistic regression was used to examine associations between demographic, clinical, and hospital characteristics and readmission.

Results: There were 836 patients with a recorded diagnosis of SPS during a 2014 hospitalization. After exclusions, 703 patients remained, 9.4% of which were readmitted within 30 days. Frequent reasons for index hospitalization were SPS (27.8%) and diabetes with complications (5.1%). Similarly, readmissions were predominantly for diabetes complications (24.2%) and SPS. Most readmissions attributed to diabetes complications (87.5%) were to different hospitals. Female sex (OR, 3.29; CI: 1.22–8.87) and routine discharge (OR, 0.26; CI: 0.10–0.64) were associated with readmission, while routine discharge (OR, 0.18; CI: 0.04–0.89) and care at for-profit hospitals (OR, 10.87; CI: 2.03–58.25) were associated with readmission to a different hospital.

Conclusions: Readmissions in SPS may result from disease complications or comorbid conditions. Readmissions to different hospitals may reflect specialty care, gaps in discharge planning, or medical emergencies. Studies are required to determine if readmissions in SPS are preventable.

Keywords: Stiff person syndrome, Inpatients, Readmission, United States, Rare disorder

Background

First described by Moersch and Woltman [1], stiff person syndrome (SPS) (formerly referred to as stiff man syndrome) is a rare and progressive autoimmune disorder that is characterized by rigidity and stiffness of axial and lower limb muscles, as well as painful involuntary spasms that may lead to patient disability [1]. Although the

pathophysiology of classic SPS remains to be fully elucidated, there are known immunological markers for SPS and an autoimmune link between diabetes mellitus (type 1) and SPS involving the neuroendocrine autoantibody specific for glutamic acid decarboxylase (65 kD isoform; GAD65) has been demonstrated [2–4]. While GAD65 positivity is common in the general population, individuals with SPS can have markedly elevated levels of GAD65 and often respond positively to immunotherapy [5, 6]. Individuals with SPS may also exhibit elevated titers for secondary SPS markers, including antibodies against gamma-aminobutyric acid A receptor protein and the glycine-alpha 1 receptor. Testing for these other antibodies is recommended, particularly in individuals with low GAD65 and symptoms of

* Correspondence: jcris021@uottawa.ca
[1]Department of Neurology, University of Pennsylvania Perelman School of Medicine, Blockley Hall, 423 Guardian Drive, Office 829, Philadelphia, PA 19104, USA
[2]Department of Biostatistics, Epidemiology and Informatics, University of Pennsylvania Perelman School of Medicine, Blockley Hall, 423 Guardian Drive, Office 811, Philadelphia, PA 19104, USA
Full list of author information is available at the end of the article

SPS [2, 5, 7]. Paraneoplastic SPS, a non-classic form of the disease reported to occur in approximately 5% of cases [4], is most common among patients with breast cancer, followed by colon cancer and lung cancer.

During a 25-year period (1984–2008), the Mayo Clinic reported caring for approximately 4 distinct individuals with classic SPS annually, two thirds of whom were women [6]. It has also been reported that 119 unique cases of SPS were identified among the entire United Kingdom population between 2000 and 2005, which coincides with prior suggestions that the prevalence of SPS is approximately 1–2 cases per million individuals [8]. To date, onset, progression, and treatment of SPS is primarily described by case reports. There is therefore a paucity of population-based data on SPS hospitalizations and subsequent readmissions.

To increase knowledge of inpatient care for SPS, we used the 2014 Healthcare Cost and Utilization Project (HCUP) Nationwide Readmission Database to identify individuals hospitalized with SPS and assess their utilization of health services. Our primary objectives were to characterize inpatients with SPS and quantify their 30-day readmission rates. Awareness of primary causes of readmission and factors associated with acute readmission may contribute to improved discharged planning, outpatient follow-up, and health outcomes. Our secondary objectives were therefore to identify primary reasons for readmission within 30 days of hospital discharge and examine whether certain demographic, clinical, and care setting characteristics were associated with inpatient readmission.

Methods
Ethics statement
This study was exempt from research ethics board review since it involved secondary analyses of de-identified health claims data and complied with conditions outlined in the United States Agency for Healthcare Research and Quality's (AHRQ) Healthcare Cost and Utilization Project (HCUP) Data Use Agreement. The HCUP Data Use Agreement prohibits reporting of cell sizes ≤10; therefore, results were suppressed as appropriate.

Data source
This study was conducted using administrative health data from the 2014 Nationwide Readmissions Database (NRD). Sponsored by the AHRQ, the NRD is a family of databases developed as part of the HCUP to support national readmission analyses. Available data include health service utilization information for all health insurance payer categories in the United States, including the uninsured. The NRD contains detailed demographic (such as age, sex, and health insurance status), clinical (such as diagnoses, procedures, and length of stay), and hospital

data (such as bed size, location, and teaching status) that may be weighted to generate nationally representative estimates of hospitalizations and subsequent readmissions for individuals of all ages. Inpatients in NRD datasets may be tracked longitudinally within but not across calendar years or states.

Study population
The 2014 NRD was queried to identify index SPS encounters, which were defined as hospitalizations where an International Classification of Diseases, Ninth Revision (ICD-9) diagnosis code for SPS (333.91) was recorded as a primary or secondary diagnosis. Encounters where length of stay was undocumented or where the patient died were then excluded. It is not possible to track individuals in the NRD across state borders; therefore, index SPS encounters occurring outside of the patient's home state were excluded. To ensure that all hospital readmissions within 30 days of the index encounter could be identified, index SPS encounters discharged in the month of December were also excluded. In instances where patients had multiple eligible SPS index encounters, a single index encounter was randomly selected for our analyses.

Inpatient demographics, comorbidities, and hospital characteristics
Demographic and clinical data extracted from index SPS encounters included patient age, sex, health insurance payer category, patient median household income, length of stay, and discharge disposition. Comorbidities recorded during the index SPS hospitalizations were ascertained using the ICD-9 Elixhauser comorbidity measures, which were previously validated in administrative claim and electronic health record data [9, 10]. A pooled morbidity score was then computed by summing the number of prevalent comorbidities measures recorded during the index hospitalization. Hospital characterisitcs examined during index encounters included hospital size, control/ownership, and teaching status.

Readmissions
Eligible readmissions included all-cause elective or non-elective readmissions within 30 days of the index encounter discharge date. For patients readmitted to hospital within 30 days, time to readmission was calculated as the number of days separating the discharge date of the index encounter and the earliest hospital readmission date. Subsequent readmissions within the 30-day follow-up period were ignored.

Statistical analyses
Nationally representative estimates of SPS index event characteristics (demographic, clinical, and hospital) and

30-day readmission (rates, reasons, and time to readmission) were calculated using survey weighting methods and reported using descriptive statistics. Primary reasons for index hospitalization and 30-day readmission were grouped using the HCUP single-level Clinical Classifications Software [11], a classification scheme that enables individual ICD-9 codes to be categorized according to clinical similarities. The 10 most common reasons for index hospitalization and readmission were reported in order of decreasing prevalence, with readmissions further categorized according to care setting (readmission to the same or to a different hospital). To examine associations between demographic, clinical, and hospital characteristics and readmission within 30 days of the index SPS encounter discharge, we fitted weighted unconditional logistic regression models to estimate the crude odds of all-cause readmission to any hospital and to a different hospital. Due to the exploratory nature of this study, adjustments were not made for multiple comparisons. Statistical analyses were performed with SAS v9.4 (SAS Institute Inc., Cary, NC, USA).

Results

Cohort and hospital characteristics

There were 836 distinct individuals with a recorded diagnosis of SPS during a 2014 hospitalization. After applying study exclusion criteria, there were 703 hospitalized individuals with SPS who were discharged between January 1, 2014 and November 30, 2014 (Table 1). Our data were consistent with previously published descriptive epidemiological data on SPS. The majority of admitted patients were 40–59 years of age (46.1%) and few patients (15.8%) were younger than 40 years of age at admission. Mean patient age was 53.7 ± 0.9 (standard error) years. Nearly two thirds of admitted patients were female (63.9%) and the majority of patients were covered by publicly funded health insurance plans (63.9%), either Medicare (53.3%) or Medicaid (10.6%). Most patients were discharged from hospital within 7 days (70.5%) and under routine circumstances (63.6%). Hospitals where inpatient care was provided were frequently large (62.3%), private non-profit (71.1%), and metropolitan teaching hospitals (72.1%).

Based on HCUP single-level Clinical Classifications Software [11], "other hereditary and degenerative nervous system conditions" was the most frequently recorded group of primary reasons for index SPS hospitalization (29.5%), with nearly all (94.2%) admissions in this group attributable to SPS (Table 2). Other leading primary reasons for index hospitalization included 'diabetes complications' (5.1%), 'septicemia' (3.9%), 'other nervous system disorders' (3.7%), and 'spondylosis, intervertebral disc disorders, and other back problems' (2.4%).

Table 1 Demographics of SPS index hospitalizations, 2014

Characteristic	Index Events n (%) n = 703
Age	
< 40	111 (15.8)
40–49	138 (19.6)
50–59	186 (26.5)
60+	268 (38.1)
Sex	
Male	254 (36.1)
Female	450 (63.9)
Primary payer[a]	
Private insurance	232 (32.9)
Medicare	375 (53.3)
Medicaid	75 (10.6)
Median household income	
$66,000+	152 (21.6)
$51,000 - $65,999	154 (21.9)
$40,000 - $50,999	192 (27.4)
$1 - $39,999	200 (28.5)
Length of stay	
0–7 days	495 (70.5)
> 7 days	208 (29.5)
Discharge disposition[a]	
Routine	447 (63.6)
Transfer: short-term hospital	**
Transfer: other type of facility	106 (15.0)
Home health care	132 (18.8)
Comorbidities	
0–2	287 (40.8)
3–4	247 (35.1)
5+	170 (24.1)
Bed size of hospital	
Small	89 (12.6)
Medium	176 (25.0)
Large	438 (62.3)
Control/ownership of hospital[a]	
Private, not-for-profit	500 (71.1)
Private, investor-owned	96 (13.7)
Teaching status of hospital[a]	
Metropolitan teaching	507 (72.1)
Metropolitan non-teaching	150 (21.3)

[a]Some categories excluded due to small sample size
**10 or fewer observations – data suppressed

Table 2 The 10 most common primary reasons for SPS index hospitalization

All Index Encounters Reason for inpatient admission (n = 703)	n (%)
Other hereditary and degenerative nervous system conditions	207 (29.5)
Diabetes mellitus with complications	36 (5.1)
Septicemia	27 (3.9)
Other nervous system disorders	26 (3.7)
Spondylosis; intervertebral disc disorders; other back problems	17 (2.4)
Complication of device; implant or graft	16 (2.3)
Meningitis	15 (2.1)
Respiratory failure; insufficiency; arrest	12 (1.7)
Other gastrointestinal disorders	12 (1.7)
Epilepsy; convulsions	11 (1.6)

Table 3 The 10 most common primary reasons for readmission within 30 days of discharge – total and by readmission hospital

All Index Encounters Reason for Readmission (n = 66 / 703; Readmission Rate = 9.4%)	n (%)
Diabetes mellitus with complications	16 (24.2)
Other hereditary and degenerative nervous system conditions	**
Other nervous system disorders	**
Residual codes; unclassified	**
Complication of device; implant or graft	**
Other nutritional; endocrine; and metabolic disorders	**
Epilepsy; convulsions	**
Septicemia	**
Mood disorders	**
Fluid and electrolyte disorders	**

Index Encounters Readmitted to Same Hospital Reason for Readmission (n = 37 / 703; Readmission Rate = 5.3%)	n (%)
Other hereditary and degenerative nervous system conditions	**
Residual codes; unclassified	**
Complication of device; implant or graft	**
Other nutritional; endocrine; and metabolic disorders	**
Septicemia	**
Fluid and electrolyte disorders	**
Pneumonia	**
Other and unspecified benign neoplasm	**
Other connective tissue disease	**
Other fractures	**

Index Encounters Readmitted to Different Hospital++ Reason for Readmission (n = 29 / 703; Readmission Rate = 4.1%)	n (%)
Diabetes mellitus with complications	14 (49.6)
Epilepsy; convulsions	**
Peri-; endo-; and myocarditis; cardiomyopathy	**
Other nervous system disorders	**
Sickle cell anemia	**
Skin and subcutaneous tissue infections	**
Mood disorders	**

**10 or fewer observations – data suppressed
++Only 7 primary reasons for hospitalization within strata

Readmissions within 30 Days

There were 66 (9.4%) patients hospitalized with SPS who were readmitted for any cause within 30-days of index encounter discharge: 5.3% of them were readmitted to the same hospital and 4.1% were readmitted to a different hospital (Table 3). Readmissions were predominantly for 'diabetes with complications' (24.2%), SPS and 'other hereditary and degenerative nervous system conditions' (% suppressed), 'unclassified events' (% suppressed), and 'complication of devices; implants or grafts' (% suppressed). Median time to the first readmission within 30 days was 10.0 days (interquartile range (IQR): 5.4–20.9). The median time to first readmission to the same hospital was 12.2 days (IQR: 3.2–22.5), whereas it was 7.7 days (IQR: 7.1–11.9) for readmissions to different hospitals. Nearly all readmissions attributed to diabetes complications (87.5%) were to different hospitals than where index inpatient care was received. Diabetes complications accounted for approximately half (49.6%) of all readmissions to different hospitals. All patients in our sample readmitted for SPS were readmitted to the same hospital from which they were previously discharged.

Factors associated with hospital readmission

Relative to males, females had an increased odds of being readmitted within 30 days of inpatient discharge (odds ratio (OR), 3.29; 95% confidence interval (CI): 1.22–8.87) (Table 4). Compared to all other discharge types, patients discharged to home under routine circumstances were significantly less likely to be acutely readmitted to any (OR, 0.26; CI: 0.10–0.64) or different hospitals (OR, 0.18; CI: 0.04–0.89). Patients who received care at private, investor-owned hospitals were significantly more likely (OR, 10.87; CI: 2.03–58.25) to be acutely readmitted to a different hospital than those receiving care at other hospitals, including non-profit care

facilities (OR, 0.26; CI: 0.05–1.41). No other demographic, clinical, or hospital characteristic was associated with all-cause readmission within 30 days of discharge.

Discussion

Stiff person syndrome is a rare and progressive neurological disorder that if left untreated may contribute to

Table 4 Odds of readmission according to demographic, clinical, and care setting characteristics

Characteristic	Any Readmission		Readmission to Different Hospital	
	p-value[b]	OR	p-value[b]	OR
Age				
< 40	0.3284	Reference	0.3284	Reference
40–49		0.31 (0.09-1.12)		0.59 (0.08–4.53)
50–59		0.52 (0.18-1.48)		0.64 (0.10–3.99)
60+		0.69 (0.21-2.34)		1.51 (0.19–12.36)
Sex				
Male	0.0231	Reference	0.0231	Reference
Female		3.29 (1.22–8.87)*		2.57 (0.52–12.65)
Primary payer[a]				
Private insurance	0.0773	0.41 (0.15–1.13)	0.0773	0.29 (0.05–1.70)
Medicare	0.2300	1.81 (0.74–4.42)	0.2300	1.88 (0.38–9.23)
Medicaid	0.6354	1.33 (0.44–3.98)	0.6354	2.13 (0.41–11.18)
Median household income[a]				
$66,000+	0.5110	Reference	0.5110	Reference
$51,000 - $65,999		1.61 (0.48–5.33)		2.10 (0.18–24.30)
$40,000 - $50,999		0.95 (0.28–3.24)		0.89 (0.05–14.82)
$1 - $39,999		2.54 (0.66–9.77)		8.87 (0.81–96.73)
Length of stay				
0–7 days	0.3016	Reference	0.3016	Reference
> 7 days		1.59 (0.65–3.90)		0.88 (0.18–4.28)
Discharge disposition[a]				
Routine	0.0244	0.26 (0.10–0.64)**	0.0244	0.18 (0.04–0.89)*
Transfer: short-term hospital	0.4935	3.28 (0.34–31.36)	0.4935	8.38 (0.73–95.73)
Transfer: other type of facility	0.0848	2.40 (0.96–5.97)	0.0848	1.14 (0.23–5.74)
Home health care	0.2774	2.63 (0.75–9.18)	0.2774	4.66 (0.71–30.70)
Comorbidities				
0–2	0.6717	Reference	0.6717	Reference
3–4		0.81 (0.34–1.97)		0.65 (0.15–2.83)
5+		1.64 (0.46–5.83)		2.90 (0.43–19.70)
Bed size of hospital				
Small	0.4433	Reference	0.4433	Reference
Medium		3.28 (0.57–18.76)		4.06 (0.33–50.36)
Large		1.62 (0.37–7.13)		0.94 (0.11–8.05)
Control/ownership of hospitala				
Private, not-for-profit	0.8673	0.89 (0.24–3.33)	0.8673	0.26 (0.05–1.41)
Private, investor-owned	0.4248	2.44 (0.53–11.25)	0.4248	10.87 (2.03–58.25)**
Teaching status of hospitala				
Metropolitan teaching	0.5039	1.38 (0.53–3.57)	0.5039	1.75 (0.35–8.77)
Metropolitan non-teaching	0.8803	1.08 (0.42–2.79)	0.8803	0.83 (0.17–4.17)

Abbreviation: OR odds ratio
[a]Some categories excluded due to small sample size. [b]Chi-square test
**p < 0.01, *p < 0.05

significant patient disability and poor quality of life. Considerable advancements have been made in understanding SPS disease etiology, with strong evidence demonstrating that GAD65 antibodies may serve as an excellent diagnostic indicator and that patients with SPS are also often diagnosed with autoimmune disorders such as diabetes, hypothyroidism, and pernicious anemia [6, 12]. Despite the pathophysiology of classic SPS not being fully understood, research has shown that the disorder may be effectively treated using pharmacotherapies, ranging from antispasticity and γ-aminobutyric acid enhancing medications to the use of immunotherapies [4]. It is widely believed that SPS is underdiagnosed [4, 13]; however, much of the current knowledge about SPS epidemiology and healthcare utilization originate from case studies and small observational studies, making it difficult to precisely estimate disease burden and health system impacts. Using NRD data, we identified more than 700 individuals who were admitted to hospital with SPS and discharged alive between January and November 2014 for the purposes of characterizing their inpatient care and readmissions within 30 days of hospital discharge. Our primary findings were that individuals with SPS are often admitted to hospital as a result of SPS and diabetes complications, and that acute readmissions among individuals with SPS are relatively common. Secondary findings include: (1) readmissions within 30 days were largely due to diabetes complications, (2) nearly all readmissions attributed to diabetes complications were to different hospitals, (3) female sex and receipt of care at private, investor-owned hospitals was associated with increased odds of being acutely readmitted and acutely readmitted to a different hospital, respectively, and (4) being discharged under routine circumstances (such as to home or self-care) was associated with decreased odds of being readmitted within 30 days. To our knowledge, this is the largest nationally representative study of SPS, which provides timely and much needed data on the epidemiology and inpatient care for this orphan disorder.

Published studies regularly report the prevalence of SPS to range from 0.5 to 2 cases per million habitants [3, 8, 14, 15]; however, to date, few population-based studies have actually been conducted to estimate the true burden of SPS [8, 13, 14]. Between 2000 and 2015, the British Neurological Surveillance Unit identified 119 individuals with SPS from the United Kingdom, suggesting a disease prevalence of 1–2 cases per million people [8]. More recently, the first reported epidemiological study of SPS in Sub-Saharan Africa estimated SPS prevalence to be 0.9 cases per 1,000,000 individuals living in the Kilimanjaro region [14]. These prevalence estimates are conservative compared to the 20 cases that were identified from a population of 2 to 3 million in the areas surrounding Heidelberg, Germany over a period of 10 years, which highlight population risk differences and

the likely underdiagnosis of SPS [13]. Our finding that 703 individuals with SPS were hospitalized between January and November 2014 in the United States suggests that the true prevalence of SPS in North America may exceed 2 cases per million habitants, which coincides with expert opinion that SPS may not be as rare as previously thought [4]. There are conflicting reports regarding SPS prevalence by sex, with some studies reporting that the disorder equally affects men and women [16] and others finding that SPS disproportionally affects women [6, 17] and men [14]. Our predominantly female (63.9%) cohort supports prior reports that nearly two thirds of SPS patients are women [6, 17]. However, it is important to acknowledge that observed sex differences in SPS prevalence may reflect underlying differences in population disease risk or health behaviors, and that additional studies are required to characterize populations at greatest risk of SPS.

Our finding that SPS and diabetes complications were the most common reasons for index hospitalization reaffirms the association and autoimmune link between SPS and type 1 diabetes (30–50% of all SPS patients are reported to have type 1 diabetes and the majority of SPS patients have elevated titer antibodies against GAD) [8, 18–20]. It is possible that acute readmissions in SPS result from planned specialty care, such as admission for intravenous immunoglobulin or plasmapheresis immunotherapies at academic medical centers, or gaps in discharge planning. However, our findings that diabetes complications were the largest driver of re-hospitalization within 30 days of inpatient discharge and that such readmissions were almost always to different hospitals suggest that these SPS readmissions resulted from medical emergencies, possibly diabetic ketoacidosis. Such emergencies have been widely reported among patients with both SPS and diabetes, and would cause individuals to seek medical care at their closest hospital [21–23].

Patients with SPS and diabetes are at risk of diabetic ketoacidosis, a preventable life-threatening condition that often leads to hospitalization [24, 25]. This raises the important question about whether a proportion of readmissions in SPS are avoidable. A recent 5-year retrospective study of 367 patients at a United States tertiary academic medical center identified history of depression or substance/alcohol abuse, and self-pay/publicly funded insurance as significant independent predictors of readmission for diabetic ketoacidosis [24]. Authors propose that readmissions for diabetes complications may be avoided by providing target interventions, including tighter glycemic control, to patients classified as high risk for recurrent diabetic ketoacidosis according to an objective scoring systems based on established risk factors [24]. Implementation of such interventions when treating inpatients with SPS and comorbid diabetes may directly translate into significant cost savings for healthcare systems, including a reduction in readmission penalties for neurology services where SPS are routinely admitted, as well as improved health outcomes and quality of life for patients.

Female sex ($p > 0.01$) and receipt of care for SPS at private, investor-owned hospitals ($p < 0.01$) were the only independent predictors that we found to be positively associated with readmission within 30 days of discharge. Small samples sizes in compared groups contributed to uncertainty around parameter estimates for examined associations, which precludes making any assertions regarding the association of these factors with readmissions in SPS. Nevertheless, these findings provide useful benchmark data for future studies that examine whether readmissions in SPS are preventable. Relative to other discharge dispositions, we found that individuals discharged under routine circumstances had decreased odds of being acutely readmitted within 30 days, including to different hospitals. This was likely attributable to this subpopulation having fewer comorbid conditions and being younger than those discharged to other facilities and with increased healthcare needs.

There are numerous strengths to our study. We used a large, nationally representative dataset of inpatient care that included longitudinal follow-up data on readmissions occurring within the same calendar year. Using these data and survey weighting methods, we were able to precisely estimate and describe annual inpatient care for SPS from a population of more than 300 million individuals. In-depth data on demographic, clinical, and hospital characteristics allowed us to describe the population with SPS that is most commonly admitted to hospital, including their primary causes of hospitalization and re-hospitalization, and factors associated with acute readmission. Inpatient care was most often received at large (62.3%) metropolitan teaching (72.1%) hospitals that are neurologist-rich and presumed leaders in adhering to best clinical practices and in leveraging advances in knowledge to improve disease diagnosis and treatment efficiencies. As such, it is likely that suspected SPS diagnoses made at these hospitals were confirmed using validated SPS diagnostic criteria and serum anti-GAD antibody testing [4, 26].

Notwithstanding our study's strengths, certain limitations should be considered when interpreting our findings. Small sample sizes precluded the reporting of most rates of primary cause of readmission and hindered us from completing adequate multivariable modeling and controlling for potential sources of confounding in our crude estimates. Study data did not permit longitudinal follow-up for individuals admitted or transferred to out-of-state hospitals, which likely resulted in our underestimation of the true number of index SPS hospitalizations. Despite these limitations, our study highlights the relatively large number of individuals, mainly women, living in the United States who

are hospitalized in a given year with SPS, and is the largest epidemiological study to characterize inpatient care and health service utilization by this population. Despite many inpatients receiving care at large, metropolitan teaching hospitals, laboratory anti-GAD antibody testing and prior medical history data were unavailable and therefore could not be used in our selection of index SPS cases, leading to possible misclassification of SPS diagnoses. Since the rarity of SPS may lead to the disorder being over- or under-diagnosed in clinical practice, it is possible that a portion of hospitalized individuals identified as having SPS in our study did not actually have SPS and that some true cases of SPS were omitted from our study cohort. Taken together, study limitations preclude us from definitively knowing the true number of SPS cases included in our study cohort or the number of cases that went undetected. Nevertheless, the demographics of our study population are consistent with those reported by other studies of SPS in the United States [6, 20].

Conclusions

In summary, using a large nationally representative readmission database from the United States, we found that readmissions in SPS are relatively common and may be attributed to complications of the disorder or associated comorbidities such as diabetes. Acute readmissions to different hospitals may result from unavoidable medical emergencies in the outpatient setting; however, may also result from planned specialty care or gaps in discharge planning. Study replication using other available health data is warranted; however, our preliminary estimates of disease burden suggest that the true prevalence of SPS may be higher than previously thought. Future studies that examine the extent to which readmissions in SPS may be prevented are required.

Abbreviations

AHRQ: Agency for Healthcare Research and Quality; CI: confidence interval; GAD: glutamic acid decarboxylase; HCUP: Healthcare Cost and Utilization Project; ICD-9: International Classification of Diseases, Ninth Revision; IQR: interquartile range; NRD: Nationwide Readmissions Database; OR: odds ratio; SPS: Stiff person syndrome

Acknowledgements

We thank Mr. Derrick Tam and Dr. Dominique Ansell for proofreading the final version of our manuscript and recommending editorial changes.

Funding

This study was supported by grants from the University of Pennsylvania Parkinson Disease and Movement Disorders Center.

Authors' contributions

All authors have read and actively contributed to the manuscript, and agree to its publication. (1) Research Project: A. Conception, B. Organization, C. Execution; (2) Statistical Analysis: A. Design, B. Execution, C. Review and Critique; (3) Manuscript Preparation: A. Writing of the First Draft, B. Review and Critique.

JAGC: 1A, 1B, 1C, 2A, 2B, 3A. AWW: 1A, 1B, 1C, 2A, 2C, 3B. DPT: 1B, 1C, 2A, 2B, 2C, 3B.YF: 1B, 2C, 3B. All authors read and approved the final manuscript.

Competing interests
The authors have no competing interest to declare.

Author details
[1]Department of Neurology, University of Pennsylvania Perelman School of Medicine, Blockley Hall, 423 Guardian Drive, Office 829, Philadelphia, PA 19104, USA. [2]Department of Biostatistics, Epidemiology and Informatics, University of Pennsylvania Perelman School of Medicine, Blockley Hall, 423 Guardian Drive, Office 811, Philadelphia, PA 19104, USA. [3]Department of Neurology Translational Center of Excellence for Neuroepidemiology and Neurological Outcomes Research, University of Pennsylvania Perelman School of Medicine, Philadelphia, PA, USA. [4]McLaughlin Centre for Population Health Risk Assessment & Interdisciplinary School of Health Science, Faculty of Health Sciences, University of Ottawa, 850 Peter Morand Crescent, Room 119, Ottawa, ON K1G 3Z7, Canada. [5]Center for Clinical Epidemiology and Biostatistics, University of Pennsylvania Perelman School of Medicine, Blockley Hall, 423 Guardian Drive, Office, Philadelphia, PA 19104, USA.

References
1. Moersch FP, Woltman HW. Progressive fluctuating muscular rigidity and spasm ("stiff-man" syndrome); report of a case and some observations in 13 other cases. Proc Staff Meet Mayo Clin. 1956;31:421–7.
2. Balint B, Bhatia KP. Stiff person syndrome and other immune-mediated movement disorders - new insights. Curr Opin Neurol. 2016;29:496–506.
3. Bhatti AB, Gazali ZA. Recent advances and review on treatment of stiff person syndrome in adults and pediatric patients. Cureus. 2015;7:e427.
4. Dalakas MC. Stiff person syndrome: advances in pathogenesis and therapeutic interventions. Curr Treat Options Neurol. 2009;11:102–10.
5. Baizabal-Carvallo JF, Jankovic J. Stiff-person syndrome: insights into a complex autoimmune disorder. J Neurol Neurosurg Psychiatry. 2015;86:840–8.
6. McKeon A, Robinson MT, McEvoy KM, Matsumoto JY, Lennon VA, Ahlskog JE, Pittock SJ. Stiff-man syndrome and variants: clinical course, treatments, and outcomes. Arch Neurol. 2012;69:230–8.
7. Hinson SR, Lopez-Chiriboga AS, Bower JH, Matsumoto JY, Hassan A, Basal E, Lennon VA, Pittock SJ, McKeon A. Glycine receptor modulating antibody predicting treatable stiff-person spectrum disorders. Neurol Neuroimmunol Neuroinflamm. 2018;5:e438.
8. Hadavi S, Noyce AJ, Leslie RD, Giovannoni G. Stiff person syndrome. Pract Neurol. 2011;11:272–82.
9. Quan H, Sundararajan V, Halfon P, Fong A, Burnand B, Luthi JC, Saunders LD, Beck CA, Feasby TE, Ghali WA. Coding algorithms for defining comorbidities in ICD-9-CM and ICD-10 administrative data. Med Care. 2005; 43:1130–9.
10. Fortin Y, Crispo JA, Cohen D, McNair DS, Mattison DR, Krewski D. External validation and comparison of two variants of the Elixhauser comorbidity measures for all-cause mortality. PLoS One. 2017;12:e0174379.
11. HCUP Clinical Classifications Software (CCS). Healthcare Cost and Utilization Project (HCUP). U.S. Agency for Healthcare Research and Quality R, MD. Updated March 2017. http://www.hcup-us.ahrq.gov/toolssoftware/ccs/ccs. jsp. Accessed August 21, 2017.
12. Pagano MB, Murinson BB, Tobian AA, King KE. Efficacy of therapeutic plasma exchange for treatment of stiff-person syndrome. Transfusion. 2014;54:1851–6.
13. Meinck HM, Thompson PD. Stiff man syndrome and related conditions. Mov Disord. 2002;17:853–66.
14. Dekker MC, Urasa SJ, Kinabo G, Maro V, Howlett WP. A report of stiff person syndrome in Tanzania with first epidemiological figures for sub-Saharan Africa. Neuroepidemiology. 2015;45:109–10.
15. Kumar MV, Savida P. Pediatric stiff-person syndrome with renal failure. J Neurosci Rural Pract. 2016;7:147–9.
16. Toro C, Jacobowitz DM, Hallett M. Stiff-man syndrome. Semin Neurol. 1994; 14:154–8.
17. Dalakas MC, Fujii M, Li M, McElroy B. The clinical spectrum of anti-GAD antibody-positive patients with stiff-person syndrome. Neurology. 2000;55: 1531–5.
18. Atkinson MA. The $64000 question in diabetes continues. Lancet. 2000;356: 4–6.
19. Murinson BB, Butler M, Marfurt K, Gleason S, De Camilli P, Solimena M. Markedly elevated GAD antibodies in SPS: effects of age and illness duration. Neurology. 2004;63:2146–8.
20. Martinez-Hernandez E, Arino H, McKeon A, Iizuka T, Titulaer MJ, Simabukuro MM, Lancaster E, Petit-Pedrol M, Planaguma J, Blanco Y, et al. Clinical and immunologic investigations in patients with stiff-person Spectrum disorder. JAMA Neurol. 2016;73:714–20.
21. Hirsch IB, D'Alessio D, Eng L, Davis C, Lernmark A, Chait A. Severe insulin resistance in a patient with type 1 diabetes and stiff-man syndrome treated with insulin lispro. Diabetes Res Clin Pract. 1998;41:197–202.
22. Enuh H, Park M, Ghodasara A, Arsura E, Nfonoyim J. Stiff man syndrome: a diagnostic dilemma in a young female with diabetes mellitus and thyroiditis. Clin Med Insights Case Rep. 2014;7:139–41.
23. Egwuonwu S, Chedebeau F. Stiff-person syndrome: a case report and review of the literature. J Natl Med Assoc. 2010;102:1261–3.
24. Bradford AL, Crider CC, Xu X, Naqvi SH. Predictors of recurrent hospital admission for patients presenting with diabetic ketoacidosis and hyperglycemic hyperosmolar state. J Clin Med Res. 2017;9:35–9.
25. Dungan KM. The effect of diabetes on hospital readmissions. J Diabetes Sci Technol. 2012;6:1045–52.
26. Sarva H, Deik A, Ullah A, Severt WL. Clinical Spectrum of stiff person syndrome: a review of recent reports. Tremor Other Hyperkinet Mov (N Y). 2016;6:340.

29

Presentation and care of a family with Huntington disease in a resource-limited community

Jarmal Charles[1†], Lindyann Lessey[1†], Jennifer Rooney[1†], Ingmar Prokop[1], Katherine Yearwood[1], Hazel Da Breo[1], Patrick Rooney[1], Ruth H. Walker[2,3] and Andrew K. Sobering[1*]

Abstract

Background: In high-income countries patients with Huntington disease (HD) typically present to healthcare providers after developing involuntary movements, or for pre-symptomatic genetic testing if at familial risk. A positive family history is a major guide when considering the decision to perform genetic testing for HD, both in affected and unaffected patients. Management of HD is focused upon control of symptoms, whether motor, cognitive, or psychiatric. There is no clear evidence to date of any disease-modifying agents. Referral of families and caregivers for psychological and social support, whether to HD-focused centers, or through virtual communities, is viewed as an important consequence of diagnosis. The experience of healthcare for such progressive neurodegenerative diseases in low- and middle-income nations is in stark contrast with the standard of care in high-income countries.

Methods: An extended family with many members affected with an autosomal dominantly inherited movement disorder came to medical attention when one family member presented following a fall. Apart from one family member who was taking a benzodiazepine for involuntary movements, no other affected family members had sought medical attention. Members of this family live on several resource-limited Caribbean islands. Care of the chronically ill is often the responsibility of the family, and access to specialty care is difficult to obtain, or is unavailable. Computed tomography scan of one patient's brain revealed severe caudate atrophy and moderate generalized cortical atrophy. Genetic diagnosis of HD was obtained.

Results: Through family recollection and by direct observation we identified four generations of individuals affected with HD. Outreach programs and collaborations helped to provide medical imaging and genetic diagnosis. Additionally these efforts helped with patient and family support, education, and genetic counseling to many members of this family.

Conclusions: Affected members of this family have limited healthcare access, and rely heavily on family support for care. Genetic and clinical diagnosis of these patients was impeded by lack of resources and lack of access to specialty care. Importantly, obtaining a definitive diagnosis has had a positive impact for this family by facilitating genetic counseling, education, community outreach, and dispelling myths regarding this hereditary disease and its progression.

Keywords: Huntington disease, Trinucleotide repeat disorder, Anticipation, Cultural competency, Resource-limited community

* Correspondence: drsobering@gmail.com
†Equal contributors
[1]New York, USA
Full list of author information is available at the end of the article

Background

Huntington disease

Huntington disease (HD) is a neurodegenerative disorder typically of adult onset, thus affected individuals typically have children before symptom manifestation. Chorea and psychiatric symptoms are typical, however, language and memory of past events may remain intact in many patients [1, 2]. In late stages patients typically require increased care as they shift from their hyperkinetic chorea state, to a rigid hypokinetic phenotype [3], leading to an increased risk for depression among caregivers due to the stress associated with care for HD patients [4].

HD is an autosomal dominant neurological disorder caused by an expanded tandem array (>35 repeats) of CAG codons within exon 1 of the *HTT* gene [5, 6]. Intermediate repeats (26–35 repeats) are termed premutations, which have the potential to expand into the pathogenic allele during gametogenesis [7, 8]. An inverse relationship exists between repeat number and onset age of symptoms. The CAG repeat length tends to expand as the trait is passed down through inheritance, accounting for the earlier onset of symptoms in successive generations, known as anticipation. Largest expansions occur through male meiosis [9]. Many reviews describing HD exist, see [10, 11] for recent summaries.

Presymptomatic genetic diagnosis may inform at-risk individuals of their future disease state [12, 13]. There is considerable debate regarding the impact of advance knowledge of a future disease such as HD, as a positive result leads to increased risk for depression and suicide [14]. When presymptomatic testing for HD first became available, it was incorrectly predicted that the majority of at-risk individuals would want to know if they had the pathogenic mutation [15]. Different studies place the actual range of test use by at-risk individuals to be in the range of 12 to 25% [16, 17]. Indeed, most individuals who are at-risk for HD opt not to pursue genetic testing [18].

Care of the HD patient in a resource-limited community

Care of a patient with HD is challenging regardless of the location and ideally should incorporate support from both public and charitable agencies [19]. Caregivers of patients with ongoing chronic disease experience stress, increasing their risk for depression due to the constant demands associated with caring for their affected loved ones. This stress is often compounded in low socio-economic status (SES) communities where healthcare systems are underfunded and not well developed [20, 21].

In this paper, we describe an extended family with many members affected with HD. The difficulties involved with care of these patients is compounded by their low SES status; barriers to access specialty, and even non-specialty, medical care; and the geographical isolation created by living on a small island nation. Apart from the initial presentation of the proband at the general hospital, all evaluations were performed on home visits which were welcomed by the patients and families. To our knowledge, this is the first report of genetically-confirmed HD in the West Indies, although three families of various ethnic backgrounds in Trinidad with clinically-diagnosed HD were reported more than 50 years ago [22]. In the broadly defined Caribbean region, the only reported genetically diagnosed cases of HD have come out of Cuba [23], and there appears to be a significant number of HD cases currently being studied in Puerto Rico (Sylvette Ayala Torres, PhD, University of Puerto Rico, and Zoé Cruz-Gil, President, Fundación Huntington Puerto Rico, personal communication). Examples of other genetic movement disorders diagnosed in the West Indies include the Huntington disease-like disorders [24], and cases of spinocerebellar ataxia [25]. Many other autosomal dominant chorea disorders are known and described in this recent comprehensive review [26].

Location

This study was approved by a local IRB which is registered with the United States National Institutes of Health: patients gave consent for medical interviews, neurologic examination, photographs, videotaping, genetic testing, and documentation of family history. To protect privacy, we will not identify the precise location of the family or the Caribbean affiliation of the authors of this manuscript. The International Monetary Fund World Economic Outlook describes this country as an emerging market with a developing economy, ranking it in the lowest 10th percentile for gross domestic product with individual income at approximately $US 8000 per capita [27]. Major sources of employment are found in tourism, fishing, agriculture, and construction. For most of the population, nutrition is good, due to ready availability of fruit, vegetables, livestock, the local fishing industry, and imported food.

Medical care is provided at a local hospital, community health centers and privately practicing physicians. The community health centers provide general health care such as medications, blood pressure testing, wound care and dressings. The centers treat medical emergencies, acute situations, and provide advice regarding preventive care for conditions such as diabetes and hypertension. Importantly, medical care for ongoing or chronic illnesses such as HD is either nonexistent or difficult to obtain. In the general hospital neurological cases are typically referred to internal medicine (generalist) or, the patient must fly off-island because the community does not have a full-time practicing neurologist. In many cases, costs of medical care are covered by the government. However, patients must pay for the majority of prescription drugs, all non-urgent testing, and imaging that is not part of hospital admission. English is the official language of these islands; however many people of the native population speak in local dialect. The evaluating physicians are not native to the island, but have spent up to 25 years practicing in the community (>75 years combined) and are fluent in the dialect. The affected patients described in this report, as well as a significant percentage of the population, live in small, wooden, single-story buildings. Electricity and running water are found in most households but might be considered more basic compared to US or UK communities; many roads are unpaved or in a state of poor repair.

Methods and Results
An overview of the family
During his initial medical evaluation and interview, the index case (III-18) described a number of other members of his extended family who also had a movement disorder. These other affected family members were sought out and three of those affected and many unaffected relatives agreed to be interviewed and examined. Based on their reported histories a detailed pedigree of the extended family was constructed (Fig. 1). All interviewed family members were asked about the possibility that they had Venezuelan heritage due to the high HD incidence in the Lake Maracaibo region [5] but we were unable to establish a connection. We note that individuals represented on this pedigree are now living on several different Caribbean islands, and also in the United States.

All affected individuals gave a similar history regarding their movement disorder in which control of their muscles seemed normal throughout childhood and early adulthood. All reported that their loss of muscle control developed at about 35 years of age. This was corroborated by unaffected family members as they recalled memories of their affected relations. During our

interviews, the affected individuals appeared euthymic and did not exhibit frank psychiatric symptoms. They were conversant and we judged them to be using language appropriate for their level of education. Initially HD was presumed to be an unlikely diagnosis. This was based upon the apparent absence of cognitive or psychiatric impairment or lack of higher cerebral functions, and also that all family members agreed that the onset of chorea occurred at a similar age.

Patient III-18
The index case was an approximately 50-year-old man who presented to the General Hospital. He had sustained a minor head injury and lacerations to the right side of his face and right arm as a result of falling while walking in the street. The patient had obvious chorea of his head and all four limbs which he said had caused him to fall. The patient insisted that falling in the street was unusual as he had learned how to live with his abnormal movements over the preceding ~20 years, and that despite his movement disorder he was usually able to maintain his balance.

The patient had been an accomplished athlete in his youth and hoped to pursue a career as a professional golfer. These aspirations were abandoned with the onset of his involuntary movements. At the time of presentation, the patient was gainfully employed as a gardener and enjoyed fishing. There was no evidence of a deterioration of performance in either work or hobbies, such as impaired ability to organize and perform specific tasks.

Cranial nerve examination revealed no abnormality apart from mild chorea of his face and his tongue. Speech was normal. His head and all four limbs displayed marked chorea. Tone was mildly reduced, and deep tendon reflexes were normal. Sensory examination was normal, and there was no evidence of cerebellar dysfunction.

The patient appeared to be oriented in time, place, and person. Based on his ability to interact and hold a

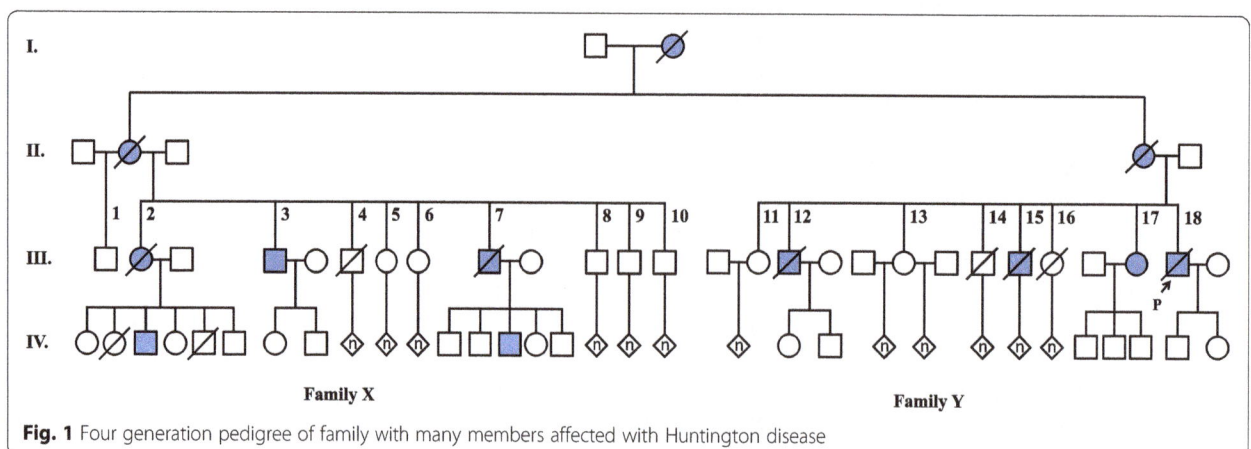

Fig. 1 Four generation pedigree of family with many members affected with Huntington disease

conversation, his cognitive skills appeared consistent with his seventh grade education. This impression was supported by his physical presentation (personal hygiene, clothing), mood, language usage, and his ability to give an apparently appropriate detailed medical history, however, formal cognitive testing was not performed. Since the patient appeared stable, and a formal psychological testing battery was not available at this time, we did not pursue further cognitive investigations. The patient died within a year of this evaluation; the cause of death remains unknown.

Patient III-17

This woman was examined initially at the age of approximately 48 years. She claimed to have developed involuntary movements approximately 12 years previously. Initially the family reported that there were no personality changes or psychiatric symptoms and her three children thought of her as a cornerstone of the family. She was regarded as a reliable, stalwart person, who could be counted on for counsel and wisdom.

On initial examination this patient had generalized chorea. Speech was fluent and not dysarthric. She was well-related, appeared to have generally high spirits, and was conversant. She was able to provide many details of the family tree, including her eight siblings and her eight cousins (the "X" family in the pedigree). Her memory appeared to be as good as, if not better than that of her unaffected relatives.

On follow-up two years later, her chorea had progressed and was so severe that it impaired her ability to perform ADLs. One year later it was clear upon casual conversation that her cognition had deteriorated. By the next year she was almost completely bedridden and markedly cachectic. She was alert and responsive but she spent most of her time lying on a mattress on the floor. She had moderately dysarthric speech, and was able to count from 1 to 10 forwards and backwards. She reported that three of her children were affected with the same movement disorder that she had, which was not accurate. She could perform simple tasks, such as finger-to-nose testing, accurately, but tended to perseverate. Power was intact in all limbs, and tone was normal. Deep tendon reflexes were increased throughout. Toes were downgoing. It was not possible to examine her eye movements due to neck chorea. She was able to push herself up to sit and stand alone, but with markedly impaired balance and required assistance for almost all ADL. She was prescribed lorazepam 1 mg b.i.d. from her family physician, which somewhat reduced the involuntary movements. We are currently considering further pharmacological strategies to control the involuntary movements, however, this is challenging due to the lack

of ongoing neurologist support and difficulty accessing medications.

Patient III-7

This patient had been employed as a caddy at the local golf course. He was well known by many in the community where most described him as a respectable, punctual, and kind person who was never talkative. On initial evaluation when he was approximately 46-years-old, he had mild chorea affecting his upper limbs and face, he was coherent and able to have a relatively normal conversation with respect to his normal non-verbal personality. On follow-up, three years later he had become severely rigid and hypokinetic, and was completely dependent for all ADLs. Even though he was always known to be reticent, by one year later he had ceased all efforts to verbally communicate and appeared apathetic.

On examination he was lethargic but arousable and somewhat attentive. With repeated questioning he would respond with one-word answers. Speech was moderately dysarthric. He was able to name his caregiver (his daughter-in-law), although he could not state her relationship to him. He was able to obey some, but not all, simple commands. He was unable to volitionally open his eyes, but actively resisted opening of his eyes by the examiner, with a Bell's phenomenon. Tone was increased throughout, and deep tendon reflexes were brisk, with downgoing toes. Both arms were held in flexion with dystonic extension of some fingers. He was unable to extend his arms to perform finger-to-nose testing. He was unable to sit without assistance. He was severely cachectic with marked difficulty with eating and swallowing. A video showing this examination may be accessed via Additional file 1: Movie S1. Shortly after this last evaluation he was brought by his family to hospital for progressive deterioration, and subsequently died, although the cause was not determined.

Brain CT scan performed approximately six months prior to death revealed marked atrophy of the caudate nucleus and putamen (Fig. 2). A Mini Mental State Examination (MMSE) was performed, modified by the examiner to fit the cultural norms of the patient [28]. The patient was unable to proceed past the third question, and of the seven separate parts of those first three questions, he only scored one correct. Concerned that the patient might not feel at ease with the formal nature of the MMSE questions, the examiner attempted to engage him in conversation around his personal life and experiences. These impromptu, personalized and culture specific questions were directed towards determining the same five levels as the MMSE; orientation, registration, attention, recall and language. Once again, the patient's responses suggested a poor level of cognitive functioning. During evaluation of this patient, we learned from another

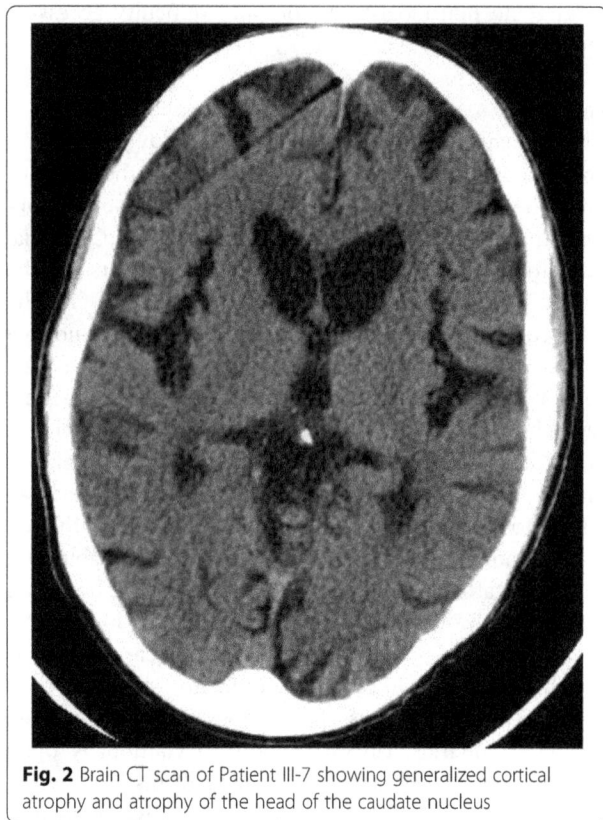

Fig. 2 Brain CT scan of Patient III-7 showing generalized cortical atrophy and atrophy of the head of the caudate nucleus

family member that when the patient first began showing movement disorder symptoms he would arrive for work at 4:00 a.m. rather than 6:30 a.m. This reported behavior is consistent with cognitive decline, specifically executive dysfunction affecting planning and decision-making [29].

Based on the family history, the phenotype of the affected family members, the CT scan, and the observed cognitive decline, we sought genetic testing to diagnose the disorder. Prior to offering the genetic test we counseled several members of the family about HD, including a discussion of possible outcomes and Mendelian genetic risk. We obtained genetic testing for HD (Neurodiagnostics Lab at Harvard Medical School) which revealed a pathogenically expanded trinucleotide repeat expansion of 47 repeats in one of the *HTT* alleles, and 17 repeats in the other.

Discussion

The Caribbean island where this family was identified is small and resource-limited. Its economy is in a state of development and is based mainly on tourism. Because of financial limitations, medical service on the island is primarily focused on acute medical care, and attention to patients with chronic conditions lags behind that provided by most Western nations. While the island is home to physicians trained in reputable institutions world-wide, the opportunity for specialization is limited due to the small economy and population.

Without exception, all members of this extended family who we spoke to understood that there was an illness that tended to affect them. However, as far as we are aware, only one patient had ever sought medical attention for treatment and no family member had access to diagnostic services. Many of the adult children of affected subjects expected to inevitably develop the illness as they entered their mid-30s. We attempted to correct this misconception, and to educate members of this family about the Mendelian risk associated with autosomal dominant inheritance. This included the implications of delayed age of onset and how recurrence risk might be estimated in the grandchild of an affected family member.

Over several generations, reports from family members consistently suggested that age of symptom onset was occurring when the affected person was in their mid-30s. This stability might be attributed to the preponderance of maternal inheritance of the preceding generations. In the current generation we have now identified an affected individual in his mid-twenties who received the HD mutation paternally. This patient has not been formally evaluated by a neurologist. Variation of onset age due to paternal transmission of the HD trait is consistent with previous observations [9].

Affected subjects were taken care of in their homes by their family members. This mode of care is consistent with the level of medical care for many other chronic conditions in this environment. While patients with medically urgent conditions receive reasonable care, illnesses which are longstanding do not receive the same level of attention. Investigations such as imaging and laboratory tests have to be paid for by patients or their families. Genetic testing is not available locally. In this case, funds for the CT scan and genetic testing were raised by community outreach projects and fundraising events.

Initially, cognitive or psychiatric impairment was not apparent in the patients who were evaluated, and impairment was not noticed or reported by family members. For these reasons, HD was at first not in the differential diagnosis. Cognitive decline was not apparent to us until approximately three years passed from our initial contact with the affected individuals. Additionally, all of the patients terminated their education in their early teenage years, and their employment did not depend upon a high level of cognitive functioning. Because of the above, we had difficulty ascertaining cognitive decline. Additionally, subject III-17, who had marked chorea, was able to give extensive information about her family history going back three generations. Although it is difficult to validate her account, her recall of family lineage appeared to be excellent, and exceeded that of several other members of her family who were unaffected. The extensive family history provided by this patient led us to believe that her cognition was intact. This observation is consistent with reports that in some cases, patients with chorea tend to have less severe cognitive impairment [30] and that older memories tend to persist better then recent [31]. It is also possible that the index case and the two other affected members of the family who were encountered by the investigators were those members whose higher cognitive functions were least impaired, and who were able to maintain employment and other social interactions for a prolonged period despite their movement disorder.

Cultural differences may have also played a role in the ability of the authors to diagnose mood and cognitive status of the patients. Although some were raised in the West Indies or have spent considerable time on the island, the clinical investigators of this case are either of European descent or from developed nations. All the patients are of African descent and were raised in a small country with a developing economy. A dramatic disparity of SES exists between the investigators and these patients; these dynamics foster changes in the doctor-patient relationship to which both clinicians and patients are accustomed [32]. Traditional values are also important when considering neurological disorders involving involuntary movements and cognition changes. Examples can be found where HD patients and families on the border of Mexico and Texas had initially sought treatment from traditional faith healers because of perceived possession [33]. Most members of this West Indian family hold strong Christian religious values, and it is possible that without a medical reason to explain the condition, there was an unconscious withholding of information pointing to cognitive issues.

A hallmark of HD is onset of mood changes, psychosis, and suicidal thoughts prior to the presentation of the movement disorder. Due to local social conventions, it is possible that these patients and their families would not recognize, or would minimize, reports of mood changes, depression, or suicidal thoughts. Although directly asked about suicidal thoughts and depression, answers might not be forthcoming unless the question is framed within a precise social context, or possibly even by the correct person, and not by a clinician. It is also known that people with HD have limited insight into the extent and nature of both their movement disorder and their psychological impairment [34, 35]. An additional possibility is that both affected and unaffected family members perceived the illness within the context of the family lore, and ignored features which were inconsistent with this. The possibility exists that they may not have wanted to admit to depression for fear that the local stigma attached to mood disorders would render them ineligible for further help. Consistent with this were

numerous reports of cognitive impairment in the affected individuals from various family members that were revealed only after the definitive diagnosis of HD was obtained. These observations included reports of sleep disturbances, paranoia, disorganization and asocial behavior that occurred at some point during the disease progression.

Following the confirmation of HD in patient III-7, several unaffected family members were informed of the diagnosis, and provided with information such as genetic features and age of onset. The response was uniformly positive, and it transpired that some had heard of HD, and this diagnosis had been discussed, although never confirmed. Even in the absence of further testing, unaffected children of affected subjects were reassured to learn that their chances of inheritance were 50:50, and that they couldn't be affected "just a little bit". Children of unaffected family members were reassured to learn that they would not develop the illness if their parent had not developed symptoms during a normal life span.

We were also able to discuss a misperception among members of the family regarding inheritance. At issue is the incorrect belief that a parent who is symptomatic during procreation or pregnancy might "cause" the trait to be passed on to her offspring. Since obtaining a definitive diagnosis, we have worked towards dispelling this myth, and to instead provide information regarding inheritance and progression of the disorder. Other at-risk individuals spoke of the disorder as being a "curse" that affects some members of the family. The idea of a curse is different from, but has parallels with how some cancer patients understand their disease [36]. Since many family members have internet access we were also able to direct family members to the appropriate on-line resources relevant to HD.

Until disease-modifying interventions for HD are identified, it could be argued that there is little benefit to confirming the diagnosis in subjects who are already affected in this population or in at-risk family members. Even when genetic diagnosis is available, many at-risk subjects choose not to learn of their carrier status. However, several family members studied here have expressed interest in learning of their carrier status and we are involved in discussions regarding the implications of presymptomatic diagnosis. This highlights the importance of cultural competency when discussing HD with at-risk individuals. The best way to discuss disorders such as HD with patients and their families in the West Indian region is currently an open question. In fact, there may not be a best practice for this region, because each island in the Caribbean archipelago is unique. In one case, we were asked about the possibility of presymptomatically providing the HD genetic test to a healthy 22-year-old woman who is at 50% risk. While we were considering how to provide the appropriate counseling services that should be associated with this test, the patient decided to opt out citing religious reasons. A secondary reason given was the idea that a consequence of testing might be manifestation of the disorder. Comparisons can be made with cancer: many studies reveal the importance of culture when discussing cancer such as the belief by some patients that talking about the disease will cause the disease [37, 38], and how family members and the community treat affected patients differently [39]. Currently no studies similar to these have been carried out in the Caribbean region with respect to Huntington disease.

Conclusions

From our dealings with this family we believe that the patients and their at-risk relations appeared to benefit from the information we were able to provide regarding mode of inheritance, genetic aspects of pathology, and the understanding that there are other people in the world with the same disorder. We believe that for this family this is timely information, since there are approximately 20 at-risk individuals who we know of, and probably more, coming of age where symptoms might manifest. The value of proper genetic investigation in this family is clear despite the outcome being less sanguine than the initial medical assessments suggested, and supports pursuing genetic diagnoses even in this resource-limited environment.

Abbreviations
ADL: Activities of daily living; HD: Huntington disease; *HTT*: Gene name abbreviation for huntingtin; MMSE: Mini mental state examination; SES: Socio economic status

Acknowledgements
We thank the local community organizations who helped us to fund this study. We also thank Winnie Xin, PhD for assistance with the genetic diagnosis, and Jennifer R. Friedman, MD, and Wendy Raskind, MD, PhD, for helpful discussions about the clinical and genetic aspects of rare movement disorders.

Funding
Self-funded.

Authors' contributions
AKS was the principal investigator. JC, LL and IP facilitated communication to family members, outreach, and pedigree construction. PR, JR, and KY contributed clinical support. HDB performed cognitive assessments. RHW acted as expert consult, examined a number of affected family members, and was instrumental with advancing this project. All authors contributed to writing this manuscript. All authors read and approved the final manuscript.

Authors' information
At the request of Institutional Review Board, the affiliation and contact information for these authors is withheld to help protect the privacy of the subjects described in this paper.

Competing interests
The authors declare that they have no competing interests.

Author details
[1]New York, USA. [2]Department of Neurology, James J. Peters Veterans Affairs Medical Center, Bronx, NY, USA. [3]Department of Neurology, Mount Sinai School of Medicine, New York City, NY, USA.

References
1.   Walker FO. Huntington's disease. Lancet. 2007;369:218–28.
2.   Tabrizi SJ, Scahill RI, Durr A, Roos RAC, Leavitt BR, Jones R, et al. Biological and clinical changes in premanifest and early stage Huntington's disease in the TRACK-HD study: the 12-month longitudinal analysis. Lancet Neurol. 2011;10:31–42.
3.   Sturrock A, Leavitt BR. The clinical and genetic features of Huntington disease. J Geriatr Psychiatry Neurol. 2010;23:243–59.
4.   Aubeeluck AV, Buchanan H, Stupple EJ. 'All the burden on all the carers': exploring quality of life with family caregivers of Huntington's disease patients. Qual Life Res. 2012;21(8):1425–35.
5.   The Huntington's Disease Collaborative Research Group. A novel gene containing a trinucleotide repeat that is expanded and unstable on Huntington's disease chromosomes. Cell. 1993;72:971–83.
6.   Brinkman RR, Mezei MM, Theilmann J, Almqvist E, Hayden MR. The likelihood of being affected with Huntington disease by a particular age, for a specific CAG size. Am J Hum Genet. 1997;60:1202–10.
7.   Yoon SR, Dubeau L, de Young M, Wexler NS, Arnheim N. Huntington disease expansion mutations in humans can occur before meiosis is completed. Proc Natl Acad Sci U S A. 2003;100:8834–8.
8.   Pearson CE. Slipping while sleeping? Trinucleotide repeat expansions in germ cells. Trends Mol Med. 2003;9:490–5.
9.   Cleary JD, Pearson CE. The contribution of cis-elements to disease-associated repeat instability: clinical and experimental evidence. Cytogenet Genome Res. 2003;100:25–55.
10. Ross CA, Aylward EH, Wild EJ, Langbehn DR, Long JD, Warner JH, et al. Huntington disease: natural history, biomarkers and prospects for therapeutics. Nat Rev Neurol. 2014;10:204–16.
11. Nopoulos PC. Huntington disease: a single-gene degenerative disorder of the striatum. Dialogues Clin Neurosci. 2016;18:91–8.
12. Williams JK, Erwin C, Juhl A, Mills J, Brossman B, Paulsen JS. Personal factors associated with reported benefits of Huntington disease family history or genetic testing. Genet Test Mol Biomarkers. 2010;14:629–36.
13. Tibben A. Predictive testing for Huntington's disease. Brain Res Bull. 2007;72:165–71.
14. Wahlin TBR. To know or not to know: a review of behaviour and suicidal ideation in preclinical Huntington's disease. Patient Educ Couns. 2007;65:279–87.
15. Hayden MR. Predictive testing for Huntington's disease: the calm after the storm. Lancet. 2000;356:1944–5.
16. Wedderburn S, Panegyres PK, Andrew S, Goldblatt J, Liebeck T, McGrath F, et al. Predictive gene testing for Huntington disease and other neurodegenerative disorders. Intern Med J. 2013;43:1272–9.
17. Morrison PJ, Harding-Lester S, Bradley A. Uptake of Huntington disease predictive testing in a complete population. Clin Genet. 2011;80:281–6.
18. Taylor SD. Predictive genetic test decisions for Huntington's disease: context, appraisal and new moral imperatives. Soc Sci Med. 2004;58:137–49.
19. Banaszkiewicz K, Sitek EJ, Rudzińska M, Sołtan W, Sławek J, Szczudlik A. Huntington's disease from the patient, caregiver and physician's perspectives: three sides of the same coin? J Neural Transm. 2012;119:1361–5.
20. Schulz R, Sherwood PR. Physical and mental health effects of family caregiving. Am J Nurs. 2008;108:23–7.
21. Cohen S, Doyle WJ, Baum A. Socioeconomic status is associated with stress hormones. Psychosom Med. 2006;68:414–20.
22. Beauburn MH. Huntington's chorea in Trinidad. West Indian Med J. 1963;12:39–46.

23. Vázquez-Mojena Y, Laguna-Salvia L, Laffita-Mesa JM, González-Zaldívar Y, Almaguer-Mederos LE, Rodríguez-Labrada R, et al. Genetic features of Huntington disease in Cuban population: implications for phenotype, epidemiology and predictive testing. J Neurol Sci. 2013;335:101–4.

24. Stevanin G, Fujigasaki H, Lebre A, Camuzat A, Jeannequin C, Dode C, et al. Huntington's disease-like phenotype due to trinucleotide repeat expansions in the TBP and JPH3 genes. Brain. 2003;126:1599–603.

25. Giunti P, Sabbadini G, Sweeney MG, Davis MB, Veneziano L, Mantuano E, et al. The role of the SCA2 trinucleotide repeat expansion in 89 autosomal dominant cerebellar ataxia families - frequency, clinical and genetic correlates. Brain. 1998;121:459–67.

26. Hermann A, Walker RH. Diagnosis and treatment of chorea syndromes. Curr Neurol Neurosci Rep. 2015;15:514–25.

27. World Economic Outlook Database. http://www.imf.org/external/pubs/ft/weo/2014/02/weodata/index.aspx. Accessed 21 May 2016.

28. Cockrell JR, Folstein MF. Mini-mental state examination. In: Copeland JRM, Abou-Saleh MT, Blazer DG, editors. Principles and practice of geriatric psychiatry. 2nd ed. John Wiley & Sons Ltd; 2002. p. 140–1.

29. Rosenblatt A. Neuropsychiatry of Huntington's disease. Dialogues Clin Neurosci. 2007;9:191–7.

30. Hart EP, Marinus J, Burgunder J, Bentivoglio AR, Craufurd D, Reilmann R, et al. Better global and cognitive functioning in choreatic versus hypokinetic-rigid Huntington's disease. Mov Disord. 2013;28:1142–5.

31. Dumas E, van den Bogaard S, Middelkoop H, Roos R. A review of cognition in Huntington's disease. Front Biosci (Schol Ed). 2013;5:1–18.

32. Willems S, De Maesschalck S, Deveugele M, Derese A, De Maeseneer J. Socio-economic status of the patient and doctor-patient communication: does it make a difference? Patient Educ Couns. 2005;56:139–46.

33. Penaranda E, Garcia A, Montgomery L. It wasn't Witchcraft-it was Huntington disease! J Am Board Fam Med. 2011;24:115–6.

34. Hoth KF, Paulsen JS, Moser DJ, Tranel D, Clark LA, Bechara A. Patients with Huntington's disease have impaired awareness of cognitive, emotional, and functional abilities. J Clin Exp Neuropsychol. 2007;29:365–76.

35. Sitek EJ, Soltan W, Wieczorek D, Schinwelski M, Robowski P, Reilmann R, et al. Self-awareness of motor dysfunction in patients with Huntington's disease in comparison to Parkinson's disease and cervical dystonia. J Int Neuropsychol Soc. 2011;17:788–95.

36. Daher M. Cultural beliefs and values in cancer patients. Ann Oncol. 2012;23:66–9.

37. Karbani G, Lim JNW, Hewison J, Atkin K, Horgan K, Lansdown M, et al. Culture, attitude and knowledge about breast cancer and preventative measures: a qualitative study of south Asian breast cancer patients in the UK. Asian Pac J Cancer Prev. 2011;12:1619–26.

38. Thomas VN, Saleem T, Abraham R. Barriers to effective uptake of cancer screening among black and minority ethnic groups. Int J Palliat Nurs. 2005;11:562–71.

39. O'Callaghan C, Schofield P, Butow P, Nolte L, Price M, Tsintziras S, et al. "I might not have cancer if you didn't mention it": a qualitative study on information needed by culturally diverse cancer survivors. Support Care Cancer. 2016;24:409–18.

30

Motor fluctuations due to interaction between dietary protein and levodopa in Parkinson's disease

Tuhin Virmani[1,2*], Sirinan Tazan[1,3], Pietro Mazzoni[1], Blair Ford[1] and Paul E. Greene[1,4]

Abstract

Background: The modulation of levodopa transport across the blood brain barrier by large neutral amino acids is well documented. Protein limitation and protein redistribution diets may improve motor fluctuations in patients with Parkinson's disease but the pharmacokinetics and pharmacodynamics of levodopa and amino acids are highly variable.

Methods: Clinical records of 1037 Parkinson's disease patients were analyzed to determine the proportion of patients with motor fluctuations related to protein interaction with levodopa. Motor fluctuations due to protein interaction with levodopa were defined as dietary protein being associated with (i) longer time to levodopa effectiveness, (ii) reduced benefit or duration of benefit, (iii) dose failures or (iv) earlier wearing off from a previously effective dose. Dose failures, sudden, painful or behavioral wearing-off periods, gait freezing, nausea, hallucinations, orthostasis, and dyskinesias were taken as markers of motor fluctuations, disease severity, and levodopa side effects potentially influenced by protein.

Results: 5.9 % of Parkinson's disease patients on levodopa, and 12.4 % with motor fluctuations on levodopa correlated their fluctuations with the relative timing of levodopa and protein intake. These patients were younger at disease onset, had worse motor fluctuations and had a higher incidence of family members with Parkinson's disease. Early wearing off or decreased dose efficacy were most commonly associated with protein interaction. 60 % of patients who modified their diets had weight loss.

Conclusions: This study suggests that clinically significant protein interaction with levodopa may occur mostly in a subset of Parkinson's disease patients with earlier disease onset and those with familial disease.

Keywords: Protein effect, Levodopa, Motor fluctuations, Parkinson disease

Background

The reduction of the response to levodopa by amino acids [1] and dietary protein [2] was first noted by Cotzias and colleagues. Dietary modifications have been tested in Parkinson's disease (PD) patients with motor fluctuations. These include low [2–5] and high protein diets [6, 7], addition of dietary large neutral amino acids (LNAAs) [1, 8, 9] and redistribution of daily protein intake [3, 7, 10–16] (the majority of dietary protein is

normally consumed with dinner). The improvement in clinical response varied from 30 % with protein redistribution [11] to 82 % with low-protein diets [5]. The ability of patients to maintain such diets long-term was variable [13, 16].

LNAAs (e.g. phenylalanine, tyrosine, and tryptophan) have been shown to compete with levodopa for absorption into the brain [17–20]. However, the data supporting a role for plasma LNAA concentrations in motor fluctuations is variable. Mean plasma levodopa levels were unchanged with low protein and protein distribution diets compared to a regular diet [3], but paradoxically higher on high protein diets [6, 7]. Peak plasma levodopa concentrations were similarly variable [4, 6, 7, 21, 22]. While

* Correspondence: TVirmani@uams.edu
[1]Department of Neurology, College of Physicians and Surgeons, Columbia University, New York, NY, USA
[2]Current addresses: University of Arkansas for Medical Sciences, 4301 W. Markham St., #500, Little Rock, AR 72205, USA
Full list of author information is available at the end of the article

levels of LNAAs are lower after meals with lower protein [3, 6, 7], the fluctuation in LNAAs with regular hospital meals was small compared to the large swings in plasma levodopa levels [9].

These studies were conducted on small populations with heterogeneous data making it difficult to recommend dietary modification to all PD patients [23]. In this study we aimed to establish the prevalence and characteristics of PD patients with clinically significant protein interaction with levodopa leading to motor fluctuations.

Methods

Of all the patients seen at the Columbia University Movement Disorders center between 2000 and 2012 by P.M., B.F. and P.E.G., with available clinical records, a total of 1037 patients with a clinical diagnosis of idiopathic PD by UK Brain bank criteria [24] were seen, and their electronic clinical notes were reviewed and the parameters described below were extracted and tabulated. Eight hundred seventy seven patients were on levodopa and 435 of these had multiple clinic visits. All available visit notes were reviewed and used to determine the presence, and in a subset, the onset of the symptoms as outlined for each parameter below.

Motor fluctuations were considered present if levodopa dosing was reported by the patient to last less than every 4 hours due to wearing off ("OFF") of the motor benefit derived from levodopa. Motor fluctuations related to protein interaction with levodopa (PIL) were considered present when meals with higher protein food groups (meat, eggs, dairy predominantly), were reported by the patient to be followed by any of (i) longer time to levodopa effectiveness, (ii) reduced benefit or duration of benefit, (iii) dose failures or (iv) earlier wearing off from a previously effective dose. Since patients may inconsistently report protein ingestion effecting levodopa effectiveness, and although all three movement disorders neurologists typically ask about protein interaction in patients with motor fluctuations, this may be an underestimate. Additionally, if patients reported that meals in general resulted in decreased effectiveness of levodopa, but did not specifically correlate this to the presence of high protein content, they were not considered to have PIL for the purpose of this study. This was done in order to try and only address protein/amino acid effects related to competing transportation with levodopa across the blood brain barrier and exclude potential issues related to any large meal leading to changes in gastric emptying and thereby altering levodopa absorption from the gut.

The age at motor onset was determined based on the year patients reported onset of their motor symptoms subtracted from their year of birth. The duration of disease was determined from the year of motor symptom onset and the year of the last (i.e. most recent) clinic note that was reviewed. The presence of freezing of gait (as a marker of disease severity) was determined based on patient report in the clinical history of the sensation of the feet sticking to the ground on initiation of gait, turning, in tight spaces or at destination or documented by the movement disorders neurologist on examination. Levodopa side effects (as potential markers influenced by PIL) of nausea, hallucinations, and orthostasis (symptomatic lightheadedness on standing) were deemed present if documented in the clinical history and dyskinesias present if documented in the clinical history or on movement disorders examination.

The year patients started levodopa therapy was available for 37/52 patients with PIL and 487/825 patients without PIL, and was used to calculate the years on levodopa based on the last recorded clinic note. In 15/52 patients the year they noted protein interaction led to motor fluctuations was documented and was used to determine the time of onset of PIL from motor symptom onset and levodopa therapy initiation. The total daily levodopa dose was calculated based on 100 % bioavailability of carbidopa/levodopa immediate release (IR) and carbidopa/levodopa/entacapone formulations [25] and an estimated 70 % bioavailability of carbidopa levodopa extended release (CR) formulation [26]. The presence of concurrent dopamine agonist use (ropinirole, pramipexole, rotigotine, pergolide or bromocriptine) or the use of deep brain stimulator (DBS) surgery for the treatment of their PD was also tabulated from the clinical charts. The report of 1st and/or 2nd degree relatives with PD in the social history was used for the calculation of the percentage with family history in the groups.

In order to exclude significant differences in age of onset or disease duration in the PIL vs no-PIL groups as a cause for the changes we observed, two subgroups of no-PIL patients were evaluated. The no-PIL group was sorted by age of onset and for each patient in the PIL group, five patients in the no-PIL group with the same age of onset were randomly included in the age of onset subgroup (no-PIL: age-ons). In the few cases where enough patients with the exact age of onset were not available, patients above and below that age were included, keeping the mean age of onset as close as possible to that of the patient with PIL. This subset of patients was then analyzed and compared to the PIL group for the other parameters described above. In a similar manner a subgroup of patients was also produced that included five randomly selected patients without PIL with the same disease duration as each patient with PIL (no-PIL: dis-dur).

The Shapiro-Wilk test was applied for data normality and statistical significance determined by chi-square or Mann–Whitney test where appropriate. SPSS version 22

(IBM) was used for statistical analysis and box plots. The study was approved by the Columbia University Institutional Review Board.

Results

Of the 1037 PD patients, 877 took levodopa, and 52/877 (5.9 %) met criteria for motor fluctuations related to PIL. Patients reporting PIL were younger at motor symptom onset, took higher maximal daily equivalent levodopa doses, used more dopamine agonists, had longer disease duration and levodopa use (Fig. 1a–e), and were younger at their last clinic visit (62.2 ± 10.8 vs. 68.8 ± 10.5 years). Gender ratio was similar in both groups (37 vs. 31 % female PIL vs. no-PIL patients). The percentage of patients who had undergone DBS was also similar in both groups (7.7 vs. 8.5 % PIL vs. no-PIL patients). PIL patients

reported more family members (first and/or second degree relatives) with PD ($p = 0.024$; OR = 1.96; 95 % CI = 1.08–3.56) (Fig. 1f). More PIL patients had dyskinesias and freezing of gait, but there was no difference in nausea, orthostasis or hallucinations (Fig. 2a).

Of the 52 patients with PIL, 26 (50 %) reported decreased efficacy of levodopa after protein intake, 15 (29 %) reported that protein intake led to wearing OFF of a previously effective dose, 9 (17 %) reported dose failures when levodopa and protein were taken concurrently, while one patient each reported delayed time to motor improvement (ON state) and decreased length of ON state time after protein. In PIL patients with data, PIL onset was 12.9 ± 6.7 years after motor onset (range 3–26 years, $N = 15$) and 7.9 ± 7.7 years after starting levodopa (range 0–25 years, $N = 8$).

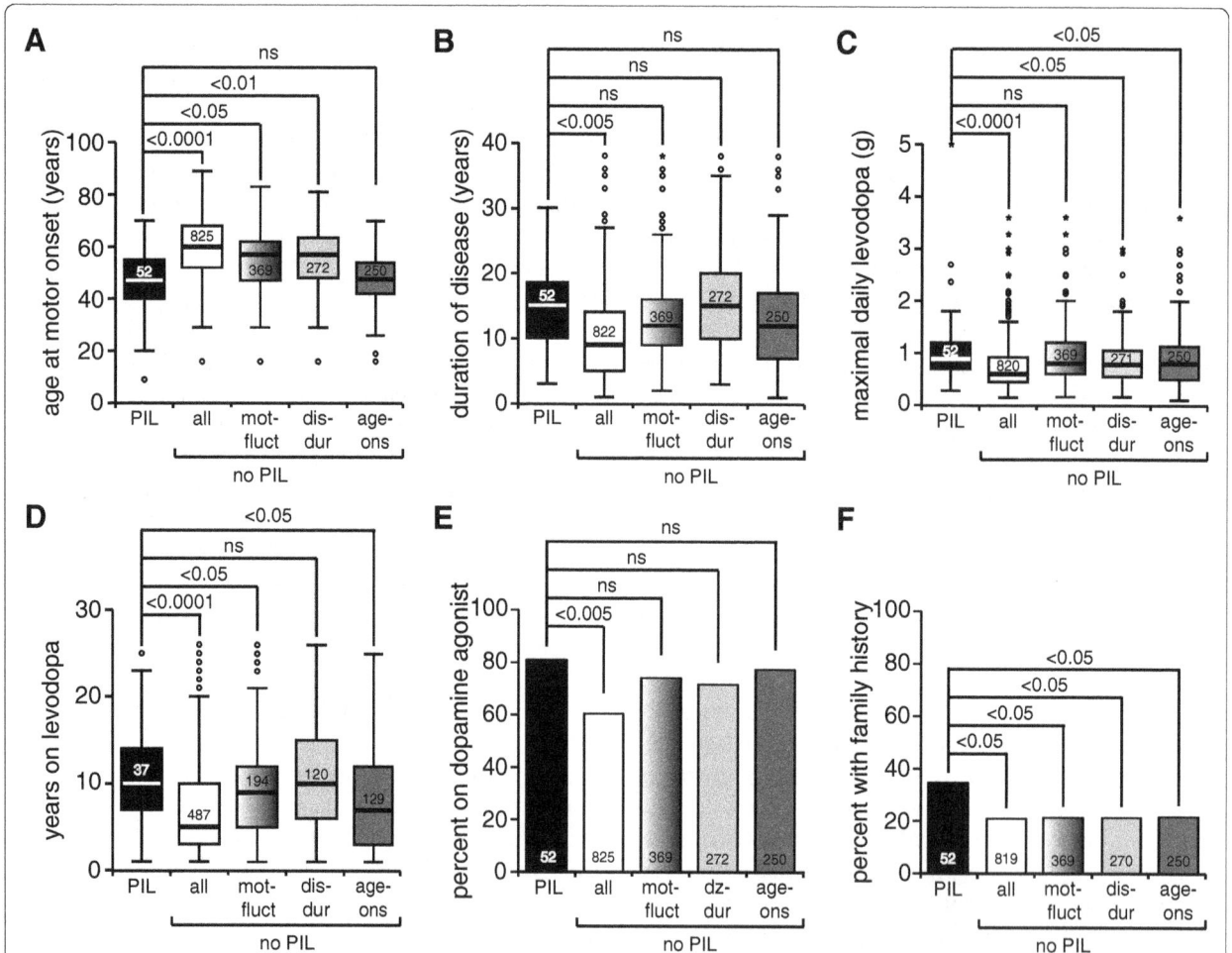

Fig. 1 General characteristics of all patients who exhibited protein interaction with levodopa **a** Age at motor onset, **b** duration of disease, **c** maximal daily levodopa dose, **d** years on levodopa, **e** percentage of patients on a dopamine agonist and **f** percentage with first or second degree relative with parkinsonism. (PIL; *black bars*) compared to those that did not (no-PIL: all; *white bars*) and subgroups of PIL patients with motor fluctuations (no-PIL:mot-fluct; *gradient bars*) and no-PIL patients matched for disease-duration (no-PIL: dis-dur; *light gray bars*) and age-at-motor-onset (no-PIL: age-ons; *dark gray bars*). The numbers of patients represented in each graph are inset. P values represent results of the chi-square or Mann–Whitney test comparing each no-PIL group to the PIL group. Legend: PIL: protein interaction with levodopa, no-PIL: no protein interaction with levodopa

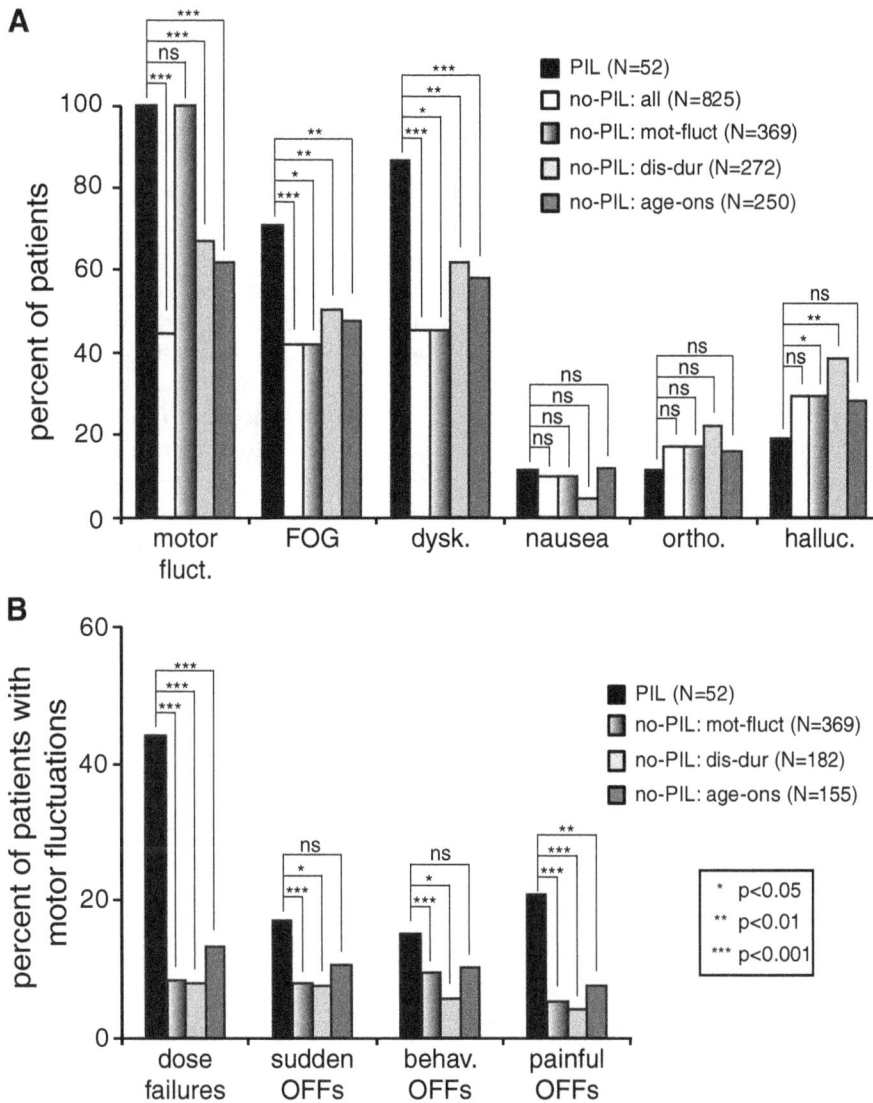

Fig. 2 a Motor and non-motor characteristics of all patients (*black bars*: PIL, *white bars*: no-PIL: all) and subgroups of no-PIL patients with motor fluctuations (no-PIL: mot-fluct; *gradient bars*), or matched for disease-duration (no-PIL:dis-dur; *light gray bars*) or age-at-motor-onset (no-PIL: age-ons; *dark gray bars*). **b** Characteristics of motor fluctuations in PIL patients compared to those with motor fluctuations in the no-PIL groups. *P* values represent results of the chi-square or Mann–Whitney test comparing each no-PIL group to the PIL group. Legend: PIL: protein interaction with levodopa, no-PIL: no protein interaction with levodopa, motor fluct: motor fluctuations, behav. OFFs: behavioral OFFs, FOG: freezing of gait, dysk: dyskinesias, ortho.:orthostasis, halluc.: hallucinations

Twenty patients had documented dietary modifications ranging from decreased total daily protein intake (15/20), redistribution of protein to the evening meal (2/20), small frequent meals (1/20), decreased total protein all taken only with the evening meal (1/20), and small frequent meals with protein in the evening meal only (1/20). Two patients had not changed their diets. The efficacy of these changes on motor fluctuations was unfortunately not adequately documented but 12/20 (60 %) reported weight loss after changing their diet.

In PD patients with motor fluctuations, a population much less likely to suffer from potential underreporting, 52/

421 (12.4 %) had PIL, with a greater frequency of dose failures, sudden OFFs, behavioral OFFs and painful OFFs compared to no-PIL patients with motor fluctuations (Fig. 2b). Hallucinations were less common in PIL patients compared to no-PIL patients with motor fluctuations (Fig. 2a). The duration of disease from time of onset of motor symptoms (Fig. 1b) and the maximal daily levodopa dose (Fig. 1c) were not statistically different between these groups. However, the duration of levodopa use was longer in PIL patients (Fig. 1d). The age at motor onset was earlier (Fig. 1a) and the percent reporting a family history of PD remained higher in PIL patients ($p = 0.037$; OR = 1.92; 95 % CI = 1.03–3.59) (Fig. 1f).

To further examine the longer disease duration in PIL patients, we performed a subgroup analysis by randomly selecting, for every PIL patient, five no-PIL patients matched for disease duration. In this subgroup (no-PIL: dis-dur), age at motor onset was again significantly lower in PIL patients (Fig. 1a), while duration of levodopa use (Fig. 1d) and percentage on dopamine agonists (Fig. 1e) were equivalent. Similarly to the whole-group results, PIL patients in this subgroup took a higher levodopa dose (Fig. 1c) and had higher frequency of motor complications (Fig. 2) and family history of PD ($p = 0.041$; OR = 1.94; 95 % CI = 1.02–3.67) (Fig. 1f). Therefore, differences in disease duration are unlikely to account for the differences between PIL and no-PIL groups.

Younger-onset patients are known to have a higher incidence of familial disease [27–29]. To determine whether there was a familial component to PIL independent of age, we matched PIL patients for age of onset (Figs. 1 and 2; no-PIL: age-ons). Similar to the whole-group comparison, the percentage of patients with PIL reporting a family history of PD was higher ($p = 0.045$; OR = 1.92; 95 % CI = 1.01–3.67) (Fig. 1f).

Discussion

A significant protein interaction with levodopa associated with motor fluctuations was reported in a small percentage of our patients: 5.9 % of our PD patients on levodopa and 12.4 % of those on levodopa with motor fluctuations. Almost 80 % of PIL patients either had decreased efficacy of their levodopa dose, or wore OFF from a prior dose after protein ingestion. PIL patients were younger at disease onset and reported a higher frequency of familial PD, even when matched for disease duration, maximal daily levodopa dose, or years of levodopa use, suggesting that PIL could be familial. The higher frequency of familial disease could not be accounted for by an earlier age of onset alone.

PIL patients also had more severe motor fluctuations with more frequent dose failures, sudden OFFs, behavioral OFFs and painful OFFs compared to no-PIL patients with motor fluctuations, which could not be accounted for by longer disease duration in the PIL group. The severity of motor fluctuations could be due to the interaction with levodopa reducing its effectiveness and therefore leading to worsened signs and symptoms of the disease. However it could potentially be a manifestation of differences in the disease process itself, as PIL patients also had a greater frequency of freezing of gait when compared with all no-PIL patients including matched for disease duration and age of onset subgroups of no-PIL patients analyzed. Additionally the mean onset of PIL from onset of motor symptoms was 12.9 years in the subset for which data was available, and the mean duration of disease in the no-PIL group with

motor fluctuations was the same suggesting that they had a long enough disease duration to develop such complications were they to occur.

In the subset of patients with both the time of levodopa initiation and the time of onset of PIL available, on average 8 years elapsed between levodopa initiation and PIL development. This suggests that allowing patients to take levodopa with meals initially, to avoid developing nausea, should not result in a significantly decreased benefit. Additionally, limiting protein in the diet or ingesting protein primarily with the evening meal led to weight loss in a majority of PIL patients. As patients with PD are already at an increased risk for weight loss [30], limiting their diet can be problematic. Apomorphine may be a better alternative to dietary protein restriction or redistribution, unless it cannot be tolerated due to nausea.

This study has the limitations of a retrospective study. We might underestimate the prevalence of PIL due to underreporting by patients or due to physicians not consistently asking about protein-levodopa effects. However the three fellowship trained movement disorders neurologist routinely ask about protein related motor OFF states, making the 12.4 % reported PIL in PD patients with motor fluctuations, less likely to be an underestimate, if at all. As patients often are not aware of the pattern of their motor fluctuations in relation to medications they may not notice the effect of meals or protein on their motor function, and therefore not report it. However the opposite is also not uncommon, whereby patients only take levodopa on an empty stomach as they are advised by their physicians or pharmacists of an interaction with protein. While this could be a significant factor in reporting by patients early in the disease course before onset of motor fluctuations, experienced patients with over 10 years disease duration, patients experiencing motor fluctuations, undergoing care at a tertiary referral center, and having their medications adjusted based upon their reports of motor fluctuations, are likely to be more aware of factors that can precipitate or worsen their motor function. In a population with over 10 years of disease, the incidence of DBS surgery was similar in both groups making it also unlikely to account for no-PIL patients not noting protein interaction due to less severe motor fluctuations from DBS therapy.

In clinical practice medications are always being adjusted based on patient's subjective reports of their motor function with levodopa dosing and would be a factor whether this were a prospective or retrospective study. While most patients reported high protein meals causing the effect and not food in general (these patients were excluded from the PIL group), we cannot account for the effect delayed gastric emptying may potentially have had in the motor response in these patients or the role fat content of meals may play in this process. However reduced benefit from a dose, earlier wearing off from a previously effective dose and decreased duration of benefit from a dose are less likely to be due to delayed gastric emptying and accounted for the majority of patients effects (79 %) in this cohort. Calculations of duration of levodopa use, time to PIL onset from motor symptom onset or levodopa initiation was limited to a subset of patients. Additionally the efficacy of dietary modifications could not be determined from records available. However, the large numbers of patient records analyzed (over 1000) and the availability of serial office notes in about 50 % of these patients helps minimize some of these concerns.

Conclusion

While it has been suggested that levodopa can be reduced in patients ingesting less protein [2, 5, 16], patients not responding to protein redistribution diets were younger at onset and had longer duration of levodopa use [16], as were our patients with PIL. This finding, together with the unclear mechanism, the small percentage of patients reporting PIL in our study, and the weight loss experienced by those changing their diets, raises the question as to whether dietary modification should be recommended to all patients reporting motor fluctuations, or as some suggest, to all patients taking levodopa.

Abbreviations
LNAA: large neutral amino acids; PD: Parkinson disease; PIL: protein interaction with levodopa.

Funding
This study had no sponsors or funding support.

Authors' contributions
TV conceived of and designed the study, collated data from clinical charts, analyzed the data, performed the statistical analysis and drafted the manuscript. ST collated data from clinical charts and helped in review and critique of the manuscript. PM and BF participated in the collection of the clinical data and critique and review of the manuscript. PEG participated in the collection of the clinical data, coordination of the study and critique and review of the manuscript. All authors read and approved the final manuscript.

Competing interests
The study has no sponsors. Dr. Virmani has no competing financial or non-financial interests related to this article. Dr. Virmani received fellowship support from the Parkinson's Disease Foundation. Dr. Tazen has no competing financial or non-financial interests related to this article. Dr. Tazen received fellowship support from the Parkinson's Disease Foundation. Dr. Mazzoni has no competing financial or non-financial interests related to this article. Dr. Ford has no competing financial or non-financial interests related to this article. Dr. Greene has no competing financial or non-financial interests related to this article. The authors declare that they have no competing interests.

Author details
[1]Department of Neurology, College of Physicians and Surgeons, Columbia University, New York, NY, USA. [2]Current addresses: University of Arkansas for Medical Sciences, 4301 W. Markham St., #500, Little Rock, AR 72205, USA. [3]Healthcare Partners, 3565 Del Amo Blvd., Ste 200, Torrance, CA 90503, USA. [4]Mt. Sinai School of Medicine, Box 1637, New York, NY 10029, USA.

References
1. Cotzias GC, Van Woert MH, Schiffer LM. Aromatic amino acids and modification of parkinsonism. N Engl J Med. 1967;276(7):374–9.
2. Mena I, Cotzias GC. Protein intake and treatment of Parkinson's disease with levodopa. N Engl J Med. 1975;292(4):181–4.
3. Carter JH, Nutt JG, Woodward WR, Hatcher LF, Trotman TL. Amount and distribution of dietary protein affects clinical response to levodopa in Parkinson's disease. Neurology. 1989;39(4):552–6.
4. Tsui JK, Ross S, Poulin K, Douglas J, Postnikoff D, Calne S, Woodward W, Calne DB. The effect of dietary protein on the efficacy of L-dopa: a double-blind study. Neurology. 1989;39(4):549–52.
5. Pincus JH, Barry K. Influence of dietary protein on motor fluctuations in Parkinson's disease. Arch Neurol. 1987;44(3):270–2.
6. Eriksson T, Granerus AK, Linde A. Carlsson A: 'On-off' phenomenon in Parkinson's disease: relationship between dopa and other large neutral amino acids in plasma. Neurology. 1988;38(8):1245–8.
7. Pincus JH, Barry K. Plasma levels of amino acids correlate with motor fluctuations in parkinsonism. Arch Neurol. 1987;44(10):1006–9.
8. Croxson S, Johnson B, Millac P, Pye I. Dietary modification of Parkinson's disease. Eur J Clin Nutr. 1991;45(5):263–6.
9. Nutt JG, Woodward WR, Carter JH, Trotman TL. Influence of fluctuations of plasma large neutral amino acids with normal diets on the clinical response to levodopa. J Neurol Neurosurg Psychiatry. 1989;52(4):481–7.
10. Barichella M, Marczewska A, De Notaris R, Vairo A, Baldo C, Mauri A, Savardi C, Pezzoli G. Special low-protein foods ameliorate postprandial off in patients with advanced Parkinson's disease. Mov Disord. 2006;21(10):1682–7.
11. Bracco F, Malesani R, Saladini M, Battistin L. Protein redistribution diet and antiparkinsonian response to levodopa. Eur Neurol. 1991;31(2):68–71.
12. Gimenez-Roldan S, Mateo D, Garcia Almansa A, Garcia Peris P. Proposal for a protein redistribution diet in the control of motor fluctuations in Parkinson's disease: acceptance and efficacy. Neurologia. 1991;6(1):3–9.
13. Karstaedt PJ, Pincus JH. Protein redistribution diet remains effective in patients with fluctuating parkinsonism. Arch Neurol. 1992;49(2):149–51.
14. Pare S, Barr SI, Ross SE. Effect of daytime protein restriction on nutrient intakes of free-living Parkinson's disease patients. Am J Clin Nutr. 1992;55(3):701–7.
15. Pincus JH, Barry K. Protein redistribution diet restores motor function in patients with dopa-resistant "off" periods. Neurology. 1988;38(3):481–3.
16. Riley D, Lang AE. Practical application of a low-protein diet for Parkinson's disease. Neurology. 1988;38(7):1026–31.
17. Leenders KL, Poewe WH, Palmer AJ, Brenton DP, Frackowiak RS. Inhibition of L-[18 F] fluorodopa uptake into human brain by amino acids demonstrated by positron emission tomography. Ann Neurol. 1986;20(2): 258–62.
18. Daniel PM, Moorhouse RS, Pratt OE. Letter: Do changes in blood levels of other aromatic aminoacids influence levodopa therapy? Lancet. 1976; 1(7950):95.
19. Oldendorf WH. Brain uptake of radiolabeled amino acids, amines, and hexoses after arterial injection. Am J Physiol. 1971;221(6):1629–39.
20. Wade LA, Katzman R. Synthetic amino acids and the nature of L-DOPA transport at the blood–brain barrier. J Neurochem. 1975;25(6):837–42.
21. Nutt JG, Fellman JH. Pharmacokinetics of levodopa. Clin Neuropharmacol. 1984;7(1):35–49.
22. Simon N, Gantcheva R, Bruguerolle B, Viallet F. The effects of a normal protein diet on levodopa plasma kinetics in advanced Parkinson's disease. Parkinsonism Relat Disord. 2004;10(3):137–42.
23. Cereda E, Barichella M, Pedrolli C, Pezzoli G. Low-protein and protein-redistribution diets for Parkinson's disease patients with motor fluctuations: a systematic review. Mov Disord. 2010;25(13):2021–34.
24. Hughes AJ, Daniel SE, Kilford L, Lees AJ. Accuracy of clinical diagnosis of idiopathic Parkinson's disease: a clinico-pathological study of 100 cases. J Neurol Neurosurg Psychiatry. 1992;55(3):181–4.

25. Hauser RA. Levodopa/carbidopa/entacapone (Stalevo). Neurology. 2004;62(1 Suppl 1):S64–71.

26. Koller WC, Hutton JT, Tolosa E, Capilldeo R. Immediate-release and controlled-release carbidopa/levodopa in PD: a 5-year randomized multicenter study. Carbidopa/Levodopa Study Group Neurol. 1999;53(5):1012–9.

27. Marder K, Levy G, Louis ED, Mejia-Santana H, Cote L, Andrews H, Harris J, Waters C, Ford B, Frucht S et al. Familial aggregation of early- and late-onset Parkinson's disease. Ann Neurol. 2003;54(4):507–13.

28. Payami H, Zareparsi S, James D, Nutt J. Familial aggregation of Parkinson disease: a comparative study of early-onset and late-onset disease. Arch Neurol. 2002;59(5):848–50.

29. Tanner CM, Ottman R, Goldman SM, Ellenberg J, Chan P, Mayeux R, Langston JW. Parkinson disease in twins: an etiologic study. JAMA. 1999; 281(4):341–6.

30. Barichella M, Cereda E, Pezzoli G. Major nutritional issues in the management of Parkinson's disease. Mov Disord. 2009;24(13):1881–92.

31

A Computerized *C*ognitive behavioral therapy *R*andomized, Controlle*d*, pilot trial for insomnia in Parkinson *D*isease (*ACCORD-PD*)

Shnehal Patel[1*], Oluwadamilola Ojo[1], Gencer Genc[1], Srivadee Oravivattanakul[1], Yang Huo[1],
Tanaporn Rasameesoraj[1], Lu Wang[2], James Bena[2], Michelle Drerup[3], Nancy Foldvary-Schaefer[4],
Anwar Ahmed[1] and Hubert H. Fernandez[1]

Abstract

Background: Parkinson disease (PD) is associated with a high prevalence of insomnia, affecting up to 88% of patients. Pharmacotherapy studies in the literature addressing insomnia in PD reveal disappointing and inconsistent results. Cognitive behavioral therapy (CBT) is a novel treatment option with durable effects shown in primary insomnia. However, the lack of accessibility and expense can be limiting. For these reasons, computerized CBT for insomnia (CCBT-I) has been developed. The CCBT-I program is a 6-week web-based course consisting of daily "lessons" providing learnable skills and appropriate recommendations to help patients improve their sleep habits and patterns.

Methods: We conducted a single-center, pilot, randomized controlled trial comparing CCBT-I versus standardized sleep hygiene instructions to treat insomnia in PD. Twenty-eight subjects with PD experiencing insomnia, with a score > 11 on the Insomnia Severity Index (ISI) were recruited. Based on a 6-point improvement in ISI in treatment group when compared to controls and an alpha = 0.05 and beta of 0.1 (power = 90%) a sample size of 11 patients (on active treatment) were required to detect this treatment effect using a dependent sample t-test.

Results: In total, 8/14 (57%) subjects randomized to CCBT-I versus 13/14 (93%) subjects randomized to standard education completed the study. Among completers, the improvement in ISI scores was greater with CCBT-I as compared to standard education (−7.9 vs −3.5; $p = 0.03$). However, in an intention-to-treat analysis, where all enrolled subjects were included, the change in ISI between groups was not significant (−.4.5 vs −3.3; $p = 0.48$), likely due to the high dropout rate in the CCBT-I group (43%).

Conclusion: This pilot study suggests that CCBT-I can be an effective treatment option for PD patients with insomnia when the course is thoroughly completed. High drop-out rate in our study shows that although effective, it may not be a generalizable option; however, larger studies are needed for further evaluation.

* Correspondence: Patels7@ccf.org
[1]9500 Euclid Ave/U2, Cleveland, OH 44195, USA
Full list of author information is available at the end of the article

Background

Parkinson Disease (PD) is associated with a high prevalence of sleep complaints, including insomnia, daytime sleepiness, sleep apnea, restless legs syndrome (RLS) and REM sleep behavior disorder (RBD) [1, 2]. The most common sleep disturbance in patients with PD is sleep maintenance insomnia, affecting up to 88% of patients [3, 4]. Sleep maintenance insomnia is characterized by a decrease in total sleep time (TST) and an increase in the number of arousals and awakenings after sleep onset. Sleep initiation insomnia affects 23% to 30% of PD patients [5, 6]. However, in controlled studies, the prevalence of sleep initiation insomnia was found to be comparable among PD patients and healthy elderly controls.

Insomnia therapy in PD has primarily consisted of pharmacotherapy using non-benzodiazepine hypnotics, sedating antipsychotics (such as quetiapine), and benzodiazepines. However, side effects, tolerance and dependency, cognitive impairment, and decreased effectiveness over time limit their use. Cognitive behavioral therapy for insomnia (CBT-I) has been shown to be more effective than pharmacotherapy long-term in primary insomnia cohorts and the NIH State-of-the-Science conference Statement identified it as the first-line approach to insomnia treatment [7]. CBT-I helps identify and modify negative thoughts about sleep and behaviors that perpetuate insomnia [8]. However, widespread use of CBT-I has been limited by lack of trained clinicians, geographical remoteness of the trained providers, stigmatization of receiving psychological service and expense. For these reasons, computerized cognitive behavioral therapy for insomnia (CCBT-I), has been developed in order to make CBT-I more convenient. The Cleveland Clinic CCBT-I program [9] consists of sleep restriction, stimulus control, cognitive restructuring, sleep hygiene, and relaxation training delivered in stages over a 6-week period [10–12]. The efficacy of CCBT-I for primary insomnia has been demonstrated in several randomized controlled trials [13–17].

Despite the high prevalence and life-quality impact of insomnia in PD, there are only a few pharmacotherapy studies specifically addressing insomnia without a focus on nocturnal motor symptoms [18–21]. Most recently, a three-arm six-week randomized pilot study comparing non-pharmacologic treatment (cognitive behavioral therapy/bright light therapy) versus doxepin 10 mg at bedtime versus inactive placebo, was published [22]. Although it was found that doxepin and non-pharmacologic treatment substantially improved insomnia, we are aware of no study on CCBT-I which provides near universal access to this patient population. Therefore, we have conducted a pilot study evaluating the effect of CCBT-I on insomnia in PD patients.

Methods

This was a 6-week pilot randomized (1:1 ratio), parallel-group, controlled study evaluating effectiveness of CCBT-I in PD patients by measuring clinical and sleep variables before and after completion of the program. PD patients with insomnia were asked to participate at their clinical visit by their current movement disorder provider. If the patient was interested, the research coordinator or investigator discussed study further with patient. Subjects meeting inclusion criteria (Table 1) were randomized to CCBT-I or standard sleep hygiene education (Table 2). Randomization was done by study coordinator who made 28 sealed envelopes containing their group designation. Once patients signed the informed consent form, they were given the sealed envelope containing their group designation.

Subjects completed questionnaires at baseline, 8 and 12 weeks after randomization, including:

1. Epworth Sleepiness Scale (ESS) —The ESS is a 4-point scale (0–3) measuring daytime sleepiness of a patient in 8 different situations or activities that most people engage in as part of their daily lives, although not necessarily every day. The total ESS score can range between 0 and 24. The higher the score, the higher the person's level of daytime sleepiness [23].
2. Pittsburgh Insomnia Rating Scale (PIRS20) —PIRS20 is a subjective measurement of the severity of insomnia that the patient rates [24].
3. Insomnia Severity Index (ISI) —ISI is a valid and reliable tool to diagnose and measure severity of insomnia. It consists of 7 questions concerning sleep onset, sleep maintenance, early awakening, level of satisfaction with sleep pattern, extent of interference with daily functioning, conspicuousness of impairment caused by sleep problem, and level of concern about current sleep problem. Each item is marked on a 5-point Likert scale (0 to 4). Total scores after evaluation ranges from 0 to 28; the higher score, the more insomnia severity. Scores 0 to 7 indicate no clinically significant insomnia, 8 to 14 sub-threshold insomnia, 15 to 21 clinically significant insomnia (moderate), and 22 to 28 clinically significant insomnia (severe) [25].
4. Fatigue Severity Scale (FSS) —FSS measures fatigue severity by measuring its effect on daily activities in patients with chronic neurologic disorders. It is measured on a 7-point scale (0–7), higher the score indicating more severe fatigue [26].
5. Unified Parkinson Disease Rating Scale (UPDRS) parts 1b and II—UPDRS 1b and II measure activities of daily living in PD evaluating motor and non-motor features. It is a 20-question

Table 1 Inclusion and Exclusion Criteria

Inclusion Criteria	Exclusion Criteria
1. 35–85 years of age	1. Dementia as defined by DSM-IV criteria
2. Diagnosis of PD by a Movement Disorders neurologist	2. Patients with suboptimally treated depression and significant depressive symptoms as defined by a PHQ-9 score of > 15. Antidepressant medications prescribed for depression or anxiety were allowed if the patient had been on a stable dose for at least 1 month.
3. On stable antiparkinsonian medications for the past 30 days	3. Significant hallucinations or psychotic symptoms requiring antipsychotic medications
4. ISI > 11	4. Presence of significant sleep disorders that could be contributing to insomnia such as known sleep apnea, RBD, RLS
5. Access to a computer and internet	5. Presence of significant motor fluctuations, especially nocturnal akinesias that could be contributing to insomnia
6. Be able to speak, read and understand English	6. Use of sedatives, benzodiazepines or sedating antidepressants (such as mirtazapine, TCAs), modafinil, stimulants, anticholinergic medications, were allowed if the patient had been on a stable dose for at least 1 month and was not taking it as a sleep aid.
	7. Significant renal, hepatic, cardiac and thyroid disease that could have interfered with protocol adherence

survey, each question with a 0–4 scale, the higher the score, the more severe the impact on the particular activity. When analysing the data, we modified the score by removing the question related to sleep to evaluate if the score change in a patient's activities of daily living that wasn't swayed by improvement in sleep.

6. Patient Health Questionnaire (PHQ-9)—The PHQ-9 is a multipurpose instrument for screening, diagnosing, and measuring severity of depression. The score ranges from 5 to 20, with the higher score suggesting more severe depression [27].

7. Parkinson Disease Questionnaire (PDQ8)—PDQ8 is an 8-question self-administered questionnaire, used to measure quality of life in persons with Parkinson's disease. Scores range from 0 to 4, the higher the score, the greater the impairment on the person's

Table 2 Sleep Hygiene Education

BEFORE GETTING INTO BED:

-Do not eat a heavy meal close to bedtime (a light bedtime s nack is OK),

-Create a positive sleep environment – cool, dark and quiet,

-Create a buffer zone – quiet time prior to bed time. During this time, you should do things that are enjoyable on their own rather than activities that are goal oriented.

WHILE IN BED:

-Avoid watching the clock. Turn your clock around (or cover it) and use your alarm if needed.

-Use your bed only for sleep and sex – Avoid TV watching, use of computer, reading, or cell phone use in bed.

IN THE MORNING AND DURING THE DAYTIME:

-Avoid naps during the day.

-Limit caffeine and consume before noon.

-Exercise regularly but not within 3–4 h of bedtime.

quality of life. The 39-point PDQ provides scores for each of the 8 domains: mobility, activities of daily living, emotional well-being, stigma, social support, cognitions, communications and bodily discomfort. Alternatively, the sum of the domain scores can be used to assess the overall health-related quality of life profile of the individual questioned [28].

CCBT-I therapy

Go! To Sleep is a 6-week online, interactive CBT-I based program designed to foster better sleep habits and help participants implement cognitive behavioral therapy for insomnia strategies. Subjects were provided with a unique password to access the program. Daily program access is encouraged via daily email reminders to complete a sleep log based on prior night's sleep pattern. After completing sleep log, the user is given individualized feedback based on their sleep log responses as well as a daily sleep efficiency score to help them track their progress through the program. There are daily "lessons" or articles that provide psychoeducation regarding insomnia and strategies to help address their sleep concerns. In addition, throughout the program they have access to relaxation/meditation practices as well as other strategies designed to improve stress management and sleep. There is a mobile application for easy sleep tracking.

Table 2 shows the sleep hygiene advice that was given to the control group.

All subjects received weekly telephone reminders from an investigator to participate in their assigned therapy. Additional telephone calls were made 8 and 12 weeks after randomization to complete the questionnaires and return to the investigators in self-addressed envelopes. Subjects were considered a dropout if they could not complete CCBT-I or if they did not return the week 8 questionnaires.

The Institutional Review Board of the Cleveland Clinic approved the project.

Statistical methods

CCBT-I has never been tested in the PD population, thus we did not have prior experience from which to perform sample size calculations. However, there is a study using ISI and advocating for a 6-point change as significant [29]. This study gives population mean value for ISI as 19.7 with standard deviation as 4.1. Another study examining the validation of the ISI as an outcome measure for insomnia research showed population mean value for ISI as 17.9 with standard deviation as 4.1 [30]. In a three-arm (cognitive behavioral therapy/bright light therapy versus doxepin versus inactive placebo), six-week, randomized study, the baseline ISI was 14.7 ± 6.1, 19.9 ± 3.7 and 16.5 ± 5.4 [22]. Based on a 6-point improvement in ISI in treatment group when compared to controls and an alpha = 0.05 and beta of 0.1 (power = 90%) a sample size of 11 patients (on active treatment) were required to detect this treatment effect using a dependent sample t-test. Assuming a dropout rate of 25%, a sample size of 14 patients on each arm were recruited.

The data are presented as mean ± standard deviation for continuous variables and N (%) for categorical variables. Comparison of demographic variables was performed by two-sample t test in continuous variables, and chi-square test or Fisher exact test in categorical variables. Change from baseline to end point was analyzed using paired t test; and compared between cases and controls by two-sample t test.

To account for the correlation among repeated measures on the same subject a mixed model assuming compound symmetry correlation structure was used to test the trend from Week 1 to Week 6 of the online program. Least square means with 95% confidence intervals were presented to show the trend. Analyses were performed based on an overall significance level of 0.05, using SAS software (version 9.4, Cary, NC).

Results

Twenty-nine subjects were screened for enrollment. One subject was not considered a candidate after screening due to low ISI score. Subsequently, 28 subjects were randomized, 14 in each group. Sample characteristics are shown in Table 3. There were no significant differences between groups except for gender, where there were more males in the CCBT-I group than in the control group.

Six subjects in the treatment group and 1 in the control group withdrew from the study. Using intention-to-treat analysis, the last available data point was used as endpoint.

Table 3 Baseline Characteristics

	Case	Control	p-value
Age (years)	63.1 ± 6.8	64.7 ± 9.5	0.62[a]
Gender			**0.022[c]**
Female	3(21.4)	9(64.3)	
Male	11(78.6)	5(35.7)	
ESS Total	11.1 ± 4.9	9.3 ± 6.2	0.39[a]
FSS Total	27.3 ± 13.1	29.1 ± 12.2	0.72[a]
ISI Total	15.7 ± 3.0	15.4 ± 2.9	0.80[a]
UPDRS1b Total	9.8 ± 4.0	9.4 ± 2.1	0.71[a]
UPDRS1b Modified	5.4 ± 3.4	5.1 ± 2.0	0.79[a]
UPDRS2 total	12.6 ± 7.9	10.4 ± 7.1	0.46[a]
PDQ Total	14.4 ± 4.4	15.2 ± 5.8	0.70[a]
PHQ9 Total	7.8 ± 5.1	7.2 ± 4.2	0.73[a]
pirs20 Total	9.1 ± 2.4	9.1 ± 2.1	0.92[a]
EQ5D Index	0.75 ± 0.15	0.79 ± 0.13	0.46[a]

p-values: [a]two-sample t test, [c]Pearson's chi-square test
Bold values are statistically significant p < 0.05

Intention-to-treat analysis showed a significant improvement in ISI ($p = 0.007$), ESS ($p = 0.048$) and PIRS20 ($p = 0.004$) and PHQ-9 ($p = 0.011$) scores in the treatment group when compared to the respective scores prior to CCBT-I treatment, as shown in Table 4. UPDRS1b scores also significantly improved after treatment, however when modifying the score by removing the sleep variables, the change was no longer significant. However, when comparing the treatment group to the control group, none of these changes were significant, including ISI (-4.5 vs -3.3; $p = 0.48$).

Per protocol analysis, i.e. only using patients who did complete treatment, is shown in Table 5. One subject in the control group who had started using a sleeping agent was excluded. A significant improvement in ISI ($p = 0.002$), ESS ($p = 0.042$), PIRS20 ($p = 0.005$) and PHQ-9 ($p < 0.001$) scores were observed in the treatment group. In addition, the change in ISI was significantly greater in the treatment group ($-7.9 ± 4.5$) compared to controls ($-3.5 ± 3.9$) ($p = 0.033$).

Five patients had a change in their medication during the trial. Two patients in the control group reported a decrease in their PD regimen, which they felt may have helped their sleep. One patient in the control group started taking a sleeping aid. Two patients (1 in treatment and 1 in control) had an increase in antidepressant medications.

Discussion

The etiology of insomnia in PD is heterogeneous and may arise from motor and non-motor features of PD such as nocturnal akinesia, nocturnal dystonia, wearing off, dyskinesias, nocturia, depression, anxiety, dementia,

Table 4 Baseline and endpoint scores per an Intention to Treat Analysis

Factor	Case(N = 14)			Control(N = 14)		
	Baseline	Endpoint	P value	Baseline	Endpoint	P value
ESS Total	11.1 ± 4.9	9.5 ± 5.8	**0.048**	9.3 ± 6.2	8.1 ± 4.8	0.25
FSS Total	27.3 ± 13.1	25.4 ± 13.6	0.20	29.1 ± 12.2	29.2 ± 12.6	0.70
ISI Total	15.7 ± 3.0	11.2 ± 5.6	**0.007**	15.4 ± 2.9	12.2 ± 5.1	**0.008**
UPDRS1b Total	9.8 ± 4.0	8.1 ± 4.2	**0.010**	9.4 ± 2.1	8.4 ± 2.5	**0.043**
UPDRS1b Modified	5.4 ± 3.4	5.0 ± 3.2	0.34	5.1 ± 2.0	4.9 ± 1.7	0.58
UPDRS2 total	12.6 ± 7.9	12.5 ± 7.0	0.93	10.4 ± 7.1	10.2 ± 8.0	0.77
PDQ Total	14.4 ± 4.4	14.2 ± 4.3	0.52	15.2 ± 5.8	14.6 ± 5.6	0.32
PHQ9 Total	7.8 ± 5.1	5.8 ± 5.5	**0.011**	7.2 ± 4.2	5.9 ± 4.1	0.14
pirs20 Total	9.1 ± 2.4	7.2 ± 3.5	**0.004**	9.1 ± 2.1	7.5 ± 3.9	0.070
EQ5D Index	0.75 ± 0.15	0.72 ± 0.16	0.23	0.79 ± 0.13	0.76 ± 0.16	0.49

Values presented as Mean ± SD. p-values: paired t test
Bold values are statistically significant $p < 0.05$

medications, punding, as well as primary sleep disorders [31, 32]. We performed the first randomized control trial to compare the effectiveness of web-based CBT-I compared to standard recommendations for insomnia in the PD population. While no significant difference in insomnia severity, as measured by the ISI, was found in the ITT analysis (likely due to the high drop out rate in the CCBT-I group), the *per protocol* analysis, amongst patients who finished the study, found significant improvement in insomnia symptoms with the CCBT-I than standard sleep hygiene education. Consistent with the improvement in ISI, subjects treated with CCBT-I also experienced significant increases in sleep efficiency that persisted to the final assessment at 12 weeks. As mentioned earlier, there are very few studies that evaluated the treatment of sleep in PD patients.

Finally, statistically significant improvements in insomnia scores observed in the control group, after receiving standard written sleep hygiene recommendations, supporting the value of simple sleep education in clinical practice. However, the degree of improvement in the ISI score was not more than 6 points to consider clinically significant improvement. This suggests that more effective treatment is still in need.

The major limitation of the study, in addition to the open-label nature of the treatment assignment, is the high dropout rate in PD population as this group had a difficult time completing the program. Dropout rates are variable across all PD clinical trials and can be up to 50%. A recently published meta-analysis on self-help CBT (via booklet, videotape, audiotape or internet) for insomnia reported an average dropout rate of 14.5% compared to 16.7% in therapist-administered CBT [33]. Our dropout rate was about 43%. While all patients had computer access, they were not used to using it on regular basis. The

Table 5 Baseline and endpoint scores Per Protocol Analysis

Factor	Case(N = 14)				Control(N = 14)			
	n	Baseline	Endpoint	P value	n	Baseline	Endpoint	P value
ESS Total	8	11.1 ± 4.9	8.4 ± 5.9	**0.042**	12	9.8 ± 6.2	9.0 ± 4.5	0.40
FSS Total	8	27.3 ± 13.1	21.3 ± 11.0	0.21	12	30.5 ± 11.5	28.2 ± 11.2	0.35
ISI Total	8	15.7 ± 3.0	7.8 ± 4.4	**0.002**	12	15.3 ± 3.0	12.2 ± 5.5	**0.033**
UPDRS1b Total	8	9.8 ± 4.0	6.9 ± 3.1	**0.004**	12	9.7 ± 1.8	8.6 ± 2.4	**0.037**
UPDRS1b Modified	8	5.4 ± 3.4	4.4 ± 2.1	0.35	12	5.4 ± 1.7	4.8 ± 1.6	0.77
UPDRS2 total	8	12.6 ± 7.9	12.3 ± 6.3	0.93	12	10.9 ± 7.1	10.6 ± 8.4	0.99
PDQ Total	7	14.4 ± 4.4	13.7 ± 3.7	0.53	11	15.6 ± 5.8	13.1 ± 3.8	0.73
PHQ9 Total	8	7.8 ± 5.1	3.5 ± 4.5	**0.005**	12	7.5 ± 4.2	5.4 ± 3.3	0.17
pirs20 Total	8	9.1 ± 2.4	5.0 ± 2.3	**<0.001**	12	9.2 ± 2.1	7.4 ± 3.9	0.14
EQ5D Index	8	0.75 ± 0.15	0.71 ± 0.17	0.24	12	0.79 ± 0.13	0.77 ± 0.17	0.55

Values presented as Mean ± SD. p-values: paired t test
Bold values are statistically significant $p < 0.05$

average age of our population was 64 years old, which is roughly 10–20 years older than prior studies that evaluated this tool for treatment for insomnia. A younger population may be more comfortable using a computer on a daily basis and therefore may achieve a higher success rate, compared to the average PD patient. Indeed, when we asked patients what were the barriers of CCBT-I that limited them from completing the program, most of them felt that the program interrupted their normal lifestyle. Patients were unable to keep up with daily logs and would have a tendency to forget to log on to computer to complete the tasks. Nonetheless, the difference in improvement of ISI scores in the *intention-to-treat* versus the *per-protocol* cohort suggests that CCBT-I treatment is only effective if patients carry it through all the way to the end.

This can be challenging for PD patients due to difficult time keeping up with daily logs and it may be helpful to decrease logging frequency to once a week. In addition, one on-line CBT-I study found that compared to physician-referred participants (46.7%), community-recruited participants were significantly less likely to drop-out (18.2%) suggesting that community based recruitment may have higher levels of pre-treatment motivation or more comfortable with technology [15]. In addition, we can consider refining the program to tailor to the unique needs PD patients, such as permitting a brief afternoon nap, if needed, to address fatigue and modification of sleep restriction and other behavioral strategies that may be more difficult for individuals with comorbid chronic health issues. The addition of periodic semi-structured video-chats or phone calls with trained personnel to monitor progress and problem-solve issues with the online program would likely decrease participant drop out as well as increase program efficacy.

In addition, 5 patients did have a change in their medication during the study. One patient, who added a sleep aid, was removed from the analysis. Changes in PD medications as well as antidepressants can certainly aid in improving sleep; however, these changes were done for PD management and treatment of depression, not necessarily to treat insomnia. Any benefit patients received in sleep is consistent with the theory that insomnia in PD population is heterogeneous and many factors are contributory.

Our observations expand the existing literature on the use of CCBT-I in clinical practice, examining its feasibility and effectiveness in an older cohort of PD patients with motor and non-motor impairments. Larger studies, with perhaps a more thoughtful construction of behavioral therapy execution and greater vigilance of its compliance, are needed to definitively compare the effectiveness on different types of insomnia therapies in PD patients.

Conclusions

This pilot study suggest that CCBT-I can be an effective treatment option for PD patients with insomnia when the course is thoroughly completed. High drop-out rate in our study shows that although effective, it may not be a generalizable option. We can tailor this program for the unique needs of PD patients and provide more trained personnel to monitor progress and problem-solve to increase program efficacy. However, larger studies are needed for further evaluation.

Abbreviations

CBT-I: Cognitive behavioral therapy for insomnia; CCBT-I: *computerized cognitive behavioral therapy for insomnia*; ESS: Epworth Sleepiness Scale; FSS: Fatigue Severity Scale; ISI: Insomnia Severity Index; PD: Parkinson Disease; PDQ8: Parkinson Disease Questionnaire; PHQ-9: Patient Health Questionnaire; PIRS20: Pittsburgh Insomnia Rating Scale; RBD: REM sleep behavior disorder; RLS: Restless legs syndrome; TST: total sleep time; UPDRS1b and II: Unified Parkinson Disease Rating Scale 1b and II

Acknowledgements

The investigators would like to thank the Cleveland Clinic Wellness Institute for providing access to the Go! To Sleep program for subject participation. In addition, we would like to thank Parkinson's Pals for their continued support in education and research.

Funding

Research and education funding from the Parkinson's Pals Organization.

Authors' contributions

SP assisted with research project conception, organization and execution, statistical analysis design and execution. He wrote the first draft of manuscript and made all edits with assistance. OO helped to recruit patients as well as execute study and assisted in reviewing and critiquing manuscript. GG and SO helped with designing the study and initial recruitment of patients. YH created and maintained database. TR helped with editing and revising manuscript. LW and JB were our statistical support for all analyses. MD, NF, AA, and HHF assisted with research project conception and organization along with statistical review and reviewing and critiquing final manuscript. All authors read and approved the final manuscript.

Competing interests

Authors have no competing interests.

Author details

[1]9500 Euclid Ave/U2, Cleveland, OH 44195, USA. [2]9500 Euclid Ave/JJN3, Cleveland, OH 44195, USA. [3]9500 Euclid Ave/P57, Cleveland, OH 44195, USA. [4]9500 Euclid Ave, Cleveland, OH 44195, USA.

References

1. Chahine LM, Amara AW, Videnovic A. A systematic review of the literature on disorders of sleep and wakefulness in Parkinson's disease from 2005 to 2015. Sleep Med Rev. 2016. doi:10.1016/j.smrv.2016.08.001. [Epub ahead of print].
2. Larsen JP, Tandberg E. Sleep disorders in patients with Parkinson's disease: epidemiology and management. CNS Drugs. 2001;15(4):267-5.
3. Oerlemans WG, de Weerd AW. The prevalence of sleep disorders in patients with Parkinson's disease: a self-reported, community-based survey. Sleep Med. 2002;3:147-9.
4. Factor SA, McAlarney T, Sanchez-Ramos JR, Weiner WJ. Sleep disorders and sleep effect in Parkinson's disease. Mov Disord. 1990;5(4):280-5.
5. Tandberg E, Larsen JP, Karlsen K. A community-based study of sleep disorders in patients with Parkinson's disease. Mov Disord. 1998;13:895-9.
6. Gjerstad MD, Wentzel-Larsen T, Aarsland D, Larsen JP. Insomnia in Parkinson's disease: frequency and progression over time. J Neurol Neurosurg Psychiatry. 07;78(5):476-479. Epub 2006 Nov 10.
7. National Institutes of Health. NIH state-of-the-science conference statement on manifestations and management of chronic insomnia in adults. NIH Consens State Sci Statements. 2005;22:1-30.
8. Morin CM. Insomnia: psychological assessment and management. New York: The Guilford Press; 1993.
9. Bearnstein A, Allexandre D, Bena J, Doyle J, Gendy G, Wang L, Fay S, Mehra R, Moul D, Foldvary-Schaefer N, Roizen M, Drerup M. "go! To sleep": a web-based therapy for insomnia. Telemedicine and e-Health. 2017;23:1-10.
10. Ritterband LM, Thorndike FP, Gonder-Frederick LA, Magee JC, Bailey ET, Saylor DK, Morin CM. Efficacy of an internet based behavioral intervention for adults with insomnia. Arch Gen Psychiatry. 2009;66:692-8.
11. Cheng SK, Dizon J. Computerised cognitive behavioural therapy for insomnia: a systematic review and meta-analysis. Psychother Psychosom. 2012;81:206-16.
12. Andrews G, Cuijpers P, Craske MG, McEvoy P, Titov N. Computer therapy for the anxiety and depressive disorders is effective, acceptable and practical health care: a meta-analysis. PLoS. 2010;5(10):e13196. doi:10.1371/journal. pone.0013196.
13. Ström L, Pettersson R, Andersson G. Internet-based treatment for insomnia: a controlled evaluation. J Consult Clin Psychol. 2004;72:113-20.
14. Suzuki E, Tsuchiya M, Hirokawa K, Taniguchi T, Mitsuhashi T, Kawakami N. Evaluation of an internet-based self-help program for better quality of sleep among Japanese workers: a randomized controlled trial. J Occup Health. 2008;50:387-99.
15. Vincent N, Lewycky S. Logging on for better sleep: RCT of the effectiveness of online treatment for insomnia. Sleep. 2009;32:807-15.
16. Riley WT, Mihm P, Behar A, Morin CM. A computer device to deliver behavioral interventions for insomnia. Behav Sleep Med. 2010;8:2-15.
17. Ritterband LM, Bailey ET, Thorndike FP, Lord HR, Farrell-Carnahan L, Baum LD. Initial evaluation of an internet intervention to improve the sleep of cancer survivors with insomnia. Psychooncology. 2012;21(7):695-705. doi:10. 1002/pon.1969. Epub 2011 Apr 29.
18. Diederich NJ, McIntyre DJ. Sleep disorders in Parkinson's disease: many causes, few therapeutic options. Neurol Sci. 2012;314(1-2):12-19. doi:10. 1016/j.jns.2011.10.025. Epub 2011 Nov 25. Review.
19. Menza M, Dobkin RD, Marin H. Treatment of insomnia in Parkinson's disease: a controlled trial of eszopiclone and placebo. Mov Disord. 2010;25:1708-14.
20. Juri C, Chaná P, Tapia J, Kunstmann C, Parrao T. Quetiapine for insomnia in Parkinson disease: results from an open-label trial. Clin Neuropharmacol. 2005;28:185-7.
21. Medeiros CA, Carvalhedo de Bruin PF, Lopes LA, Magalhães MC, de Lourdes Seabra M, de Bruin VM. Effect of exogenous melatonin on sleep and motor dysfunction in Parkinson's disease. A randomized, double blind, placebo-controlled study. J Neurol. 2007;254:459-64.
22. Rios Romenets S, Creti L, Fichten C, Bailes S, Libman E, Pelletier A, Postuma RB. Doxepin and cognitive behavioural therapy for insomnia in patients with Parkinson's disease - A randomized study. Parkinsonism Relat Disord. 2013. doi:10.1016/j.parkreldis.2013.03.003.
23. Johns MW. A new method for measuring daytime sleepiness: the Epworth sleepiness scale. Sleep. 1991;50:5.
24. Moul DE, Pilkonis PA, Miewald JM, Carey TJ, Buysse DJ: Preliminary study of the test-retest reliability and concurrent validities of the Pittsburgh Insomnia Rating Scale (PIRS). Sleep 25 Abstract Supplement, A246-A247, 2002.
25. Smith MT, Wegener ST. Measures of sleep: the insomnia severity index, medical outcomes study (MOS) sleep scale, Pittsburgh sleep diary (PSD), and Pittsburgh sleep quality index (PSQI). Arthritis Rheum. 2003; 49(Suppl 5):S184-96.
26. Krupp LB, LaRocca NG, Muir-Nash J, Steinberg AD. The fatigue severity scale: application to patients with multiple sclerosis and systemic lupus erythematosis. Arch Neurol. 1989;46:1121-3.
27. Kroenke K, Spitzer R, Williams W. The PHQ-9: Validy of a brief depression severity measure. JGIM. 2001:606-16.
28. Jenkinson C, Fitzpatrick R, Peto V, Greenhall R, Hyman N. The PDQ-8: development and validation of a short-form Parkinson's disease questionnaire. Psychol Health. 1997;12(6):805-14.
29. Yang M, et al. Interpreting score differences in the insomnia severity index: using health-related outcomes to define the minimally important difference. Journal Curr Med Res Opin. 2009;25(10):2487-94.
30. Bastien CH, Vallières A, Morin CM. Validation of the insomnia severity index as an outcome measure for insomnia research. Sleep Med. 2001;2(4):297-307.
31. Adler CH, Thorpy MJ. Sleep issues in Parkinson's disease. Neurology. 2005;64(12 Suppl 3):S12-20.
32. Kaynak D, Kiziltan G, Kaynak H, Benbir G, Uysal O. Sleep and sleepiness in patients with Parkinson's disease before and after dopaminergic treatment. Eur J Neurol. 2005;12(3):199-207.
33. Yan-Yee Ho F, Chung K-F, Yeung W-F, et al. Self-help cognitive-behavioral therapy for insomnia: A meta-analysis of randomized controlled trials. Sleep Med Rev. 2015;19:17-28.

32

Depressive symptoms can amplify embarrassment in essential tremor

Elan D. Louis[1,2,3*], Stephanie Cosentino[4,5] and Edward D. Huey[4,5,6,7]

Abstract

Background: Embarrassment can be a considerable problem for patients with essential tremor (ET) and is a major motivator for treatment. Depression is also a common feature of ET; as many as 35 % of patients report moderate to severe depressive symptoms. Our goal was to assess the associations between these motor and psychosocial factors (tremor, depression, embarrassment) in ET, with a particular interest in more fully assessing the possible association between depression and embarrassment.

Methods: Ninety one ET cases (age 70.4 ± 12.8 years) enrolled in a prospective, clinical-epidemiological study. Depressive symptoms were assessed with the Center for Epidemiological Studies Depression Scale (CESD-10, 0–30 [maximum]), embarrassment, with the Essential Tremor Embarrassment Assessment (ETEA, 0–70 [maximum]), and action tremor, with a detailed in-person neurological examination.

Results: Higher CESD-10 score was significantly associated with higher ETEA score ($p = 0.005$), but not with increasing tremor severity ($p = 0.94$). In stratified analyses, cases with no or minimal depressive symptoms had the lowest ETEA scores, cases with moderate depressive symptoms had intermediate ETEA scores, and cases with severe depressive symptoms had the highest ETEA scores ($p = 0.01$). Furthermore, at each level of tremor severity, cases with more depressive symptoms had more embarrassment.

Conclusions: Depressive symptoms seem to be more than a secondary response to the tremor in ET; they seem to amplify the level of embarrassment and, in addition to their own importance, seem to be a driver of other important clinical outcomes. Earlier treatment of depressive symptoms in ET patients could lessen the burden of secondary embarrassment.

Keywords: Essential tremor, Non-motor, Depression, Embarrassment, Clinical, Treatment

Background

According to some estimates, 60 % of essential tremor (ET) patients report embarrassment surrounding their tremor [1]. Embarrassment, classified as a "self-conscious" emotion along with shame and guilt, and in contrast to "basic" emotions such as anger and joy [2], often arises when someone violates a social rule or expectation [3]. Embarrassment is associated with autonomic reactivity including increased heart rate, blood pressure, and sweating and behavioral reactions including gaze avoidance, regret

signaling, and avoidance of others [3]. Embarrassment about tremor is a considerable problem for patients with ET [1, 4–7]. It is one of the two main motivators for ET patients to initiate medical therapy [1, 4–6] and it is a particularly strong predictor of receptivity to deep brain stimulation (DBS) surgery among patients with ET [8]. Moreover, feelings of embarrassment can lead to avoidance of social situations and social isolation [9]. Indeed, handling embarrassment and the social effects of tremor has been highlighted by ET patients as one of the top issues not being addressed in their care [10].

Depressive symptoms and depression have been associated with ET in numerous case–control studies [11–17]; according to some estimates, as many as 35 % of patients report moderate to severe depressive symptoms [17]. Similar to embarrassment, depression in ET is often

---

* Correspondence: elan.louis@yale.edu
[1]Division of Movement Disorders, Department of Neurology, Yale School of Medicine, Yale University, LCI 710, 15 York Street, PO Box 208018, New Haven, CT 06520-8018, USA
[2]Department of Chronic Disease Epidemiology, Yale School of Public Health, Yale University, New Haven, CT, USA
Full list of author information is available at the end of the article

viewed as a secondary response to the disabling condition [11, 14]. Overall; however, depression has not been well studied in ET [11], and there is emerging evidence that depression may be a primary feature of the disease, preceding motor symptoms [18]. This suggests that depression itself could drive other clinical outcomes in ET, such as embarrassment, rather than representing a passive response to the motor symptoms.

Although tremor, embarrassment, and depression may all occur in ET, and likely impact one another, the associations among them have not been the subject of previous analyses. The goal of these analyses was to assess the associations between these motor and psychosocial factors (ie, tremor, embarrassment, and depression) in individuals with ET, with a particular interest in more fully assessing the possible association between depression and embarrassment.

Methods

Participants and evaluation

As described previously, ET cases were enrolled in a clinical-epidemiological study of the epidemiology of movement disorders at Columbia University Medical Center (CUMC) [19, 20]. The large majority of cases were derived from two sources: (1) a computerized billing database of ET patients at the Neurological Institute of New York, CUMC, and (2) advertisements to members of the International Essential Tremor Foundation. One-hundred-forty-one cases were enrolled (2009–2014). During that time period, a formal assessment of embarrassment was added. Ninety-one cases were enrolled after the embarrassment assessment was added. Cases had all received a diagnosis of ET from their treating neurologist and were confined to a geographical area within 2 h driving distance of CUMC. Prior to enrollment, one of the authors (E.D.L.) reviewed the office records of identified patients; those with diagnoses of or physical signs consistent with other movement disorders were excluded.

The CUMC Internal Review Board approved of all study procedures. Written informed consent was obtained upon enrollment. Analysis of data was also approved by the Internal Review Board at Yale School of Medicine.

During the in-person evaluation, the trained research worker administered a series of structured clinical questionnaires (demographics, clinical features, medications, family history). The research worker also administered the Center for Epidemiological Studies Depression Scale (CESD-10) (0–30 [higher scores indicate greater depressive symptoms]) [21]. The CESD is a self-report measure of 10 questions about the frequency of experiencing (0 to 3 for each item) different depressive symptoms. It is a reliable and valid instrument [22]. In addition, the Essential Tremor Embarrassment Assessment (ETEA), an assessment of tremor-related embarrassment (range = 0–70 [maximal embarrassment]) [15] was administered to ET

patients [4]. The ETEA, which is a valid and reliable instrument [4], comprises 14 questions that assess overall embarrassment and its effects on the patient's desire for tremor medication, as well as embarrassment in a variety of situations (eg, eating in public, speaking in front of a group, social situations). Each item is rated from 0 to 5, with higher scores indicating greater embarrassment [4].

All cases underwent a standardized videotaped tremor examination, which included tests of postural and kinetic tremors and assessments for the presence of other involuntary movements. The aim was to use the videotape to carefully validate ET diagnoses using rigorous research-grade diagnostic criteria [23]. Thus, each videotape was reviewed by a senior neurologist specializing in movement disorders (E.D.L.) who confirmed the ET diagnoses using Washington Heights-Inwood Genetic Study of ET (WHIGET) diagnostic criteria (moderate or greater amplitude kinetic tremor [tremor rating ≥2] during three or more tests or a head tremor, in the absence of Parkinson's disease, dystonia or another cause) [23]. The neurologist also rated postural and kinetic tremor (range = 0–3) during 12 videotaped tests and computed a total tremor score (range = 0–36).

Statistical analyses

Data were analyzed in SPSS (Version 22.0). Chi-square tests were used to assess associations within categorical data. Total tremor score, ETEA score and CESD-10 score were all normally distributed (Kolmogorov-Smirnov Test p values = 0.67, 0.70, 0.35, respectively); hence, parametric tests (eg, Pearson's r) were used when assessing these variables.

Several CESD-10 cut-offs have been recommended for depression, including a score ≥10 [21], and a more conservative score ≥20 [24]. To incorporate both sets of recommendations, as in a prior set of analyses [25], we divided cases into three groups based on their CESD-10 score: 0–9 (no or minimal depressive symptoms), 10–19 (moderate depressive symptoms), ≥20 (severe depressive symptoms). Scores > 20 have high sensitivity and specificity for the diagnosis of Major Depressive Disorder as defined in the DSM [26–28]. To derive strictly mathematical cut-points, CESD-10 scores were also stratified into quartiles (≤3, 4–7, 8–12, ≥13).

Linear regression models were used to assess the associations between variables.

Results

The 91 ET cases had a mean age of 70.4 ± 12.8 years and a mean tremor duration of 36.9 ± 18.7 years. The mean CESD-10 score was 9.5 ± 6.2 (range = 0–26) (Table 1), with 47 (51.6 %) having no or minimal depressive symptoms, 37 (40.7 %) having moderate depressive symptoms and 7 (7.7 %) having severe depressive symptoms. Six (6.6 %) cases had CESD-10 scores > 20, of whom one (1.1 %) was

Table 1 Demographic and clinical characteristics of 91 ET cases

Age in years	70.4 ± 12.8 (range = 33–96)
Female gender	47 (51.6)
Education in years	16.2 ± 2.8
Non-Hispanic white race	86 (94.5)
Age of onset of tremor in years	37.7 ± 18.1
Tremor duration in years	36.9 ± 18.7
Family history of:	
ET	28 (30.8)
ET or tremor	58 (63.7)
Total tremor score	20.6 ± 5.9
Head (neck) tremor on examination	32 (35.2)
Voice tremor on examination	24 (26.4)
CESD-10 score	9.5 ± 6.2 (range = 0–26)
CESD-10 score	
0–9 (no or minimal depressive symptom category)	4.7 ± 2.7 (n = 47)
10–19 (moderate depressive symptom category)	13.0 ± 2.5 (n = 37)
≥ 20 (severe depressive symptom category)	23.1 ± 2.3 (n = 7)
CESD-10 score	
≤ 3 (lowest quartile)	1.4 ± 1.2
4–7 (second quartile)	5.4 ± 1.2
8–12 (third quartile)	10.2 ± 1.2
≥ 13 (highest quartile)	17.1 ± 4.1
ETEA score	24.2 ± 16.9 (range = 0–61)

Values represent mean ± standard deviation or number (percentage)
CESD-10 (Center for Epidemiological Studies Depression Scale), ETEA (Essential Tremor Embarrassment Assessment)

also taking an antidepressant medication. The mean ETEA score was 24.2 ± 16.9 (range = 0–61).

Higher total tremor score was associated with higher ETEA score (Pearson's $r = 0.27$, $p = 0.016$ and see Fig. 1); however, higher total tremor score was not associated with higher CESD-10 score (Pearson's $r = 0.008$, $p = 0.94$).

Higher CESD-10 score was associated with higher ETEA score (Pearson's $r = 0.29$, $p = 0.005$, Fig. 2). Furthermore, cases with no or minimal depressive symptoms had the lowest ETEA scores, cases with moderate depressive symptoms had intermediate ETEA scores, and cases with severe depressive symptoms had the highest ETEA scores ($p = 0.01$, Table 2). Similarly, there was a significant association between CESD-10 score quartile and ETEA score ($p = 0.001$, Table 2).

At each level of tremor severity (ie, at each total tremor score), higher level of depressive symptoms was associated with more embarrassment; thus, cases in the lowest CESD-10 quartile (ie, fewest depressive symptoms) had the lowest levels of embarrassment and cases in the highest CESD-10

quartile (ie, most depressive symptoms) had the highest levels of embarrassment (Fig. 1).

Cases with severe depressive symptoms (CESD-10 score ≥20) had higher ETEA scores than those with fewer depressive symptoms, despite the fact that they had similar levels of tremor severity (Table 3). Indeed, mean level of embarrassment was 50 % higher in cases with severe depressive symptoms than those with no or minimal depressive symptoms (31.4 vs. 19.9, Table 3) despite nearly identical total tremor scores (19.0 vs. 19.6, Table 3). This was associated with greater medication usage; 7 of 7 (100 %) cases with severe depressive symptoms had taken medication for tremor vs. 28/47 (59.6 %) of those with no or minimal depressive symptoms (chi-square test = 4.37, $p = 0.037$, Table 3).

In a subgroup analysis of 58 patients with family history of ET or tremor, higher CESD-10 score was associated with higher ETEA score (Pearson's $r = 0.30$, $p = 0.02$). Furthermore, cases with no or minimal depressive symptoms had the lowest ETEA scores ($n = 28$, 21.9 ± 17.6), cases with moderate depressive symptoms had intermediate ETEA scores ($n = 25$, 28.6 ± 16.4), and cases with severe depressive symptoms had the highest ETEA scores ($n = 5$, 36.8 ± 18.2) (linear regression analysis, $p = 0.04$).

Discussion

Tremor, depression, and embarrassment may co-occur in many ET patients, making this an important constellation of motor and psychosocial factors. Hence, it is surprising that the associations between these factors have not been delineated previously. In the current study, higher depressive symptom scores were associated with significantly greater levels of embarrassment ($p = 0.005$). Indeed, cases with no or minimal depressive symptoms had the lowest embarrassment scores, cases with moderate depressive symptoms had intermediate embarrassment scores, and cases with severe depressive symptoms had the highest embarrassment scores ($p = 0.01$). Cases with severe depressive symptoms (CESD-10 score ≥20) had higher ETEA scores than those with fewer depressive symptoms, despite the fact that they had similar levels of tremor severity. Indeed, level of embarrassment was 50 % higher in cases with severe depressive symptoms than those with minimal depressive symptoms despite nearly identical total tremor scores.

As noted above, at each level of tremor severity, cases who had more depressive symptoms had more embarrassment. While it is conceivable that greater embarrassment could lead to more depression, it is more plausible that the converse is the case, that is, that depressive symptoms are amplifying the level of embarrassment. The CESD-10 scale measures the full range of depressive symptoms including somatic symptoms such as poor appetite, decreased energy, psychomotor retardation, and insomnia. Embarrassment is unlikely to be the direct cause of any of

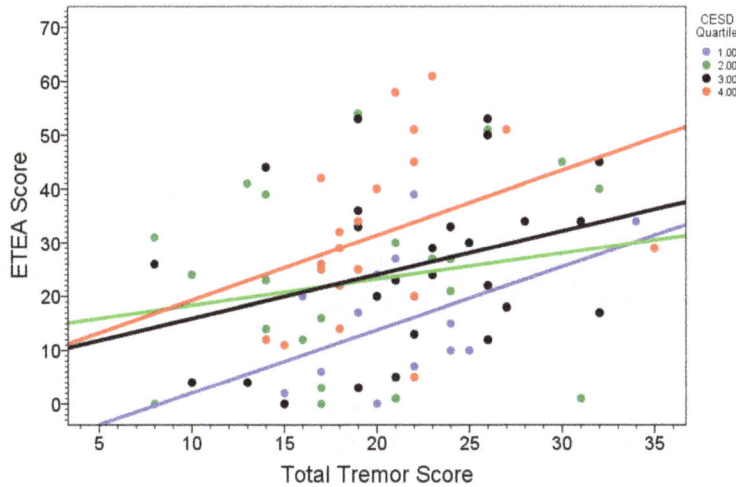

Fig. 1 ETEA score by total tremor score in each CESD-10 quartile. At each level of tremor severity (ie, at each total tremor score), higher level of depressive symptoms was associated with more embarrassment; thus, cases in the lowest CESD-10 quartile (ie, fewest depressive symptoms) had the lowest levels of embarrassment and cases in the highest CESD-10 quartile (ie, most depressive symptoms) had the highest levels of embarrassment

these depressive symptoms. Depression often acts as an amplifier of related symptoms in psychiatric disorders. Depression is associated with an increase in the distress and disability associated with chronic pain [29]. Self-conscious emotions including shame, guilt, and embarrassment increase, often dramatically, during an episode of major depressive disorder [30].

More broadly, these data also suggest that depressive symptoms are a driver of other important clinical outcomes in ET rather than merely a passive, secondary response to tremor. Depressive symptoms and/or depression have been reported as more prevalent in ET cases than controls in numerous studies [11–17]. Indeed, in the current study, more than half of the cases had moderate or severe depressive symptoms. Despite its high prevalence,

the causes, effects and natural history of depression in ET have not been studied in any detail [11], although in a prior set of analyses, we showed that depressive symptoms were a strong predictor of tremor-related quality of life in ET [25]. Furthermore, its relationship to the motor features of ET may be complex. Emerging evidence suggests that depression may even be a primary feature of ET, preceding the motor features [18]. This finding has precedent in other movement disorders, including Huntington's disease and Parkinson's disease [31, 32]. Studies that examine the clinical correlates of depression and its relationships with other disease features in ET are therefore of importance.

Table 2 Association between CESD-10 and ETEA scores in 91 ET cases

	ETEA score
CESD-10 score category	
0–9 (no or minimal depressive symptoms)	19.9 ± 16.4
10–19 (moderate depressive symptoms)	28.4 ± 16.4
≥ 20 (severe depressive symptoms)	31.4 ± 17.6
	$p = 0.01$[a]
CESD-10 score quartiles	
≤ 3 (lowest quartile)	15.3 ± 12.2
4–7 (second quartile)	20.2 ± 17.3
8–12 (third quartile)	26.6 ± 16.5
≥ 13 (highest quartile)	31.6 ± 16.7
	$p = 0.001$[b]

Values represent mean ± standard deviation or number (percentage)
CESD-10 (Center for Epidemiological Studies Depression Scale), ETEA (Essential Tremor Embarrassment Assessment)
[a]Linear regression analysis with ETEA score as dependent variable and CESD score category as the independent variable
[b]Linear regression analysis with ETEA score as dependent variable and CESD score quartile as the independent variable

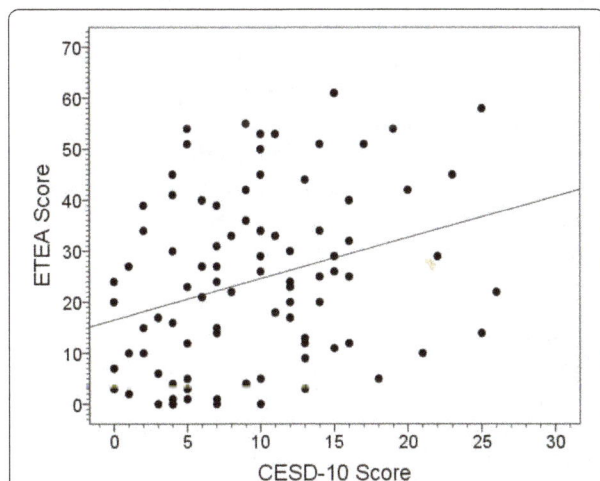

Fig. 2 ETEA score by CESD-10 score. Higher CESD-10 score was associated with higher ETEA score (Pearson's $r = 0.29$, p = 0.005)

Table 3 CESD-10 score category, total tremor score, ETEA score and medication usage in 91 ET cases

CESD-10 score category	n	Total tremor score	ETEA score	Number (%) who had been prescribed medication for tremor
0–9 (no or minimal depressive symptoms)	47	19.6 ± 6.2	19.9 ± 16.4	28 (59.6)
10–19 (moderate depressive symptoms)	37	22.1 ± 5.8	28.4 ± 16.4	24 (64.9)
≥20 (severe depressive symptoms)	7	19.0 ± 2.0	31.4 ± 17.6	7 (100)
		$p = 0.36^a$	$p = 0.01^b$	

Values represent mean ± standard deviation or number (percentage)
CESD-10 (Center for Epidemiological Studies Depression Scale), ETEA (Essential Tremor Embarrassment Assessment)
[a]Linear regression analysis with total tremor score as dependent variable and CESD score category as the independent variable
[b]Linear regression analysis with ETEA score as dependent variable and CESD score category as the independent variable

One clinical implication of the current findings is that they increase the importance of treating depressive symptoms in patients with ET as, in addition to reducing depressive symptoms, it may reduce embarrassment as well. Embarrassment is a considerable problem for ET patients [1, 4–6]. It is one of the two main motivators for initiating medical therapy [1, 4–6] and can further lead to avoidance of social situations and social isolation [9]. Indeed, handling the embarrassing social effects of tremor has been highlighted by patients as one of the top issues not being addressed in their current care [10]. While the effect of depression treatment has not been specifically studied in ET patients, the effect size for the treatment of depressive symptoms with antidepressant medication in patients with Parkinson's disease is moderate [33]. The findings of the current study also suggest that the treatment of depression with psychotherapy in patients with ET should assess and target embarrassment as well as the more usual depressive symptoms. In ET patients with depression and prominent embarrassment, referral to a psychotherapist who utilizes a symptom-based therapy method such as Cognitive-Behavioral Therapy (CBT) or Problem-Solving Therapy (PST) could be preferable to insight-oriented psychodynamic therapy.

Our cases had a mean CESD-10 score of 9.5 ± 6.2. A feature of this clinical-epidemiological study, but not of these analyes, was the enrollment of control subjects of similar age ($n = 177$, 74.9 ± 9.5 years). The mean CESD-10 score of these controls was only 6.7 ± 4.6, a value that was lower than that of our cases (t test = 3.84, p <0.001), indicating a higher burden of depressive symptoms among our cases, as has been reported in ET in the past [11–17].

This study should be interpreted within the context of certain limitations. First, the study was cross-sectional, so that we are not able to directly address issues of causality. Second, the sample size was modest and this may have limited our ability to detect associations. However, the study was able to detect significant main effects between several of the key variables. Third, depressive symptoms were assessed with a brief, validated screening instrument; it is possible that more in-depth psychiatric assessments

could have uncovered additional associations of interest. For example, the relationship between symptoms of anxiety, including social anxiety, and embarrassment and the relationship between ET and other self-conscious emotions. In particular, anxiety is also a common feature of patients with ET [9, 17] and it could impact upon levels of embarrassment. Future studies could further assess such relationships. Fourth, we did not collect data on past history of depression in our cases; such information could have supplemented the data we collected on current depressive symptoms.

The study also had several strengths. First, to our knowledge, it is the only study to have assessed this particular gap in knowledge and these particular associations. Second, this was not a retrospective study or chart review; the study cohort was enrolled prospectively, with a standardized assessment.

Conclusions

In summary, we found that cases with severe depressive symptoms had higher embarrassment scores than those with fewer depressive symptoms, despite the fact that they had similar levels of tremor severity. Furthermore, greater tremor severity was not associated with more depressive symptoms. One interpretation of these data is that depressive symptoms are more than a secondary response to the tremor in ET; in addition to being clinically important in themselves, they also seem to drive other important outcomes such as embarrassment. Earlier treatment of depressive symptoms in ET patients might be a strategy to lessen the burden of secondary embarrassment.

Abbreviations
(CES-D), Center for Epidemiological Studies Depression Scale; (CBT), Center for Epidemiological Studies Depression Scale; (CUMC), Columbia University Medical Center; (DBS),Deep brain stimulation; (ET), Essential tremor; (ETEA), Essential Tremor Embarrassment Assessment; (PST), Essential Tremor Embarrassment Assessment; (WHIGET), Washington Heights-Inwood Genetic Study of ET

Acknowledgements
None.

Funding
Dr. Louis has received research support from the National Institutes of Health: NINDS #R01 NS086736, #R01 NS094607 and #R01 NS076837. This funding body played no role in the design of the study, the collection, analysis, and interpretation of data, or the writing of the manuscript.

Authors' contributions
EDL designed the study, over-saw the collection of data, obtained funding, performed the initial statistical analyses, and prepared the initial manuscript. SC participated in the design of study, design of additional analyses, interpretation of data, and manuscript preparation. EDH participated in the design of study, design of additional analyses, interpretation of data, and manuscript preparation. All authors read and approved the final manuscript.

Competing interests
The authors declare that they have no competing interest.

Author details
[1]Division of Movement Disorders, Department of Neurology, Yale School of Medicine, Yale University, LCI 710, 15 York Street, PO Box 208018, New Haven, CT 06520-8018, USA. [2]Department of Chronic Disease Epidemiology, Yale School of Public Health, Yale University, New Haven, CT, USA. [3]Center for Neuroepidemiology and Clinical Neurological Research, Yale School of Medicine, Yale University, New Haven, CT, USA. [4]Department of Neurology, College of Physicians and Surgeons, Columbia University, New York, NY, USA. [5]Division of Geriatric Psychiatry, Department of Psychiatry, College of Physicians and Surgeons, Columbia University, New York, NY, USA. [6]G.H. Sergievsky Center, College of Physicians and Surgeons, Columbia University, New York, NY, USA. [7]Taub Institute for Research on Alzheimer's Disease and the Aging Brain, Columbia University, New York, NY, USA.

References
1. Louis ED, Rios E. Embarrassment in essential tremor: prevalence, clinical correlates and therapeutic implications. Parkinsonism Relat Disord. 2009;15:535–8.
2. Lewis M, Haviland-Jones JM, editors. Handbook of Emotions. New York: The Guilford Press; 2000. p. 623–36.
3. Keltner D, Buswell BN. Embarrassment: its distinct form and appeasement functions. Psychol Bull. 1997;122:250–70.
4. Traub RE, Gerbin M, Mullaney MM, Louis ED. Development of an essential tremor embarrassment assessment. Parkinsonism Relat Disord. 2010;16:661–5.
5. Holding SJ, Lew AR. Relations between psychological avoidance, symptom severity and embarrassment in essential tremor. Chronic Illn. 2015;11:69–71.
6. Louis ED. Clinical practice. Essential tremor. N Engl J Med. 2001;345:887–91.
7. Koller W, Biary N, Cone S. Disability in essential tremor: effect of treatment. Neurology. 1986;36:1001–4.
8. Louis ED, Gillman A. Factors associated with receptivity to deep brain stimulation surgery among essential tremor cases. Parkinsonism Relat Disord. 2011;17:482–5.
9. Schneier FR, Barnes LF, Albert SM, Louis ED. Characteristics of social phobia among persons with essential tremor. J Clin Psychiatry. 2001;62(5):367–72.
10. Louis ED, Rohl B, Rice C. Defining the treatment gap: what essential tremor patients want that they are not getting. Tremor Other Hyperkinet Mov (N Y). 2015;5:331. doi:10.7916/D87080M9. eCollection 2015.
11. Louis ED. Non-motor symptoms in essential tremor: A review of the current data and state of the field. Parkinsonism Relat Disord. 2016;22 Suppl 1:S115–8.
12. Dogu O, Louis ED, Sevim S, Kaleagasi H, Aral M. Clinical characteristics of essential tremor in Mersin, Turkey–a population-based door-to-door study. J Neurol. 2005;252:570–4.
13. Li ZW, Xie MJ, Tian DS, Li JJ, Zhang JP, Jiao L, et al. Characteristics of depressive symptoms in essential tremor. J Clin Neurosci. 2011;18:52–6.
14. Chandran V, Pal PK, Reddy JY, Thennarasu K, Yadav R, Shivashankar N. Non-motor features in essential tremor. Acta Neurol Scand. 2012;125:332–7.
15. Fabbrini G, Berardelli I, Falla M, Moretti G, Pasquini M, Altieri M, et al. Psychiatric disorders in patients with essential tremor. Parkinsonism Relat Disord. 2012;18:971–3.
16. Lee SM, Kim M, Lee HM, Kwon KY, Koh SB. Nonmotor symptoms in essential tremor: Comparison with Parkinson's disease and normal control. J Neurol Sci. 2015;349:168–73.
17. Sengul Y, Sengul HS, Yucekaya SK, Yucel S, Bakim B, Pazarci NK, et al. Cognitive functions, fatigue, depression, anxiety, and sleep disturbances: assessment of nonmotor features in young patients with essential tremor. Acta Neurol Belg. 2014;115:281–7.
18. Louis ED, Benito-Leon J, Bermejo-Pareja F. Self-reported depression and anti-depressant medication use in essential tremor: cross-sectional and prospective analyses in a population-based study. Eur J Neurol. 2007;14:1138–46.
19. Louis ED, Rao AK. Functional aspects of gait in essential tremor: a comparison with age-matched parkinson's disease cases, dystonia cases, and controls. Tremor Other Hyperkinet Mov (N Y). 2015;27:5. doi:10.7916/D8B27T7J. eCollection 2015.
20. Louis ED, Factor-Litvak P, Michalec M, Jiang W, Zheng W. Blood harmane (1-methyl-9H-pyrido[3,4-b]indole) concentration in dystonia cases vs. controls. Neurotoxicology. 2014;44:110–3.
21. Andresen EM, Malmgren JA, Carter WB, Patrick DL. Screening for depression in well older adults: evaluation of a short form of the CES-D (Center for Epidemiologic Studies Depression Scale). Am J Prev Med. 1994;10:77–84.
22. Bjorgvinsson T, Kertz SJ, Bigda-Peyton JS, McCoy KL, Aderka IM. Psychometric properties of the CES-D-10 in a psychiatric sample. Assessment. 2013;20:429–36.
23. Louis ED, Ottman R, Ford B, Pullman S, Martinez M, Fahn S, et al. The Washington Heights-Inwood Genetic Study of Essential Tremor: methodologic issues in essential-tremor research. Neuroepidemiology. 1997;16:124–33.
24. Kirsch-Darrow L, Fernandez HH, Marsiske M, Okun MS, Bowers D. Dissociating apathy and depression in Parkinson disease. Neurology. 2006;67:33–8.
25. Louis ED, Huey ED, Gerbin M, Viner AS. Depressive traits in essential tremor: impact on disability, quality of life, and medication adherence. Eur J Neurol. 2012;19:1349–54.
26. Lyness JM, Noel TK, Cox C, King DA, Conwell Y, Caine ED. Screening for depression in elderly primary care patients. A comparison of the Center for Epidemiologic Studies-Depression Scale and the Geriatric Depression Scale. Arch Intern Med. 1997;157:449–54.
27. Irwin M, Artin KH, Oxman MN. Screening for depression in the older adult: criterion validity of the 10-item Center for Epidemiological Studies Depression Scale (CES-D). Arch Intern Med. 1999;159:1701–4.
28. Louis ED, Huey ED, Gerbin M, Viner AS. Apathy in essential tremor, dystonia, and Parkinson's disease: a comparison with normal controls. Mov Disord. 2012;27:432–4.
29. Von Korff M, Simon G. The relationship between pain and depression. Br J Psychiatry Suppl. 1996;101–8.
30. Buist-Bouwman MA, Ormel J, de Graaf R, de Jonge P, van Sonderen E, Alonso J, et al. Mediators of the association between depression and role functioning. Acta Psychiatr Scand. 2008;118:451–8.
31. Tabrizi SJ, Scahill RI, Owen G, Durr A, Leavitt BR, Roos RA, et al. Predictors of phenotypic progression and disease onset in premanifest and early-stage Huntington's disease in the TRACK-HD study: analysis of 36-month observational data. Lancet Neurol. 2013;12:637–49.
32. Chen JJ, Marsh L. Depression in Parkinson's disease: identification and management. Pharmacotherapy. 2013;33:972–83.
33. Troeung L, Egan SJ, Gasson N. A meta-analysis of randomised placebo-controlled treatment trials for depression and anxiety in Parkinson's disease. PLoS One. 2013;8:e79510.

33

Characterization of vitamin D supplementation and clinical outcomes in a large cohort of early Parkinson's disease

Nijee S. Luthra[1*], Soeun Kim[2], Yunxi Zhang[2], Chadwick W. Christine[1,3] and On behalf of the NINDS NET-PD Investigators

Abstract

Background: Vitamin D (VitD) deficiency is common in Parkinson's disease (PD) and has been raised as a possible PD risk factor. In the past decade, VitD supplementation for potential prevention of age related conditions has become more common. In this study, we sought to characterize VitD supplementation in early PD and determine as an exploratory analysis whether baseline characteristics or disease progression differed according to reported VitD use.

Methods: We analyzed data from the National Institutes of Health Exploratory Trials in Parkinson's Disease (NET-PD) Long-term study (LS-1), a longitudinal study of 1741 participants. Subjects were divided into following supplement groups according to subject exposure (6 months prior to baseline and during the study): no VitD supplement, multivitamin (MVI), VitD ≥400 IU/day, and VitD + multivitamin (VitD+MVI). Clinical status was followed using the Unified Parkinson's Disease Rating Scale, Symbol Digit Modalities Test, total daily levodopa equivalent dose, and Parkinson's Disease Questionnaire.

Results: About 5% of subjects took VitD alone, 7% took VitD+MVI, 34% took MVI alone, while 54% took no supplement. Clinical outcomes at 3 years were similar across all groups.

Conclusion: This study shows VitD supplementation ≥400 IU/day was not common in early PD and that its use was similar to that seen in the US population. At 3 years, there was no difference in disease progression according to vitamin D supplement use.

Keywords: 1,25-dihydroxyvitamin D, Parkinson's disease

Background

Numerous reports have shown that vitamin D (VitD) insufficiency is common in aging, is associated with greater risk of falls and fractures, and that VitD supplementation may reduce the risk of fractures [1]. Because of this observation, and possibly because of numerous studies showing associations of D deficiency with diseases in adults, VitD supplementation has become common. A cross-sectional survey from 2011 to 12 found that about 21% of adults aged 40–64 and 38% of those > 65 take a separate VitD supplement [2].

A relationship of VitD levels and Parkinson's disease (PD) was first recognized in 1997 when Sato and colleagues reported a higher prevalence of VitD deficiency and reduced bone mass in PD [3]. Since then, a number of studies have confirmed these findings [4] and that a mutation in the VitD receptor is associated with an increased risk of developing PD [5]. Studies in experimental animal models of PD have demonstrated neuroprotective effects of VitD [6], lending support to the hypothesis that VitD status may influence PD pathogenesis. The Mini-Finland Health Survey provided additional support of this hypothesis by showing a greater risk for PD in those with lower VitD levels [7].

Because these studies raise the question as to whether VitD supplementation affects PD progression,

* Correspondence: nijee.luthra@ucsf.edu
[1]Department of Neurology, University of California, 1635 Divisadero, Suite 520-530, San Francisco, CA 94115, USA
Full list of author information is available at the end of the article

we performed a study to characterize contemporary VitD supplementation in a large, longitudinal cohort of early PD patients from the National Institutes of Health Exploratory Trials in Parkinson's Disease (NET-PD) Long-term study (LS-1) which enrolled subjects from the United States and Canada from 2007 to 2010. As a an exploratory outcome, we also determined whether baseline characteristics or disease progression outcomes differed according to reported VitD supplement use prior to baseline and during the study observation period.

Methods

The NET-PD LS-1 study was a large randomized multi-center, double-blind, placebo-controlled study of creatine monohydrate. As previously described, eligible subjects had diagnosis of PD for < 5 years and had started treatment with levodopa or dopamine agonist for ≥90 days but < 2 years prior to the baseline visit [8]. Subjects were monitored with annual visits for up to 6 years. The study was halted before completion after it was determined no difference would emerge between the treatment arms [8].

At study entry, subjects were required to report all medications and supplements used in the prior 180 days, although many provided much longer histories of supplement use. We reviewed the concomitant medication records for VitD and multivitamin (MVI) use including supplement brand name (when available), dose, frequency, start date and end date. Of the 1956 records of supplement use (separate records were created for each supplement), 620 (31%) documented supplement use starting prior to 2005. For those taking specified supplements, the published dose was used. The daily dose was calculated according to dose and frequency. Subjects were stratified according to the following VitD exposure groups: no VitD or MVI supplement (NoSupp), multivitamin where dose of VitD was assumed (if not specified) to be 400 IU/dose (MVI group), ≥ 400 IU/day of VitD (VitD group), or multivitamin plus ≥ of 400 IU/day of VitD (VitD+MVI group).

In order to construct defined groups of participants with different dose and longitudinal VitD exposures, subjects were included in the analysis if they had been taking supplements for ≥90 days prior to baseline and continued that supplement for at least 1.5 years of the first 3 years of the study or their records indicated no D supplementation or MVI during this timeframe (NoSupp group). Subjects who took VitD for shorter durations during the study period or at lower doses were excluded.

Assessments

Because a significant fraction of subjects did not complete the 5-year visit due to early study termination, we calculated mean study outcomes at baseline and the change from baseline in outcomes at 3 years. Outcomes included demographics, Unified Parkinson's Disease Rating Scale (UPDRS) total score and its subscores obtained in the practically defined "On-medication" state, [mental (Part 1), activities of daily living (Part 2), and motor (Part 3)], Parkinson's Disease Questionnaire (PDQ39), Scales for Outcomes in Parkinson's Disease-Cognition (SCOPA--COG; only performed at baseline and 5 year visit), Symbol Digit Modalities Test (SDMT), and total daily levodopa equivalent dose (LED).

Statistical analysis

To investigate baseline characteristics for each group, means and standard deviations were calculated for continuous variables, and percentages were computed for categorical variables. NoSupp, MVI, VitD, VitD+MVI groups were compared using Analysis of variance (ANOVA) test for continuous variables, and Chi-square tests and Fisher's exact tests for categorical variables. Baseline age and age at PD diagnosis was summarized by performing subgroup analyses on males and females, using ANOVA test within each gender group. Pairwise comparisons were assessed using the Hochberg's multiple testing method. Changes from baseline in the outcomes were computed at the third year visit, and mean changes were compared for four groups using ANOVA test. The ANOVA test was used to compare mean age at diagnosis for the four supplement groups, within each age categories. In order to adjust for baseline morbidity, we also performed the outcome analysis using mixed models, adjusting for baseline age and the corresponding baseline score as fixed effects and including site as a random effect. SAS 9.4 was used for the analyses.

Results

Of the 1741 subjects who enrolled in the study, 943 subjects had been taking MVI, VitD, or VitD+MVI for ≥90 days prior to baseline and at least 1.5 years of duration of the study or reported no supplement use (NoSupp group) during this timeframe. Of these subjects, 54% of subjects took NoSupp, 34% took MVI, 5% took VitD, and 7% took VitD+MVI (where for VitD, the dose was > 400 IU/day).

Although disease severity as measured by rating scales was similar between the groups at baseline, the age at baseline, and the related age at diagnosis of PD, was higher in subjects taking supplements [MVI (60.2 ± 8.7), VitD (63.9 ± 6.6) and VitD+MVI (64.1 ± 7.7)] compared to subjects in NoSupp (58.5 ± 9.7) group (Table 1). In order to address whether supplement use differed according to age, we then performed an analysis segregated according to age range (< 50, 50-59, 60–69, ≥70) at PD diagnosis (Table 2). This analysis confirmed that VitD use was higher in older patients and that when sorted by age range, the mean ages at diagnosis were not different. Time

Table 1 Baseline Characteristics

	No Supplement (N = 511)	MVI (N = 322)	D (N = 42)	D + MVI (N = 68)	P value
	Mean (SD)				F test
Age in years	60.1 (9.7)	61.8 (8.6)*	65.3 (6.4)*	65.5 (7.7)*	< 0.0001
Age at PD Dx	58.5 (9.7)	60.2 (8.7)*	63.9 (6.6)*	64.1 (7.7)*	< 0.0001
Yrs since Dx	1.6 (1.1)	1.7 (1.2)	1.3 (1.0)	1.4 (0.8)	0.07
Years since Dx to D-treatment	1.1 (1.1)	1.3 (1.2)	0.9 (1.0)	1.0 (0.8)	0.08
UPDRS total	25.1 (10.3)	25.4 (10.3)	25.1 (11.4)	24.5 (9.8)	0.92
UPDRS mental	1.2 (1.3)	1.2 (1.3)	1.4 (1.4)	1.2 (1.3)	0.85
UPDRS ADL	6.8 (3.7)	6.8 (3.6)	6.2 (3.9)	6.4 (3.4)	0.66
PDQ 39 summary	12.9 (10.4)	11.5 (8.7)	12.5 (9.6)	10.5 (8.3)	0.08
SCOPA COG	30.4 (5.1)	30.4 (5.2)	30.9 (4.6)	31.1 (5.0)	0.71
SDMT	45.1 (11.1)	44.4 (10.9)	45.2 (11.4)	45.9 (11.4)	0.71
Total daily LED	374.9 (224.9)	371.3 (232.8)	390.0 (208.0)	367.4 (355.4)	0.96
	Frequency (%)				X^2test[a]
Female %	144 (28.2%)	94 (29.2%)	27 (64.3%)	38 (55.9%)	< 0.0001
Non-Hispanic white	448 (87.7%)	303 (94.1%)	41 (97.6%)	66 (97.1%)	0.001
Education > 17 years[a]	149 (29.2%)	118 (36.7%)	16 (38.1%)	18 (26.5%)	0.08

Abbreviations: PD Parkinson's disease, *Dx* diagnosis, *yrs* years, *D-treatment* dopaminergic treatment (dopamine agonist or levodopa), *UPDRS* Unified Parkinson's Disease Rating Scale, *ADL* activities of daily living, *PDQ* Parkinson's disease questionnaire, *SCOPA COG* Scales for outcomes of Parkinson's disease-Cognition, *SDMT* symbol digit modalities test, *LED* levodopa equivalent dose
*$p < .05$ compared to NoSupp, according to pairwise comparisons Hochberg method
[a]X^2 test was calculated by Fisher's exact test

from diagnosis to start of dopaminergic treatment was not different in subjects taking supplements (Table 1). The percentage of females and non-Hispanic whites was higher in the VitD and VitD+MVI groups.

No differences in mean clinical outcomes were noted between groups at 3 years (Table 3). An analysis using mixed models, adjusted for baseline age and corresponding baseline scores as covariates, also failed to show a difference in outcomes according to supplement use (Table 4).

Discussion

In this analysis of the NET-PD LS1 cohort, we found that about 12% of subjects took >400 IU/day of VitD

supplementation while 34% took a MVI estimated to contain 400 IU/day of VitD. Disease progression as measured by a variety of rating scales at 3 years was similar in all 4 groups. Although methods of ascertainment were quite different, these rates of MVI and VitD use are in line with rates reported in the United States population from the large cross-sectional NHANES study of 34% for MVI use and 11% for separate VitD supplement use from 2007 to 8 [2].

Our finding that the age at diagnosis of PD was older in the MVI group, VitD and VitD plus MVI groups could suggest a disease delaying effect. However, further analysis of this data segregated according to age range of onset showed that VitD supplementation was higher in

Table 2 Analysis of Supplement Use by Age Range

Age at Diagnosis	Statistics	No Supp (N = 511)	MVI (N = 322)	VitD (N = 42)	VitD + MVI (N = 68)	p-value
< 50	Freq (%)	91 (70%)	35 (27%)	1 (1%)	2 (2%)	
	Mean (SD)	44.04 (4.54)	44.63 (5.07)	45.00 (NA)	46.50 (3.54)	0.83
50–59	Freq (%)	182 (58%)	106 (34%)	10 (3%)	17 (5%)	
	Mean (SD)	54.85 (2.73)	54.87 (2.96)	56.70 (3.09)	56.06 (2.88)	0.08
60–69	Freq (%)	164 (46%)	139 (39%)	23 (6%)	30 (9%)	
	Mean (SD)	63.81 (2.90)	64.12 (2.85)	64.83 (3.16)	64.13 (2.76)	0.42
≥70	Freq (%)	74 (52%)	42 (29%)	8 (6%)	19 (13%)	
	Mean (SD)	73.54 (3.21)	73.29 (2.62)	72.38 (1.06)	73.37 (3.92)	0.78

Table 3 Mean Change in Outcomes and at 3-year Visit

	No D Supplement (N = 511) Mean (SD)	MVI (N = 322)	D (N = 42)	D + MVI (N = 68)	P value F test
Change in UPDRS total	5.5 (11.8)	6.2 (12.0)	4.9 (9.8)	9.2 (14.3)	0.12
Change in UPDRS mental	0.5 (1.5)	0.5 (1.5)	0.6 (2.0)	0.6 (1.8)	0.83
Change in UPDRS ADL	2.0 (4.4)	2.3 (4.5)	1.9 (3.6)	3.0 (4.7)	0.30
Change in PDQ 39 summary	4.6 (10.4)	4.3 (9.6)	4.0 (11.3)	4.8 (10.5)	0.96
Change in SDMT	0.002 (9.5)	−0.2 (9.4)	−1.6 (11.0)	−0.8 (13.3)	0.73
Change in Total daily LED	294.6 (367.1)	268.4 (339.8)	220.6 (244.5)	271.5 (346.4)	0.48

Abbreviations: UPDRS Unified Parkinson's Disease Rating Scale, *ADL* activities of daily living, *PDQ* Parkinson's disease questionnaire, *SDMT* symbol digit modalities test, *LED* levodopa equivalent dose

older participants (suggesting reverse causation), and that mean age at diagnosis was no longer significantly different between groups.

Our finding that VitD supplementation did not affect PD progression is consistent with observations from the

Table 4 Change in Outcomes at 3-year Visit according to mixed models[a]

Outcome	Group	Estimate	P value
Change in UPDRS total	No Supplement	.	.
	MVI	0.248	0.77
	D	−1.517	0.43
	D + MVI	2.540	0.10
Change in UPDRS ADL	No Supplement	.	.
	MVI	0.117	0.70
	D	−0.555	0.43
	D + MVI	0.469	0.41
Change in UPDRS mental	No Supplement	.	.
	MVI	−0.058	0.58
	D	0.083	0.73
	D + MVI	0.083	0.67
Change in PDQ39	No Supplement	.	.
	MVI	−0.571	0.43
	D	−0.986	0.55
	D + MVI	−0.422	0.75
Change in SDMT	No Supplement	.	.
	MVI	−0.041	0.95
	D	−0.654	0.67
	D + MVI	0.871	0.48
Change in Total daily LED	No Supplement	.	.
	MVI	−23.174	0.34
	D	−63.506	0.25
	D + MVI	−19.346	0.66

Abbreviations: UPDRS Unified Parkinson's Disease Rating Scale, *ADL* activities of daily living, *PDQ* Parkinson's disease questionnaire, *SDMT* symbol digit modalities test, *LED* levodopa equivalent dose
[a]Model controlled for baseline age and the corresponding baseline score as fixed effects and including site as a random effect

DATATOP study of early PD in which no correlation was seen between VitD levels and disease progression [9]. However, a more recent 3-year study did find a small, but significant association between VitD levels measured at baseline and motor progression [10], raising the possibility that the amount of VitD supplementation by the NET-PD LS1 participants was inadequate to provide benefit.

Although there is evidence of high prevalence of VitD deficiency in early PD [9] and established PD [11], there is currently little published regarding the effect of VitD supplementation in PD. Suzuki et al. conducted a randomized, placebo-controlled study examining the effect supplementation with 1200 IU/day of vitamin D3/d for 12 months [12]. They found that D supplementation was associated with smaller changes in a number of outcomes measures including the Hoehn and Yahr stage, UPDRS part II and total, and some domains of the PDQ39 as well as the participants' VitD receptor genotype. Their study differed from our study in a number of ways since it was randomized, larger doses of VitD were specified, and because subjects started treatment after baseline while our study followed subjects on established VitD supplementation for a longer duration of time. Their design examines both potential treatment and neuroprotective effects of D supplementation while our study more specifically examined baseline characteristics of supplemented patients and their progression.

Our study has several limitations. As it is a secondary analysis, subjects were not randomized to treatment. Also, subjects were analyzed according to reported supplement dose with no independent measurements of serum VitD levels nor were we able to account for differing levels of sunlight exposure. Moreover although many subjects provided information regarding supplement use for years prior to study entry, study procedures only required report of supplement use in the 180 days prior to baseline, which for the majority of subjects was after their PD diagnosis. There were also lower numbers of subjects taking VitD or VitD+MVI compared to the other groups. Finally, while this study did not show differences in disease progression in the first three years after starting dopaminergic treatment, it is possible that D supplementation could affect later PD progression.

Conclusion

Although VitD insufficiency is common in PD, this study shows VitD >400 IU/day supplementation was not common and was similar to the rate observed in cross-sectional studies of the general US population according to age group. Although no difference in early disease progression was observed in patients taking VitD supplementation, it remains possible that consistent VitD supplementation could reduce the development of disability related to bone health, since osteoporosis is more common in PD and the risk of falls and bone fracture increase with disease duration. These data may be helpful in the design of studies testing the effect of vitamin D supplementation over a longer time frame.

Abbreviations

ANOVA: Analysis of variance; LED: Levodopa equivalent dose; LS-1: Long-term study; MVI: Multivitamin; NET-PD: National Institutes of Health Exploratory Trials in Parkinson's Disease; NoSupp: No supplement; PD: Parkinson's disease; PDQ39: Parkinson's Disease Questionnaire; SCOPA-COG: Scales for Outcomes in Parkinson's Disease-Cognition; SDMT: Symbol Digit Modalities Test; UPDRS: Unified Parkinson's Disease Rating Scale; Vitamin D: VitD

Acknowledgements

We gratefully acknowledge patients and their families for participation in the NET-PD LS-1 clinical trial.

Funding

The NET-PD LS-1 trial received funding support from the National Institute for Neurological Disorders and Stroke (U01NS43128 and U01 NS043127). For the current report, a secondary analysis of trial data, the authors received no specific funding to support this work.

Authors' contributions

NL and CC made substantial contributions to conception, design, analysis and interpretation of data, drafting the manuscript and gave final approval of the version to be published. SK and YZ made substantial contributions to acquisition of data, statistical analysis and interpretation of data. Each author has participated sufficiently in the work to take public responsibility for appropriate portions of the content and agreed to be accountable for all aspects of the work in ensuring that questions related to the accuracy or integrity of any part of the work are appropriately investigated and resolved. All authors read and approved the final manuscript.

Competing interests

The authors declare that they have no competing interests.

Author details

[1]Department of Neurology, University of California, 1635 Divisadero, Suite 520-530, San Francisco, CA 94115, USA. [2]Department of Biostatistics and Data Science, University of Texas Health Center, 1200 Pressler Street, Houston, TX 77030, USA. [3]Department of Neurology, University of California San Francisco, 400 Parnassus Ave Box 0348, San Francisco, CA 94122, USA.

References

1. Rosen CJ. Clinical practice Vitamin D insufficiency. N Engl J Med. 2011. https://doi.org/10.1056/NEJMcp1009570.
2. Kantor ED, Rehm CD, Du M, White E, Giovannucci EL. Trends in dietary supplement use among US adults from 1999-2012. JAMA. 2016. https://doi.org/10.1001/jama.2016.14403.
3. Sato Y, Kikuyama M, Oizumi K. High prevalence of vitamin D deficiency and reduced bone mass in Parkinson's disease. Neurology. 1997. https://doi.org/10.1212/WNL.49.5.1273.
4. Wang L, Evatt ML, Maldonado LG, Perry WR, Ritchie JC, Beecham GW, et al. Vitamin D from different sources is inversely associated with Parkinson disease. Mov Disord. 2015. https://doi.org/10.1002/mds.26117.
5. Han X, Xue L, Li Y, Chen B, Xie A. Vitamin D receptor gene polymorphism and its association with Parkinson's disease in Chinese Han population. Neurosci Lett. 2012. https://doi.org/10.1016/j.neulet.2012.07.033.
6. Deluca GC, Kimball SM, Kolasinski J, Ramagopalan SV, Ebers GC. Review: the role of vitamin D in nervous system health and disease. Neuropathol Appl. 2013. https://doi.org/10.1111/nan.12020.
7. Knekt P, Kilkkinen A, Rissanen H, Marniemi J, Sääksjärvi K, Heliövaara M. Serum vitamin D and the risk of Parkinson disease. Arch Neurol. 2010. https://doi.org/10.1001/archneurol.2010.120.
8. Kieburtz K, Tilley BC, Elm JJ, Babcock D, Hauser R, Ross GW, Augustine AH, et al. Effect of Creatine monohydrate on clinical progression in patients with Parkinson disease. JAMA. 2015. https://doi.org/10.1001/jama.2015.120.
9. Evatt ML, DeLong MR, Kumari M, Auinger P, McDermott MP, Tangpricha V. High prevalence of hypovitaminosis D status in patients with early Parkinson disease. Arch Neurol. 2011. https://doi.org/10.1001/archneurol.2011.30.
10. Sleeman I, Aspray T, Lawson R, Coleman S, Duncan G, Khoo TK. The role of vitamin D in disease progression in early Parkinson's disease. J Parkinsons Dis. 2017. https://doi.org/10.3233/JPD-171122.
11. Wang L, Evatt ML, Maldonado LG, Perry WR, Ritchie JC, Beecham GW, et al. Vitamin D from different sources is inversely associated with Parkinson disease. Mov Disord. 2014. https://doi.org/10.1002/mds.26117.
12. Suzuki M, Yoshioka M, Hashimoto M, Murakami M, Noya M, Takahashi D, et al. Randomized, double-blind, placebo-controlled trial of vitamin D supplementation in Parkinson disease. Am J Clin Nutr. 2013. https://doi.org/10.3945/ajcn.112.051664.

Permissions

List of Contributors

Brian W Starr and Alberto J Espay
Gardner Family Center for Parkinson's Disease and Movement Disorders, Department of Neurology, University of Cincinnati, 260 Stetson St, Suite 2300, Cincinnati, OH 45267-0525, USA

Matthew C Hagen
Department of Pathology, Division of Neuropathology, University of Cincinnati, Cincinnati, OH, USA

Giuseppe Frazzitta, Davide Ferrazzoli and Rossana Bera
Department of Parkinson Disease Rehabilitation, Moriggia-Pelascini Hospital, Gravedona ed Uniti, Fondazione Europea Ricerca Biomedica FERB, "S.Isidoro"Hospital, Trescore Balneario, Italy

Roberto Maestri
Department of Biomedical Engineering, Scientific Institute of Montescano, S. Maugeri Foundation IRCCS, Montescano, Italy

Giulio Riboldazzi
Center for Parkinson's Disease, Macchi Foundation, Varese and Department of Rehabilitation, "Le Terrazze" Hospital, Cunardo, Italy

Cecilia Fontanesi
Department of Physiol. Pharmacol. and Neuroscience, CUNY Medical School, Harris Hall 08, CCNY, 160 Convent Ave, New York, NY 10031, USA
The Graduate Center, Biology - Neuroscience PhD Program, CUNY, New York, NY, USA

Roger P Rossi and Maria F Ghilardi
Department of Physical Medicine and Rehabilitation, JFK Johnson Rehabilitation Institute, Edison, NJ, USA
NYU Movement Disorder Center, New York University, New York, NY, USA

Gianni Pezzoli
Parkinson Institute, Istituti Clinici di Perfezionamento, Milano, Italy

Giuseppe Frazzitta
Department of Parkinson Rehabilitation, Ospedale Moriggia Pelascini, Via Pelascini 3, Gravedona ed Uniti, Como 22015, Italy

Kazumi Iseki, Hidenao Fukuyama, Naoya Oishi, Hidekazu Tomimoto, Yoshinobu Otsuka and and Takashi Hanakawa
Human Brain Research Center, Kyoto University Graduate School of Medicine, 54 Kawahara-cho, Shogoin, Sakyo-ku, Kyoto 606-8507, Japan

Kazumi Iseki, David Benninger and Mark Hallett
Human Motor Control Section, Medical Neurology Branch, National Institute of Neurological Disorders and Stroke, National Institutes of Health, Bethesda, MD, USA

Kazumi Iseki
Department of Behavioral Neurology and Cognitive Neuroscience, Tohoku University, Graduate School of Medicine, Sendai, Miyagi, Japan
Department of Neurology, Sakakibara-Hakuho Hospital, Tsu, Mie, Japan

Hidekazu Tomimoto
Department of Neurology, Mie University, Graduate School of Medicine, Tsu, Mie, Japan

Manabu Nankaku
Department of Physical Therapy, Kyoto University Hospital, Kyoto, Japan

Takashi Hanakawa
Department of Advanced Neuroimaging, Integrative Brain Imaging Center, National Center of Neurology and Psychiatry, Kodaira, Japan
PRESTO, JST, Kawaguchi, Saitama, Japan

Amar Patel and Steven J Frucht
Department of Neurology, Icahn School of Medicine at Mount Sinai, 5 E 98th Street, New York, NY 10029, USA

William G Ondo
University of Texas Health Science Center at Houston, 6410 Fannin Street, Suite 1010, Houston, TX 77030, USA

Neal Hermanowicz
University of California Irvine Movement Disorders Program, 100 Irvine Hall, Irvine, CA 92697, USA

Diego García Borreguero
Sleep Research Institute, Alberto Alcocer 19, 28036 Madrid, Spain

Mark J Jaros
Summit Analytical, LLC, 2422 Stout Street, Denver, CO 80205, USA

Richard Kim and Gwendoline Shang
XenoPort, Inc., 3410 Central Expressway, Santa Clara, CA 95051, USA

André Lee, Shinichi Furuya and Eckart Altenmüller
Inistitute of Music Physiology and Musicians' Medicine, Hannover University of Music, Drama and Media, Hannover, Germany

William G. Ondo and Sana Sarfaraz
Department of Neurology, Methodist Neurological Institute, 6560 Fannin, Ste 802, Houston, TX 77030, USA

MinJae Lee
Biostatistics/Epidemiology/Research Design (BERD) Core, Center for Clinical and Translational Sciences, The University of Texas Health Science Center at Houston and Division of Clinical
and Translational Sciences, Houston, TX 77030, USA Department of Internal Medicine, The University of Texas Medical School at Houston Center for Clinical and Translational Sciences, University of Texas Health Science Center at Houston, Houston, TX 77030, USA

Charles Ellis, Yolanda F Holt and Thomas West
Department of Communication Sciences and Disorders, East Carolina University, 3310H Health Sciences Building, MS 668, Greenville, NC 27834, USA

Peter W. Iltis
Department of Kinesiology, Gordon College, Wenham, MA, USA

Jens Frahm, Dirk Voit and Arun Joseph
Biomedizinische NMR Forschungs GmbH am Max-Planck-Institut für biophysikalische Chemie, Göttingen, Germany

Eckart Altenmüller and Peter W. Iltis
Hochshule für Musik, Theater und Medien, Hannover, Germany

André Lee and Eckart Altenmüller
Institute of Music Physiology and Musicians' Medicine, Hannover University of Music, Drama and Media, Emmichplatz 1, 30175 Hannover, Germany

Pichet Termsarasab, Donald R Tanenbaum and Steven J Frucht
Department of Neurology, Movement Disorders Division, Icahn School of Medicine at Mount Sinai, 5 East 98th St, first floor, New York, NY 10029, USA

Fumihito Yoshii, Yusuke Moriya, Tomohide Ohnuki, Masafuchi Ryo and Wakoh Takahashi
Department of Neurology, Tokai University Oiso Hospital, 21-1 Gakkyou, Oiso, Naka-gun, Kanagawa 259-0198, Japan

Elizabeth L Stegemöller and Jennifer Uzochukwu
Department of Kinesiology, Iowa State University, 235 Forker, Ames, IA 50011, USA

Elizabeth L Stegemöller, Mark D Tillman and Chris J Hass
Department of Applied Physiology and Kinesiology, University of Florida, Gainesville, USA

Elizabeth L Stegemöller, Nikolaus R McFarland, SH Subramony, Michael S Okun and Chris J Hass
Center for Movement Disorders and Neurorestoration, Department of Neurology, University of Florida, McKnight Brain Institute, Gainesville, USA

Mark D Tillman
Department of Kinesiology and Health Promotion, Troy University, Troy, USA

Raja Mehanna
University of Texas Health Science Center, 6410 Fannin Street, Suite 1014, Houston, TX 77030, USA

Kathy M Wilson, Scott E Cooper, Andre G Machado and Hubert H Fernandez
Cleveland Clinic Foundation, Cleveland, Ohio, USA

Megan H Trager, Anca Velisar, Mandy Miller Koop, Lauren Shreve, Emma Quinn and Helen Bronte-Stewart
Department of Neurology and Neurological Sciences, Stanford University, 300 Pasteur Drive, Stanford, CA 94305, USA

Helen Bronte-Stewart
Department of Neurosurgery, Stanford University, Stanford, CA, USA

Dawit Kibru Worku
Addis Ababa, Ethiopia

Yared Mamushet Yifru
Department of Neurology, Addis Ababa University, Addis Ababa, Ethiopia

Douglas G Postels
International Neurologic and Psychiatric Epidemiology Program, Michigan State University, Michigan, USA

Fikre Enquselassie Gashe
Department of Community Health, Addis Ababa University, Addis Ababa, Ethiopia

Hatice N. Eken and Elan D. Louis
Department of Neurology, Yale School of Medicine, Yale University, LCI 710, 15 York Street, New Haven, CT 06520-8018, USA

Elan D. Louis
Department of Chronic Disease Epidemiology, Yale School of Public Health, Yale University, New Haven, CT, USA
Center for Neuroepidemiology and Clinical Neurological Research, Yale School of Medicine, Yale University, New Haven, CT, USA

Celia Faye Stewart
New York University, Steinhardt School of Culture, Education, and Human Development, 665 Broadway, Suite 900, New York NY 10012, USA

Catherine F. Sinclair
IcahnSchool of Medicine at Mount Sinai, 425 West 59th Street, New York NY 10019, USA

Irene F. Kling
Mannes College the New School for Music, 55 West 13th St, New York 10011, USA
Adelphi University, 75 Varick St, New York 10013, USA

Beverly E. Diamond
Clinical Endocrinology and Metabolism, Endocrine Society, 2055 L Street NW, Suite 600, Washington, DC 20036, USA

Andrew Blitzer
Columbia University College of Physicians and Surgeons, Neurology, Icahn School of Medicine at Mt. Sinai, Center for Voice and Swallowing Disorders, 425 West 59th Street, New York NY 10019, USA

Debra J. Ehrlich and Steven J. Frucht
Icahn School of Medicine at Mount Sinai, 5 East 98th Street, 1st Floor, Box 1637, New York, NY 10029, USA

Daniele Volpe, Leila Bakdounes, Chiara Sorbera and Maria Giulia Giantin
Department of Physical Medicine and Rehabilitation, Neurorehabilitation Unit "Villa Margherita, ", Via Costacolonna n.6 Arcugnano, Vicenza, Italy

Elisa Pelosin
Department of Neuroscience, University of Genoa, Genoa, Italy

Stefano Masiero
School of Physical Medicine and Rehabilitation, University of Padua, Padua, Italy

Giannettore Bertagnoni
Department of Physical Medicine and Rehabilitation, S. Bortolo Hospital, Vicenza, Italy

Ali Amouzandeh, Michael Grossbach and Eckart Altenmüller
1Institute of Music Physiology and Musicians' Medicine (IMMM), University of Music, Drama and Media, Emmichplatz 1, 30175 Hannover, Germany

Joachim Hermsdörfer
Institute of Human Movement Science, Department of Sport and Health Sciences, Technical University of Munich, Munich, Germany

Steven J Frucht
East 98th Street, New York, NY 10029, USA

Emma M. Coppen and Raymund A. C. Roos
Department of Neurology (J3-R-162), Leiden University Medical Center, 2300 RC Leiden, The Netherlands

Jeroen van der Grond
Department of Radiology, Leiden University Medical Center, Leiden, The Netherlands

Paola Ortelli, Marianna Zarucchi, Veronica Cian, Elisa Urso, Francesca Giacomello, Davide Ferrazzoli and Giuseppe Frazzitta
Department of Parkinson's disease, Movement Disorders and Brain Injury Rehabilitation, "Moriggia-Pelascini" Hospital, Via Pelascini, 3, Gravedona ed Uniti, 22015 Como, Italy

Roberto Maestri
Department of Biomedical Engineering, Istituti Clinici Scientifici Maugeri Spa Società Benefit, IRCCS, Via per Montescano 31, Montescano, 27040 Pavia, Italy

Martje E. van Egmond, Hendriekje Eggink, Anouk Kuiper, Marina A. J. Tijssen and Tom J. de Koning
Department of Neurology, University of Groningen, University Medical Center Groningen, Groningen, the Netherlands

Martje E. van Egmond
Department of Neurology, Ommelander Ziekenhuis Groningen, Delfzijl and Winschoten, 9700, RB, Groningen, the Netherlands

Deborah A. Sival and Tom J. de Koning
Department of Pediatrics, University of Groningen, University Medical Center Groningen, Groningen, the Netherlands

Corien C. Verschuuren-Bemelmans and Tom J. de Koning
Department of Genetics, University of Groningen, University Medical Center Groningen, Groningen, the Netherlands

Dirk Dressler and Fereshte Adib Saberi
Movement Disorders Section, Department of Neurology, Hannover Medical School, Carl-Neuberg-Str. 1, D-30625, Hannover, Germany

Clara Warden
Department of Psychology, Stanford University, Stanford, CA, USA

Clara Warden, Jaclyn Hwang, Anisa Marshall, Michelle Fenesy and Kathleen L. Poston
Department of Neurology and Neurological Sciences, Stanford University, Stanford, CA, USA

Anisa Marshall
Department of Neuroimaging, King's College London, London, UK

Michelle Fenesy
Department of Psychology, University of California, Los Angeles, CA, USA

Kathleen L. Poston
Department of Neurosurgery, Stanford University, Stanford, CA, USA

James A. G. Crispo, Dylan P. Thibault and Allison W. Willis
Department of Neurology, University of Pennsylvania Perelman School of Medicine, Blockley Hall, 423 Guardian Drive, Office 829, Philadelphia, PA 19104, USA

James A. G. Crispo, Dylan P. Thibault and and Allison W. Willis
Department of Biostatistics, Epidemiology and Informatics, University of Pennsylvania Perelman School of Medicine, Blockley Hall, 423 Guardian Drive, Office 811, Philadelphia, PA 19104, USA

Dylan P. Thibault and and Allison W. Willis
Department of Neurology Translational Center of Excellence for Neuroepidemiology and Neurological Outcomes Research, University of Pennsylvania Perelman School of Medicine, Philadelphia, PA, USA

Yannick Fortin
McLaughlin Centre for Population Health Risk Assessment and Interdisciplinary School of Health Science, Faculty of Health Sciences, University of Ottawa, 850 Peter Morand Crescent, Room 119, Ottawa, ON K1G 3Z7, Canada

Allison W. Willis
Center for Clinical Epidemiology and Biostatistics, University of Pennsylvania Perelman School of Medicine, Blockley Hall, 423 Guardian Drive, Office, Philadelphia, PA 19104, USA

Jarmal Charles, Lindyann Lessey, Jennifer Rooney, Ingmar Prokop, Katherine Yearwood, Hazel Da Breo, Patrick Rooney and Andrew K. Sobering
New York, USA

Ruth H. Walker
Department of Neurology, James J. Peters Veterans Affairs Medical Center, Bronx, NY, USA
Department of Neurology, Mount Sinai School of Medicine, New York City, NY, USA

Tuhin Virmani, Sirinan Tazan, Pietro Mazzoni, Blair Ford and Paul E. Greene
Department of Neurology, College of Physicians and Surgeons, Columbia University, New York, NY, USA

Tuhin Virmani
Current addresses: University of Arkansas for Medical Sciences, 4301 W. Markham St., #500, Little Rock, AR 72205, USA

Sirinan Tazan
Healthcare Partners, 3565 Del Amo Blvd., Ste 200, Torrance, CA 90503, USA

Paul E. Greene
Mt. Sinai School of Medicine, Box 1637, New York, NY 10029, USA

Shnehal Patel, Oluwadamilola Ojo, Gencer Genc, Srivadee Oravivattanakul, Yang Huo, Tanaporn Rasameesoraj, Anwar Ahmed and Hubert H. Fernandez
9500 Euclid Ave/U2, Cleveland, OH 44195, USA

Lu Wang and James Bena
9500 Euclid Ave/JJN3, Cleveland, OH 44195, USA

Michelle Drerup
9500 Euclid Ave/P57, Cleveland, OH 44195, USA

Nancy Foldvary-Schaefer
9500 Euclid Ave, Cleveland, OH 44195, USA

Elan D. Louis
Division of Movement Disorders, Department of Neurology, Yale School of Medicine, Yale University, LCI 710, 15 York Street, PO Box 208018, New Haven, CT 06520-8018, USA
Department of Chronic Disease Epidemiology, Yale School of Public Health, Yale University, New Haven, CT, USA

Center for Neuroepidemiology and Clinical Neurological Research, Yale School of Medicine, Yale University, New Haven, CT, USA

Stephanie Cosentino
Department of Neurology, College of Physicians and Surgeons, Columbia University, New York, NY, USA Division of Geriatric Psychiatry, Department of Psychiatry, College of Physicians and Surgeons, Columbia University, New York, NY, USA

Edward D. Huey
G.H. Sergievsky Center, College of Physicians and Surgeons, Columbia University, New York, NY, USA Taub Institute for Research on Alzheimer's Disease and the Aging Brain, Columbia University, New York, NY, USA

Nijee S. Luthra and Chadwick W. Christine
Department of Neurology, University of California, 1635 Divisadero, Suite 520-530, San Francisco, CA 94115, USA

Soeun Kim and Yunxi Zhang
Department of Biostatistics and Data Science, University of Texas Health Center, 1200 Pressler Street, Houston, TX 77030, USA

Chadwick W. Christine
Department of Neurology, University of California San Francisco, 400 Parnassus Ave Box 0348, San Francisco, CA 94122, USA

Index